Health Informatics

T0075989

Sajeesh Kumar • Ellen R. Cohn

Editors

Telerehabilitation

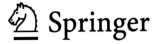 Springer

Editors
Sajeesh Kumar, Ph.D.
Department of Health Informatics &
Information Management
UT Health Science Center
Memphis
Tennessee
USA

Ellen R. Cohn, Ph.D.
School of Health and Rehabilitation
Sciences
University of Pittsburgh
Pittsburgh
USA

ISBN 978-1-4471-6030-4   ISBN 978-1-4471-4198-3 (eBook)
DOI 10.1007/978-1-4471-4198-3
Springer London Heidelberg New York Dordrecht

Springer is part of Springer Science+Business Media (www.springer.com)

Foreword

Telerehabilitation, the most recent evolution in the larger realm of "Telehealth," is a rapidly evolving discipline. A contemporary visualization of a word describing a process preceded by the prefix *tele-* is almost certain to be based on electronic transmission; however, there is credible evidence that the practice of telehealth has roots in antiquity. Such means as signal fires and drum messages were used to warn of danger from plague and other health threats. The initiation of telehealth in the form of telemedicine in the 'modern' era is often attributed to Willem Einthoven who transmitted electrocardiograph signals via telephone in 1905. In contrast to these venerable historic events, my first occasion to see the term *telerehabilitation* in print was in a published comment by Katherine "Kate" Seelman circa 1992 near the beginning of her incumbency as Director of the National Institute on Disability and Rehabilitation Research (NIDRR). Kate, who is one of the distinguished contributors to this book, can reasonably be credited with initiating significant advances in telerehabilitation by making it a NIDRR research and development priority.

Presently viewed as an emerging discipline and area of practice in the larger and more familiar domains of telemedicine and telehealth, telerehabilitation is a rapidly developing technology that enables the extension of rehabilitation expertise and services to remote and underserved areas. Telerehabilitation is equally effective in providing specific health, medical and rehabilitation expertise from comprehensive medical centers of excellence to homes and small clinics in metropolitan areas effectively and efficiently.

The rate of development and expansion in a field of endeavor is generally proportional to its contribution to knowledge and practices. Telerehabilitation is still a nascent field, but intellectual and technical development are proceeding apace. The latter are reflected in a growing literature that has been enhanced with the establishment of the *International Journal of Telerehabilitation* (*IJT*). The *IJT* was initiated by Dr. Ellen Cohn, Associate Dean for Instructional Development in the School of Health and Rehabilitation Sciences, and is published by the University Library System of the University of Pittsburgh and co-sponsored by the University Press. The *IJT* was launched with a Special Prepublication Issue in November, 2008.

As with most new endeavors, telerehabilitation is experiencing growing pains. A main deterrent to current expansion and development is gaining approval for reimbursement for services delivered to remote sites and patients. This is particularly true for the delivery of health care over political boundaries.

I believe the case for telerehabilitation has been elegantly presented in the course of articles by pioneering contributors to this field. *Telerehabilitation* provides a history, authoritative information and serves a foundation for future development.

In closing I shall paraphrase Abraham Lincoln's 'book review.' If you find telerehabilitation to be of interest and relevance, then *Telerehabilitation* is indeed a book you will like.

Pittsburgh, USA   Clifford E. Brubaker, Ph.D.

Preface

Telerehabilitation (a subset of telehealth) is the use of telecommunications to deliver rehabilitation services at a distance. Who might benefit from telepractice? There are 50 million children and adults with disabilities, many of whom might be candidates for telerehabilitation services. Moreover, there are conservatively 430,000 potential providers of telerehabilitation (TR) in the USA.

Telepractice can bridge the gaps created by personnel shortages that exist in underserved and remote areas, as well as serve persons in urban settings who cannot easily leave their homes or offices to seek care. Given the mobile nature of our society, telerehabilitation can enable continuity of care while persons travel for work, vacation and/or education.

While the technical capacities to conduct telerehabilitation have surged ahead in the past 10 years, there has been slower, yet ongoing progress in the development of the policies (e.g., legislation; state licensure; reimbursement) that will be required to actualize wide-spread telepractice service delivery. Most promising is that consumers of all ages are increasingly adopting the electronic delivery of many kinds of services.

As book editors, we recognize that it is a weighty responsibility to put forth one of the first books on a topic as complex as telerehabilitation. We have taken that responsibility seriously – striving to make wise selections of the content and the outstanding authors therein, and to act as diligent stewards of their work. *We therefore dedicate this work, with gratitude, to our foreword and chapter authors.*

We appreciate the wise efforts of Springer's Senior Editor–Medicine, Grant Weston, and his superb production team, and are honored that this work resides within Springer's Health Informatics Series. The diligent efforts of Editorial Assistant Ms. Latika Hans in the pre-production phase cannot be overstated.

The expertise showcased in this book was drawn heavily from the American Telemedicine Association's Special Interest Group in Telerehabilitation. Moreover, the work of the editors and several chapter authors was supported in part by the Rehabilitation Engineering and Research Center on Telerehabilitation; H133E090002, National Institute on Disability and Rehabilitation Research (NIDRR); and US Department of Education, led by Principal Investigators

Drs. David Brienza and Michael McCue. Colleagues at the University of Pittsburgh's School of Health and Rehabilitation Sciences, under the leadership of Dean Clifford E. Brubaker, offered ongoing encouragement and support, and we thank them as well.

Telerehabilitation consists of 21 chapters, which, taken together, present a wide-angle view of telerehabilitation at a seminal time in its development. The book includes authors from multiple disciplines, as well as a consumer-based perspective. We trust that we have much to learn from each other, and humbly suggest that our authors' collective contributions will contribute to the current understanding of telerehabilitation, as well as elucidate the immense potential for telerehabilitation-based service delivery to benefit persons with disabilities.

Pittsburgh, USA

Tennessee, USA

Ellen R. Cohn, Ph.D.

Sajeesh Kumar, Ph.D.

Contents

Contributors

Nancy A. Baker Department of Occupational Therapy, School of Health and Rehabilitation Sciences, University of Pittsburgh, Pittsburgh, PA, USA

David M. Brienza Department of Rehabilitation Science and Technology, School of Health and Rehabilitation Sciences, University of Pittsburgh, Pittsburgh, PA, USA

Anthony L. Brooks Director SensoramaLab, AD:MT, School of ICT, Aalborg University, Esbjerg, Esbjerg, Denmark

Janet E. Brown American Speech-Language-Hearing Association, Rockville, MD, USA

Clifford E. Brubaker School of Health and Rehabilitation Sciences, University of Pittsburgh, Pittsburgh, PA, USA

Jana Cason Auerbach School of Occupational Therapy, Spalding University, Louisville, KY, USA

S.V.G. Cobb Human Factors Research Group, University of Nottingham, Nottingham, UK

Ellen R. Cohn School of Health and Rehabilitation Sciences, University of Pittsburgh, Pittsburgh, PA, USA

Paco Dionisio Technology and Health Department, The Italian National Institute of Health, Rome, Italy

Donald B. Egolf Department of Communication, University of Pittsburgh, Pittsburgh, PA, USA

Daniele Giansanti Technology and Health Department, The Italian National Institute of Health, Rome, Italy

Philip Girard Department of Clinical Initiatives, Defense and Veterans Brain Injury Center, Walter Reed Army Medical Center, Washington, DC, USA Manchester VA Medical Center, Manchester, NH, USA

Nancy D. Harada Department of Health Services,
Fielding School of Public Health, Los Angeles, CA, USA

Karen Jacobs Department of Occupational Therapy,
College of Health and Rehabilitation Sciences: Sargent College,
Boston University, Boston, MA, USA

Jongbae Kim National Rehabilitation Center Research Institute,
Seoul, South Korea

Mark Krumm Northeast Ohio Au.D. Consortium,
Kent State University, Kent, OH, USA

Sajeesh Kumar Department of Health Informatics & Information Management,
UT Health Science Center, Memphis, TN, USA

Alan Chong W. Lee Physical Therapy Program, Mount St. Mary's College,
Los Angeles, CA, USA

Giovanni Maccioni Technology and Health Department,
The Italian National Institute of Health, Rome, Italy

Kristina Martinez Tele-Rehabilitation Services, Henry M. Jackson
Foundation CTR for Defense and Veterans Brain Injury Center,
James A. Haley Veterans' Hospital, Tampa, FL, USA

Michael McCue Department of Rehabilitation Science and Technology,
School of Health and Rehabilitation Sciences, University of Pittsburgh,
Pittsburgh, PA, USA

Sohrab Moeini Department of Health Information Management,
School of Health and Rehabilitation Sciences,
University of Pittsburgh, Pittsburgh, PA, USA

Sandra Morelli Technology and Health Department,
The Italian National Institute of Health, Rome, Italy

Suzanne Paone eHealth Services Information Services Division,
University of Pittsburgh Medical Center, Pittsburgh, PA, USA

Tammy Richmond Go 2 Care, Inc., Los Angeles, CA, USA

Katherine D. Seelman Department of Rehabilitation Science and Disorders,
School of Health and Rehabilitation Sciences, University of Pittsburgh,
Pittsburgh, PA, USA

Paul M. Sharkey University of Reading, Reading, UK

Grant Shevchik Health-UPMC, University Center at Level Green,
Level Green, PA, USA

Jenifer Simpson American Association of People with Disabilities,
Washington, DC, USA

Katie Ambrose Stout Department of Tele-Health, Tele-Rehabilitation Chief, Kimbrough Ambulatory Care Center, Fort Meade, MD/Rosslyn, VA, USA

Deborah Theodoros Division of Speech Pathology, Telerehabilitation Research Unit, School of Health and Rehabilitation Sciences, The University of Queensland, St. Lucia, Brisbane, QLD, Australia

Lyn R. Tindall Physical Medicine and Rehabilitation, Department of Veterans Affairs Medical Center, Lexington, KY, USA

Michael Towey Voice and Swallowing Center of Maine, Waldo County General Hospital, Belfast, ME, USA

Barbara A. Vento Department of Communication Science and Disorders, School of Health and Rehabilitation Sciences, University of Pittsburgh, Pittsburgh, PA, USA

Valerie J.M. Watzlaf Department of Health Information Management, School of Health and Rehabilitation Sciences, University of Pittsburgh, Pittsburgh, PA, USA

Jack M. Winters Department of Biomedical Engineering, Marquette University, Milwaukee, WI, USA

Chapter 1
Introduction to Telerehabilitation

David M. Brienza and Michael McCue

Abstract Telerehabilitation (TR) is an important subdiscipline of telemedicine. Although its history is relatively brief compared to other areas of telemedicine, it has quickly emerged as an area of practice where communication and information technology can have a large positive impact on the health and well-being of those capitalizing on its advantages. Comparison of TR with traditional, in-person rehabilitation service reveals that costs may be reduced and the effectiveness may be improved with use of TR. The potential for improvements and cost reductions are particularly high for rehabilitation services that involve prolonged interventions, as is the case for people with permanent disabilities and chronic conditions, or who are context or environmentally sensitive, such as in vocational and educational applications. This chapter summarizes the development of TR as a discipline, describes its current scope and its position relative to other telemedicine disciplines.

1.1 Development of Telerehabilitation as a Discipline

The term *telerehabilitation* (TR) is relatively new, but applications in telemedicine go as far back as the 1880s when some physicians experimented with telecommunication technologies after the invention of the telephone in 1876 [24]. The U.S. government first supported telemedicine through services provided by agencies such as the

---

D.M. Brienza (✉)
RERC on Telerehabilitation, University of Pittsburgh,
6425 Penn Ave., Suite 401, Pittsburgh, PA 15206, USA
e-mail: dbrienza@pitt.edu

M. McCue
Department of Rehabilitation Science and Technology, School of Health
and Rehabilitation Sciences, University of Pittsburgh,
5050 Forbes Tower, 3600 Forbes Avenue, Pittsburgh, PA 15260, USA
e-mail: mmccue@pitt.edu

S. Kumar, E.R. Cohn (eds.), *Telerehabilitation*, Health Informatics,
DOI 10.1007/978-1-4471-4198-3_1, © Springer-Verlag London 2013

1

Department of Veterans Affairs (VA). The first recorded use of telemedicine by the VA was in 1957 for a telemental health project in Nebraska [5]. Other projects followed with notable success over the subsequent 20 years, leading the VA to begin a systematic implementation of telemedicine in 1997. The VA adopted the broader, more encompassing term *telehealth* in lieu of *telemedicine* in 2003. Telemedicine is now considered a subset of VA telehealth, with VA telehealth incorporated as one part of the wider rubric of VA care coordination. By 2005, many of the Veteran's Health Administration's (VHA) 21 Veteran's Integrated Service Networks (VISNs) were using some form of TR technology at VA medical centers and health-care systems. These facilities use TR to augment services to community-based outpatient clinics (CBOCs) and Veterans Center programs.

In 1998, The National Institute for Disability and Rehabilitation Research (NIDRR) in the United States Department of Education funded the nation's first Rehabilitation Engineering Research Center on TR to initiate research on TR as a complement to telemedicine and in an effort to address a service delivery gap that emerged when managed-care policies truncated the allowable duration for inpatient rehabilitation. NIDRR also recognized the potential benefits of TR in the areas of primary and secondary prevention across the lifespan in people with disabilities, cost containment, and vocational rehabilitation.

Through 2010, most non-veteran, federally funded telehealth programs have targeted rural populations, often with an emphasis on older adults (U.S. Department of Health and Human Services Health Resources and Services Administration). For example, the Office for the Advancement of Telehealth in the Health Resources and Services Administration supports the Telehealth Network Grant Program's efforts to develop capacity for telehealth in medically underserved rural areas to improve and coordinate health-care services. The Office of Rural Health Policy supports rural health-care services through outreach grant programs.

1.2 Policy Issues

Public policy plays an important role in the implementation of telemedicine, and by association, TR [34, 39]. Seelman and Hartman [26] conducted a comprehensive review of the literature on TR policy and research tools, and concluded that rigorous and comprehensive outcome studies are needed to drive reimbursement policy. Government health policy addresses quality, cost, and access to health service resources. The U.S. government and the research community both employ policy analysis and evaluation to determine the efficacy and efficiency of policies as a basis for decisions about resource allocations.

Theodoros and Russell [28] observed that while it may be technically possible to deliver rehabilitation services across the world, many key policy issues must be addressed. These issues include: (a) licensure across state and national borders; (b) equivalence of international clinical standards; (c) regulation on privacy issues and the access and protection of patient health information; (d) issues on costs and remuneration of services; (e) liability and accountability; and (f) unification of international rules effecting clinical consultations. Theodoros and Russell also noted that while a number of international organizations, such as the World Health Organization and the World Trade Organization, are entering the debate, there is a lack of leadership on e-health policy.

Seelman's review of remote home care found that authors expressed the need for policy guidance that addresses function and quality-of-life factors in clinical assessments. She recommended that technical and clinical systems be held accountable through scrutiny of reports on service delivery and technology performance. Kaplan and Litewka [13] identified the following policy-related problem areas: (a) abridgement of privacy from combining and mining data and the influences of new technology on informed consent; (b) inaccurate and obsolete data; (c) security breaches; (d) usability and user friendliness; (e) data standards and integration for linking patient and personal information to achieve interoperability of individual records, personal health management, and public health; (f) systems design and deployment decisions; and (g) tradeoffs between social isolation and enhanced care.

Cost and reimbursement dominate the TR policy literature. Roine et al. [21] conducted a systematic review of telemedicine literature using economic assessment as one of their inclusion criteria. However, of the 50 articles reviewed, they identified few comprehensive economic analyses, and the quality of the analyses was described as relatively poor. With few exceptions, they reported that studies lacked empirical background about the costs and benefits included in the studies. Because costs varied considerably among studies, the authors concluded that comparison of the cost estimates might not be feasible in many cases [25]. The Center for Telemedicine and e-Health Law (CTeL) has studied telehealth reimbursement and published an independent sourcebook for telemedicine. The *CTeL Reimbursement Sourcebook* and *State Telemedicine Reimbursement Guide* address a broad range of legislative and regulatory issues involving telemedicine reimbursement policies at the federal for Medicare, Medicaid, and private insurance—all of which pay for telehealth to varying degrees. According to Robert Waters [33], telemedicine reimbursement in the United States may be provided by: (a) public payers, Medicare, and Medicaid; (b) private payers and fee for service; (c) managed care, both public and private; and (d) special payers such as government and worksite. Medicare reimbursement-related issues include criteria for eligible sites, geographic coverage, and services; store and forward technology; facility fees and co-payments; and home health durable medical equipment [33].

1.3 Rehabilitation in the Natural Environment

The primary barriers for early implementations and studies on TR have been to determine if it can be an effective alternative to face-to-face rehabilitation approaches, can reduce costs, can increase geographic accessibility, or can extend limited resources to justify its general applicability and use. However, the potential benefits of TR are greater than these goals when it is applied to rehabilitation of people in the *natural* environment. The reasoning for providing rehabilitation services in the environment that the client lives, works, and/or interacts socially and recreationally is compelling.

The World Health Organization has focused attention on the ability of individuals to function effectively in their own environments [14, 34]. Both behavioral therapy and vocational rehabilitation literatures support a *natural environment* model of TR. Evidence from these two bodies of literature suggests that the delivery of a wide range of rehabilitation services and interventions can be more effective if deployed in the natural environment rather than in a clinical environment [7, 16, 18, 23, 29–31, 41].

Some aspects of rehabilitation are not particularly well suited to TR, but a growing body of evidence proves that there is substantial value in providing interventions and services that can be delivered effectively in the home. Some reported benefits include increased functional outcomes [36], enhanced patient satisfaction [15], and self-directed goal setting for post-stroke patients [32]; minimizing problems with generalization and contextualization for patients with brain injury [37, 40]; and reducing duration and costs of rehabilitation for TBI and elderly populations [3]. Combining the best technologies for an efficient service delivery with the most effective rehabilitation treatments will ensure the success of TR in the natural environment.

1.4 Self-Management of Chronic Conditions

Management of chronic conditions, especially self-management of these conditions, is another application area where TR has the potential to exceed that of traditional care and management strategies. Although advances in medical care have increased life expectancy in individuals with disabilities, evidence points to chronic conditions and their associated complications as the primary cause of premature death. A recent prospective study has identified infections, amputations, surgeries for pressure ulcers, and depression as the strongest predictors of risk for premature death among spinal cord-injured (SCI) persons. Similar predictors of morbidity and mortality have been identified in the medically complex populations (e.g., adults with spina bifida and wheelchair-dependent persons with chronic edema/lymphedema of the lower extremities). This evidence echoes the larger picture of the global disease burden associated with chronic conditions. Chronic conditions are currently responsible for 60% of the global disease burden, which may become 80% by 2020 in developing countries [35].

Fortunately, advances in biomedical and behavioral management have increased our ability to prevent and/or control chronic conditions effectively, i.e., prolonged physical or mental impairments, diabetes, cardiovascular disease, cancer, and HIV/AIDS. Many of the complications of chronic conditions (secondary conditions) can also be prevented. In fact, growing evidence from around the world suggests that persons with chronic conditions improve when they receive effective treatments, regular follow-up, and self-management support in their living and working, or "natural," environments. The global shortage of health-care workers coupled with increasing life expectancy has made the development of innovative strategies to improve care for chronic conditions and prevent secondary complications one of the highest priorities of health-care systems worldwide [35].

Health-care providers, public health personnel, and health-care organizations need new models and evidence-based skills for managing chronic conditions. Care for chronic conditions must be reoriented around the disabled person and their family with support from their communities. Support must extend beyond clinic walls and infuse the disabled person's natural environments. Advanced communication abilities, behavior change techniques, education, and counseling skills are also necessary to help persons with chronic problems. Clearly, providers of rehabilitation services are particularly well positioned to support this paradigm shift. TR is poised to provide a high-reach, cost-efficient means of delivering rehabilitation services when and where they are needed most.

Eighty percent of the world's population now lives in an area with mobile phone coverage and that figure is expected to rise to 85% by 2010. By 2012, 50% of all individuals in remote areas of the world will have mobile phones. This has important implications for our future application of TR for self-management because even though most of clinical TR efforts in this arena will likely have tremendous impact on and application for limited-resource environments worldwide.

1.5 TR Informatics Overview

TR is experiencing rapid growth and is fast becoming a significant segment of telemedicine and e-health [19]. The field of TR existed under the assumption that the barriers imposed by distance could be minimized, thus enhancing access and introducing new possibilities for delivering intervention strategies across the continuum of care. The distance barriers are overcome by applying a variety of telecommunications, including voice, video, and virtual reality. Previously, TR was viewed as a field that focused heavily on real-time interactivity (synchronous interaction) rather than a store-and-forward approach (asynchronous interaction) [38]. As a result, most studies and developments presented in the literature focus on devices that can mimic face-to-face interactivity in a telesetting. The categories of services found in the literature include teleconsultation, telemonitoring, telehomecare, and teletherapy. Winters [38] defined teleconsultation as a standard "face-to-face" telemedicine model using interactive videoconferencing between a local provider (and client) and a remote rehabilitation expert to gain access to specialized expertise. Telehomecare service delivery occurs when a clinician (usually a nurse or technician) coordinates a rehabilitation service delivery from various providers to the client's home. For example, Hoenig et al. [11] described a protocol to deliver in-home teletraining to adults with mobility impairments. Telemonitoring is a clinical application wherein the rehabilitation provider sets up

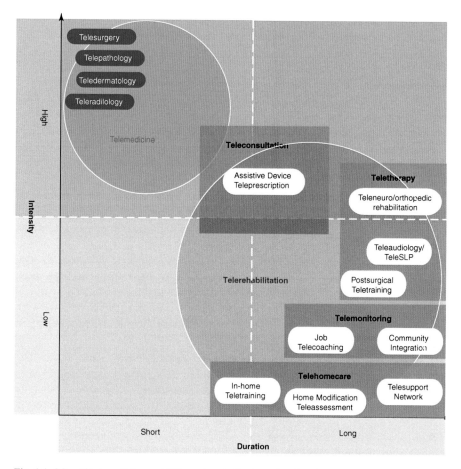

Fig. 1.1 Map of telemedicine and TR services in the intensity-duration space

unobtrusive monitoring or assessment technology for the client. Teletherapy is defined as a model of TR service delivery wherein the client conducts therapeutic activities in the home setting using a therapy protocol that is remotely managed by the therapist. There are numerous examples of applications in this area, including teleneuro and teleorthopedic rehabilitation, teleaudiology and speech-language pathology, and postsurgical teletraining [8–10, 20].

TR service is generally characterized by repetitive encounters over a long time period. This is in contrast to other telehealth applications such as in telesurgery, telepathology, and teledermatology that require short-duration, high-intensity interactions. The nature of the informatics infrastructure must take into account the nature of the interactions. Parmanto [19] has mapped the various types of telehealth on a relative intensity and duration space, as shown in Fig. 1.1. The mapping shows the relative differences between representative telemedicine and TR applications. This figure shows the four quadrants of telemedicine applications. These range from a short-duration process with low intensity to a long-duration process with high intensity. Most TR services are of long duration with a relatively low intensity [19].

As an example of how these differences impact the requirements of the informatics infrastructure consider that the many repeated TR encounters over long periods of time result in an accumulation of information that needs to be stored and organized for use by therapists. Managing a wealth of information in complex forms (e.g., video, sound, text, and still images) poses a challenge in TR. However, the reward for doing so in an efficient manner may be the creation of opportunities that do not exist for traditional face-to-face encounters. For example, clinical outcomes may be extracted from the data, or recorded videos of the interactions between therapists and patients can be used to educate future therapists. Data mining may be employed to learn and characterize the wealth of information that was previously not available.

Teletechnologies allow for remote access to professional expertise [2, 38]. However, unlike telemedicine where interventions require one or two types of technologies and single populations, the TR environment requires the integration of multiple specialists, technologies, and delivery settings with a highly variable population. Numerous professional considerations shape the use of technology in rehabilitation services requiring a review of current TR technologies, including their strengths and limitations as they relate to accessibility and usability.

The Internet is not merely a source of information; it increasingly has become the medium for social networking. The Internet has been transformed from a static media delivering information, commonly known as Web 1.0 [1], into a dynamic platform where users can share and publish their information and connect with other users, commonly known as Web 2.0 [6, 17]. The most well-known examples of Web 2.0 technology are the social networking sites (SNSs) such as Facebook and MySpace. With more than 200 million active users as of April 2009 and an annual growth of 125% (adding more than half a million users a day), Facebook is arguably the fastest growing medium in human history. The importance of social networking to our health and our lives cannot be underestimated. A recent analysis of the famous Framingham study conducted using data collected from 1971 to 2003, involving 12,067 volunteers [4, 5], found that social distance, as opposed to geographical distance, was much more important in mapping the spread of obesity or the habit of smoking. Similarly important roles of social networks have been reported in rehabilitation [27, 33].

An information and communications technology (ICT) device that combines a mobile cellular phone with Internet access, commonly known as the smartphone, is another important, fast-growing technology. The popularity of the iPhone has boosted the growth rate of smartphones to 30%. Sales of smartphones surpassed that of laptops and other mobile phones in 2007 [12]. We will see even more exciting developments with the roll-out of 4 G to replace the current 3 G connections. Providers such as Sprint started rolling out earlier this year while Verizon intends to do so at the end of 2009. The 4 G speed of 100 Mbps (while moving) is capable of delivering high-definition television. But the most important potential for TR is the fact that the stationary speed of 4 G is 1 Gbps and improves quality of service (more stable connections). This will allow delivery of very high-quality videoconferencing to almost anywhere.

The rapid progress in ICT has effectively blurred the old categories of telemonitoring, telehomecare, telemedicine, and e-health [38]. The oft-cited definition of TR as the delivery of rehabilitation services over a distance via telecommunication [22] may no longer be a valid representation of the potential, challenge, and utility of TR for the next decade. Advancements in ICT make it possible for TR to not only replicate existing rehab services over a distance, but also create new types of rehabilitation. An example of a new type of rehabilitation is job coaching using a mobile phone for individuals with cognitive disabilities who require constant monitoring. Technologies make it possible to deliver rehabilitation that otherwise is prohibitively expensive. The technologies can also potentially bridge the gulf between the "clinical/health" and the "consumer" model of rehabilitation.

Finally, an ideal TR infrastructure should be scalable. That is, instead of developing individual applications for every TR service, a scalable underlying infrastructure that can easily be adjusted to different types of TR services is desirable. To be cost effective, the use of inexpensive equipment and components already available in typical health-care environments is desirable. Protecting the confidentiality of the electronic health record (EHR) is critical.

1.6 Conclusion

TR has emerged as a methodology to address obstacles to rehabilitation through cost-effective alternatives to face-to-face and clinic-based care. In addition, TR has been demonstrated as an effective and satisfactory (from both the consumer and the clinician perspective) means of accessing necessary services in rural areas where specialized rehabilitation services and resources have not been available. Finally, TR offers a unique clinical advantage of enabling intervention and support to take place within the natural context of the individual's home, workplace, and community setting. This potential for "in vivo" intervention is of particular value in addressing the needs of individuals with disabilities. Technological advances, guided by consumer and clinician input, have made TR significantly more robust, accessible, usable, and adaptable. The potential to enhance rehabilitation service provision, rather than simply offering a more convenient or economical alternative, has been realized.

Summary

- TR is an important subdiscipline of telemedicine, where communication and information technology can have a large positive impact on the health and well-being of those capitalizing on its advantages.
- The primary barriers for early implementations and studies on TR have been to determine if it can be an effective alternative to face-to-face rehabilitation approaches, can reduce costs, can increase geographic accessibility, or can extend limited resources to justify its general applicability and use. However, the potential

benefits of TR are greater than these goals when applied to rehabilitation of people in the natural environment.

- Self-management of chronic conditions is another application area where TR has the potential to exceed that of traditional care and management strategies.
- TR is experiencing rapid growth and is fast becoming a significant segment of telemedicine and e-health. Advancements in ICT make it possible for TR to not only replicate existing rehab services over a distance, but also create new types of rehabilitation.
- Technological advances guided by consumer and clinician input, have made TR significantly more robust, accessible, usable, and adaptable.

Abbreviations/Acronyms

CBOC   Community-based outpatient clinic
CTeL   Center for Telemedicine and e-Health Law
EHR   Electronic health record
ICT   Information and communications technology
NIDRR   National Institute for Disability and Rehabilitation Research
SCI   Spinal cord injury
SNS   Social networking site
TBI   Traumatic brain injury
TR   Telerehabilitation
VA   Veterans Affairs
VHA   Veteran's Health Administration
VISN   Veteran's Integrated Service Network

References

1. Al-Khalifa HS, Al-Salman AS. From Web 1.0 to Web 2.0 and beyond: is the Web becoming more accessible for people with visual impairments? In: International conference on information integration and web-based applications, Austrian Computer Society, Yogyakarta, 2006.
2. Bashshur RL. Telemedicine and health care. Telemed J E Health. 2002;8(1):5–12.
3. Caplan GA, Coconis J, Board N, et al. Does home treatment affect delirium? A randomised controlled trial of rehabilitation of elderly and care at home or usual treatment (The REACH-OUT trial). Age Ageing. 2006;35(1):53–60.
4. Christakis NA, Fowler JH. The spread of obesity in a large social network over 32 years. N Engl J Med. 2007;357(4):370–9.
5. Christakis NA, Fowler JH. The collective dynamics of smoking in a large social network. N Engl J Med. 2008;358(21):2249–58.
6. Cormode G, Krishnamurthy B. Key differences between Web 1.0 and Web 2.0. First Monday. 2008;13(6).
7. de Beurs E, van Balkom AJ, Lange A, et al. Treatment of panic disorder with agoraphobia: comparison of fluvoxamine, placebo, and psychological panic management combined with exposure and of exposure in vivo alone. Am J Psychiatry. 1995;152(5):683–91.

8. Feng X, Winters JM. An interactive framework for personalized computer-assisted neurorehabilitation. IEEE Trans Inf Technol Biomed. 2007;11(5):518–26.

9. Heuser A, Kourtev H, Winter S, et al. Telerehabilitation using the Rutgers Master II glove following carpal tunnel release surgery: proof-of-concept. IEEE Trans Neural Syst Rehabil Eng. 2007;15(1):43–9.

10. Hill AJ, Theodoros DG, Russell TG, et al. An internet-based telerehabilitation system for the assessment of motor speech disorders: a pilot study. Am J Speech Lang Pathol. 2006; 15(1):45–56.

11. Hoenig H, Sanford JA, Butterfield T, et al. Development of a teletechnology protocol for in-home rehabilitation. J Rehabil Res Dev. 2006;43(2):287–98.

12. In-Stat. Size and growth of smartphone market will exceed laptop market for next five years. 2007. Available at: http://www.instat.com/newmk.asp?ID=2149. Accessed 18 Oct 2011.

13. Kaplan B, Litewka S. Ethical challenges of telemedicine and telehealth. Camb Q Healthc Ethics. 2008;17(4):401–16.

14. Kuipers P, Foster M, Smith S, et al. Using ICF – environment factors to enhance the continuum of outpatient ABI rehabilitation: an exploratory study. Disabil Rehabil. 2009;31(2):144–51.

15. Legg L, Langhorne P. Therapy-based rehabilitation for stroke patients living at home. Stroke. 2004;35(4):1022.

16. Mersch PP. The treatment of social phobia: the differential effectiveness of exposure in vivo and an integration of exposure in vivo, rational emotive therapy and social skills training. Behav Res Ther. 1995;33(3):259–69.

17. O'Reilly T. What is Web 2.0: design patterns and business models for the next generation of software. O'Reilly Network; 2005. Available at: http://oreilly.com/web2/archive/what-is-web-0.html.

18. Ost L-G, Thulin U, Ramnerö J. Cognitive behavior therapy vs exposure in vivo in the treatment of panic disorder with agoraphobia. Behav Res Ther. 2004;42(10):1105–27.

19. Parmanto B, Saptono A. Telerehabilitation: state-of-the-art from an informatics perspective. Int J Telerehabil. 2008;1(1):73–84 (Special Prepublication Issue).

20. Placidi G. A smart virtual glove for the hand telerehabilitation. Comput Biol Med. 2007; 37(8):1100–7.

21. Roine R, Ohinmaa A, Hailey D. Assessing telemedicine: a systematic review of the literature. CMAJ. 2001;165(6):765–71.

22. Russell TG. Telerehabilitation: a coming of age. Aust J Physiother. 2009;55(1):5–6.

23. Salaberria K, Echeburua E. Long-term outcome of cognitive therapy's contribution to self exposure in vivo to the treatment of generalized social phobia. Behav Modif. 1998; 22(3):262–84.

24. Scalvini S, Vitacca M, Paletta L, et al. Telemedicine: a new frontier for effective healthcare services. Monaldi Arch Chest Dis. 2004;61(4):226–33.

25. Seelman KD. Converging, pervasive technologies: chronic and emerging issues and policy adequacy. Assist Technol. 2008;20(3):126–37. quiz 138.

26. Seelman KD, Hartman L. Telerehabilitation: policy issues and research tools. Int J Telerehabil (Special Prepublication Issue). 2008:37–48.

27. Stalnacke BM. Community integration, social support and life satisfaction in relation to symptoms 3 years after mild traumatic brain injury. Brain Inj. 2007;21(9):933–42.

28. Theodoros D, Russell T. Telerehabilitation: current perspectives. Stud Health Technol Inform. 2008;131:191–209.

29. Vlaeyen JW, de Jong J, Geilen M, et al. Graded exposure in vivo in the treatment of pain-related fear: a replicated single-case experimental design in four patients with chronic low back pain. Behav Res Ther. 2001;39(2):151–66.

30. Vlaeyen JWS, de Jong J, Geilen M, et al. The treatment of fear of movement/(re)injury in chronic low back pain: further evidence on the effectiveness of exposure in vivo. Clin J Pain. 2002;18(4):251–61.

31. Vlaeyen JWS, De Jong JR, Onghena P, et al. Can pain-related fear be reduced? The application of cognitive-behavioural exposure in vivo. Pain Res Manag. 2002;7(3):144–53.

32. von Koch L, Wottrich AW, Holmqvist LW. Rehabilitation in the home versus the hospital: the importance of context. Disabil Rehabil. 1998;20(10):367–72.

33. Ware NC, Hopper K, Tugenberg T, et al. A theory of social integration as quality of life. Psychiatr Serv. 2008;59(1):27–33.

34. Weinstein RS, Lopeez AM, Krupinski EA, et al. Integrating telemedicine and telehealth: putting it all together. In: Current principles and practices of telemedicine and e-health. Amsterdam: IOS Press; 2008. p. 23–38.

35. WHO. Innovative care for chronic conditions: building blocks for action: global report. Geneva: WHO Health Care for Chronic Conditions Team, World Health Organization; 2002. p. 1–99.

36. Widen Holmqvist L, von Koch L, Kostulas V, et al. A randomized controlled trial of rehabilitation at home after stroke in southwest Stockholm. Stroke. 1998;29(3):591–7.

37. Willer B, Corrigan JD. Whatever it takes: a model for community-based services. Brain Inj. 1994;8(7):647–59.

38. Winters JM. Telerehabilitation research: emerging opportunities. Annu Rev Biomed Eng. 2002;4:287–320.

39. Wipf KR, Langner B. Policy approaches to chronic disease management. Home Health Care Manag Pract. 2006;18:452–62.

40. Ylvisaker M. Context-sensitive cognitive rehabilitation: theory and practice. Brain Impairment. 2003;4(1):1–16.

41. Zitrin CM, Klein DF, Woerner MG. Treatment of agoraphobia with group exposure in vivo and imipramine. Arch Gen Psychiatry. 1980;37(1):63–72.

Chapter 2
Challenges and Trends Driving Telerehabilitation

Jenifer Simpson

Abstract With broadband Internet devices and applications exploding into the marketplace for all kinds of business and residential uses, we should expect to see uses of these devices in areas such as rehabilitation. Although we are a long way from ubiquitous use of all the new technologies in rehabilitation activities and programs, we can start to see what this emergent technology ecosystem, telerehabilitation, will look like. This chapter discusses the challenges of telerehabilitation in light of the circumstances for people with disabilities and the current trends in technology.

2.1 Introduction

Generally, the rehabilitation of individuals with disabilities is about all the programmatic efforts aimed at maintaining and improving their lives from birth through adulthood, with a focus on their employment. Technology has surely been a part of that for many years. However, we are at the beginning of our understanding of how the rehabilitation system is taking up and expanding capacity to improve the lives of people with disabilities by using all the new information technology and communications tools available. Telerehabilitation is where intersects with broadband technologies, with the purpose of enhancing independent living and community integration for people with disabilities.

There is much to explore in telerehabilitation as a way to improve the everyday lives of individuals with disabilities. Surely new technology systems in health care, independent living, employment, communications, transportation, and civic participation could untether rehabilitation from on-the-spot geographically bound service

J. Simpson
American Association of People with Disabilities,
1629 K Street NW, Suite 950, Washington, DC 20006, USA
e-mail: jsimpson@aapd.com

S. Kumar, E.R. Cohn (eds.), *Telerehabilitation*, Health Informatics,
DOI 10.1007/978-1-4471-4198-3_2, © Springer-Verlag London 2013

to reach a greater number of people in more diverse and interesting ways and, at the same time, promote and facilitate more independent living by people with disabilities. This paper looks at some of the elements influencing this telerehabilitative direction and offers some views on where it might lead us. First, there are many challenging circumstances for people with disabilities in regard to rehabilitation. However, on the brighter side, there are several trends within the overall technology ecosystem that could drive to more and better solutions and support a vibrant telerehabilitation ecosystem.

2.2 The Challenges

2.2.1 Disability Is Everywhere

In the United States, nearly one in eight people has a disability. Statisticians reported that, in 2008, over 36 million people, or 12.1% of the civilian non-institutionalized population, had a disability. Nearly 19 million people reporting disabilities (i.e., 10.1% of the civilian non-institutionalized population), are of working age (18–64 years old). Over 4 million working-age people report having difficulty hearing, 3.4 million report vision difficulty, and 7.7 million report cognitive difficulties [25]. However, many believe that the census and other statistics [21] undercount people with disabilities and that the real number of people with disabilities in the United States is closer to 20% of the population.

The tools for telerehabilitation efforts need to be flexible, open, and responsive to meet the needs of the people with disabilities. While much of this will be market driven, some adaptations and custom technology applications will also be needed.

2.2.2 Disability is Diverse

It is important to note the diversity within disability. The working-age population with disability experiencing unemployment may have various functional limitations depending on their underlying physical, mental, or medical condition, or may have multiple conditions. They may have at least one of the following conditions or limitations: deaf or serious difficulty hearing; blind or serious difficulty seeing even when wearing glasses; serious difficulty concentrating, remembering, or making decisions because of a physical, mental, or emotional condition; serious difficulty walking or climbing stairs; difficulty dressing or bathing; or difficulty doing errands alone such as visiting a doctor's office or shopping because of a physical, mental, or emotional condition [3].

These functional limitations may be the result of a particular medical condition or disability, or may be age or injury related. Telerehabilitation should focus on the functional manifestations of people with disabilities rather than on medical diagnoses. This is because telerehabilitation technologies are all about the human involvement, or the interface, with information, communication, and medical systems that simply do not need to know how the medical record describes the condition.

2.2.3 People with Disabilities Experience High Unemployment Rates

Despite years of efforts to expand employment opportunities for people with disabilities, and because of the more recent economic downturn, the unemployment rate for people with disabilities remains high. Approximately 60.9% of working-age people with disabilities are not employed compared to 22.3% of those without disabilities [19]. Millions of people with disabilities are not working and in need of jobs and services, if they wish to return to or secure employment.

There are critical transition-to-employment barriers for these millions of people with disabilities who are unemployed today. Employment-related tools and programming using new technologies and those that are developed by telerehabilitation practitioners are likely to be critical to addressing the employment needs of people with disabilities.

2.2.4 People with Disabilities Are Among the Poorest

The economic status of people with disabilities—something that rehabilitation can surely change if outcomes shift to greater employment—is another long-term challenge. In 2007, a study by the National Council on Disability found high poverty rates for people with disabilities. Of the households having one or more persons with disabilities, 16.8% reported receiving food stamps in the previous 12 months versus 6% of households without disabilities. People with disabilities are more likely to have income below the poverty level (25.5% versus 10.4%), with median earnings lagging those without disabilities by more than $10,000 [19]. People with disabilities are nearly three times more likely to live in poverty—the same ratio as existed before the Americans with Disabilities Act was passed [19].

For consumers interfacing with telerehabilitation, technology solutions that are cheap, easy to use, and as much as possible involve items found in the mainstream will surely be helpful. While there will be a need for some more expensive specially designed custom technologies or applications, the income issue is not going to be resolved soon and, if we are to engage people with disabilities directly in telerehabilitation, the cost of devices will be important.

2.2.5 People with Disabilities Have Less Access to the Internet

Less usage and lower rates of adoption of broadband—or higher-speed Internet access—by people with disabilities are a challenge for telerehabilitation practitioners.

2.2.5.1   Persistence of the Digital Divide

In November 2010, the U.S. Commerce Department's Economics and Statistics Administration released a report, "Exploring the Digital Nation: Home Broadband Internet Adoption in the U.S." [26]. Based on the data collected from 54,000 households in October 2009, the report showed that 7 out of 10 American households used the Internet in 2009 and that broadband Internet use among these households increased from 9 to 64% between 2001 and 2009. However, this new report detailed more information about the digital divide for people with disabilities, among other groups looked at. They noted that differences in *socioeconomic* and *geographic* characteristics explain a substantial portion of the broadband adoption lag among people with disabilities.

One section of the report, "Disability and Broadband Internet Use," examined data collected on broadband Internet usage among people with disabilities. They found that among non-users of broadband Internet, people with disabilities tended to be older, earn less income, have lower rates of educational attainment, and live in rural areas. As each of these characteristics is generally associated with lower Internet access and usage, they represent a pressing problem when looked at for the purposes of telerehabilitation activities.

Such reports are likely to facilitate greater awareness about how to develop telerehabilitation approaches within the overall context of broadband adoption programs if there is to be a positive impact for people with disabilities seeking rehabilitation programs and services. It also emphasizes the need for remote connections and telepresence as a way to serve people with disabilities.

2.2.5.2   Disability Correlated with Lower Levels of Online Activity

Similar studies reflect similar data. The Federal Communications Commission conducted a survey in late 2009 to estimate how many people use broadband Internet. The survey asked questions about Internet use in general, and used six separate questions to determine if respondents had a disability. Even after accounting for advanced age and lower income, the proportion of people having a disability is significantly correlated with lower levels of online activity. The results showed less access for people with disabilities [16]. They found that 56% of people with disabilities use the Internet, compared to 78% of all people. Among the people who do not use the Internet at all, 47% have some sort of disability; 39% of people who do not use broadband have a disability compared to 15% of people who do use broadband. Senior citizens with disabilities are 76% less likely to have broadband than those without a disability [16].

An even more recent survey in 2011 by the Pew Foundation—based on a telephone survey that might have missed out inclusion of people with speech, language, and hearing disabilities—found that 54% of adults living with a disability use the Internet, compared with 81% of adults who report none of the disabilities listed in the survey [11]. Two percent of American adults may have a disability or illness that makes it very difficult or impossible for them to use the Internet.

The persistence of this gap points to the need for relevance of applications, devices, and services as broadband capacity grows. Telerehabilitation can be seen as a very relevant set of applications that will benefit people with disabilities directly.

2.2.6 Need for Vocational Rehabilitation

Over 615,000 people applied for vocational rehabilitation in 2008, the most recent year reported by the Rehabilitation Services Administration [23]—a clear statement of the need for such services. While many state vocational rehabilitation agencies allow online application for their services, it is not clear how well this technology-based approach is working and or how effective it is.

More research is needed to clarify better how information technology infrastructure transformations at state agencies could lead to more effective outcomes. There can and should be many more opportunities for telerehabilitation to connect and work with these systems as they develop. Opportunities may arise to integrate case management or other follow-up work that could, on an ongoing basis, connect directly with individuals needing rehabilitation services.

2.3 The Trends

There are, according to the experts, apparently over 35 billion devices attached already to the Internet [7]. The same experts predict that in the next 10 years there are likely to be well over a trillion devices with network potential. This may include cars, home appliances, tags for livestock and pets [7], and anything else we care to think of that can be "hooked up" to the Internet. Adding in any of the other new startling statistics from the business sector about how the Internet is transforming, we can really start imagining how the Internet can change forever rehabilitation and outcomes for people with disabilities.

According to the experts, it is likely that by 2020 a $1,000 PC will have the raw processing power of the human brain and that by 2013 wireless network traffic will reach 400 petabytes a month, compared to today when the entire global network transfer is only 9 exabytes per month [7]. There is no doubt that the general technology infrastructure is growing and transforming rapidly. Similarly, there is little doubt that growth of telerehabilitation will be directly influenced by many of the trends that are within this larger technology ecosystem. Several of these trends are discussed below.

2.3.1 Growth of the Internet and its Importance

The Internet has grown exponentially and will likely continue to do so. In 1997, about 19 million Americans were using the Internet. That number tripled in 1 year and passed 100 million in 1999. In the first quarter of 2000, more than five million Americans joined the online world—roughly 55,000 new users each day. Every 24 h, the Internet is enriched with more than 3.2 million web pages and more than 715,000 images. The number of electronic mailboxes worldwide reached almost 570 million in 1999. In 1998, the U.S. Postal Service delivered 101 billion pieces of paper mail; the number of e-mails transmitted that year was estimated to be as high as 4 trillion [24]. And these are old statistics!

As the Internet continues to grow and becomes a large part of Americans' lives, more and more activities migrate online. People now find jobs, attend schools, entertain themselves, bank, buy and sell, and interact with the government online, among many other activities. There is little doubt that some forms of rehabilitation processes will also have to migrate online simply because of consumer expectations and familiarity with electronic processes.

2.3.2 Wireless Migration

The July–December 2008 National Health Interview Survey (NHIS) indicated that the number of American homes with only wireless telephones continued to grow. More than one of every five American homes (20.2%) had only wireless telephones (also known as cellular telephones, cell phones, or mobile phones) during the second half of 2008, an increase of 2.7% since the first half of 2008. This is the largest 6-month increase observed since NHIS began collecting data on wireless-only households in 2003. In addition, one of every seven American homes (14.5%) received all or almost all calls on wireless telephones, despite having a landline telephone at home [2]. The shift from wireline to wireless phone use is a trend that will impact telerehabilitation.

Furthermore, wireless connection to broadband technology is also growing rapidly. As experts predict, by 2015, the number of wireless broadband connections will increase from 12.4 to 49 million in the United States [4] and there will be nearly one mobile device per capita worldwide [5].

What all this wireless connectivity means for telerehabilitation is that more and more devices will be available in the marketplace for use in rehabilitation activities. And, with the advent of mobile broadband capacities by more and more major providers in the United States, such as via 4 G wireless networks, there are some clear opportunities to find ways to shift some, if not many, aspects of rehabilitation programs and services into the electronic environment.

2.3.3 More Affordable Computers

Boding well for people with disabilities—and the people who serve them in the rehabilitation field—is the increasing ability to buy an essential tool of modern life, a computer, at a cheap price. It is a very positive trend for people with disabilities that the prices of devices such as computers, laptops, desktops, tablets, smart phones, net books, etc. have become more affordable [20]. These mainstream devices are the key to accessing the Internet and the myriad of services, programs, information, and applications that make up the entire technology ecosystem. Activities that were unthinkable as online activities even a few short years ago are now common every-day occurrences. Refinancing a house, applying to college, buying stocks, purchasing plane tickets, searching and securing a job, reading a downloaded book or magazine, downloading songs, and accessing thousands of applications or "apps" are but the tip of the iceberg, as the Internet's capabilities mirror our society's previous paper-based processes and systems.

Rehabilitation activities such as assessment, evaluation, reviewing, training, cueing, reminding, and other processes are surely candidates for transfer to information technology processes. Medical and therapeutic actions will also be transferred to some degree, as well as the business and reimbursement processes that support such activities.

2.3.4 Cloud Computing

While the term "cloud computing" [31] is popular, there is little doubt that this is an ongoing trend that will drive broadband deployment expansion and availability. This is because purchasing services "in the cloud" will free up budgets that are currently used for ongoing in-house information technology expenses. For instance, instead of purchasing software licenses and hardware for new employees and locations, businesses will simply add cloud-based service accounts to expand computing capacity. This will increase availability of free or low-cost services and may offer a way to do business better, cheaper, and faster, and perhaps more effectively, for rehabilitation services providers.

This is surely the path for rehabilitation experts to provide a greater amount of services to a greater number of people over a wider range of locations. It is not unreasonable to assume that electronic outsourcing of some aspects of rehabilitation will also be driven by this general business trend.

2.3.5 Growth in Online Learning

Higher education is trending online, with more students taking online courses than before. A November 2010 report by the Sloan Foundation found that for the fall term in 2009, 5.6 million students who enrolled in higher education took at least one online course, which is a 21% increase from the prior year. The study also found that traditional classroom enrollment in higher education increased by 2% for the same period and that nearly 30% of higher education students now take at least one course online [1]. While some of this increase is likely due to the economic down-turn, it indicates a path open for telerehabilitation. In fact, 63% of the academic officers in this Sloan report said that their long-term strategy included expansion of online education. Officers from publicly funded educational institutions were more likely than others to say this was part of their long-term strategy [1].

This is important to look at because more and more students with disabilities are receiving and completing more education [18,22][1] and they will have greater expectations for entering the mainstream of society, and in particular, will expect to secure and retain employment. It is also likely that they will expect to use the tools of technology in any rehabilitation activity associated with securing employment.

2.3.6 More Video on the Internet

Nowadays, more videos are available on the Internet than ever before. This will continue to increase and will have an impact on how we use and interact with the technologies that broadband brings to us. If the number of people viewing video clips and other video material is any indication, recent data show that Internet users expect and view a lot of online video material. For instance, in March 2010, U.S. Internet users watched 31.2 billion videos, with Google's YouTube site ranking at the top with 13.1 billion videos, representing 41.8% of all videos viewed online. Hulu ranked second with 1.1 billion videos, or 3.4% of all online videos viewed in 1 month's period. Microsoft sites ranked third with 655 million (2.1%), followed by Yahoo! sites with 478 million (1.5%) and CBS Interactive with 457 million (1.5%) [6]. Long-time Internet users will no doubt recall when there was little, if any, such material available because of lack of broadband availability.

The implications for telerehabilitation are clear. Consumers expect to find material in video format online, and if rehabilitation experts expect to serve consumers using the tools that consumers use, video applications must surely be at the forefront.

2.3.6.1 Automated Accessibility is Nascent

For people with sensory disabilities to access video material, the key to equality is both captioning and audio description of video. However, there is a long way to go before accessibility of video media is the norm and not the exception. Some not-yet-high-quality automated accessibility (e.g., a beta version of automatic captioning) is available on Google's YouTube service [13]. There is little to no automated video description available, although it is clear that most video has a "text version" some-where that could be transformed into audio output.

---

[1]Alexa Posny, Assistant Secretary for Special Education and Rehabilitative Services: "School grad-uation rates—where students with disabilities receive regular diplomas—have increased 45% since 1995, with an associated decrease in dropout rates for students with disabilities." She also noted that enrollment into college has doubled for students with disabilities and more students have jobs than ever before.

Some believe that cloud computing offers a way to provide the necessary artificial intelligence or electronic infrastructure that will permit the automatic adjustment to the means of accessibility and usability an individual user may need. A system such as a global public inclusive infrastructure (GPII) has been proposed and may support this type of automatic accessibility [12].

Nevertheless, the overall trend of more video viewing via the Internet in general indicates how people like to use the Internet and offers potentialities for telerehabilitation activities. Making such material accessible and usable to the widest number of potential users will be a challenge that rehabilitation can take up as it moves out of the downtown clinic and into any living room, anywhere.

2.3.6.2 Video Conferencing

Part of this trend is the increasing availability of two-way conferencing and video presence, which has increased dramatically in the past decade due to the greater availability of faster broadband Internet access. Video conferencing allows face-to-face interaction between a person with disability and another person, such as a colleague or an expert. The rapid uptake of Video Relay Service by sign language users is one technology example of how the availability of ever-cheaper computers, web cams, and microphones made "phone calls" possible. Video Remote Interpreting as a solution for lack of available sign language interpreters is another similar example.

Some believe that two-way video over the Internet removes many barriers to access for people with disabilities (including speech disability), seniors, and people who work out of their home, allowing them to connect for educational, medical, or professional purposes. There is little doubt that these video-conferencing technologies offer much potential for exploitation by telerehabilitators if privacy and security concerns can be addressed at the outset.

2.3.7 Health Information Technology

National policy is establishing specific targets for health information technology initiatives. As and if they are implemented, these will spur other efforts to ensure more broadband-based health-care services delivery, which can partner with rehabilitation efforts. These include implementation of the national broadband plan and greater deployment of electronic health records (EHRs) and systems such as health information exchanges (HIEs).

2.3.7.1 National Broadband Plan

In the National Broadband Plan, several provisions focused on health-care and services delivery [8]. These included the following: (1) ensuring that all health-care providers have access to affordable broadband, by revamping the Rural Health Care

Program; (2) upgrading Indian Health Services' broadband network to meet their health information technology needs; (3) creating economic incentives for broader health information technology adoption and innovation; (4) unlocking the power of health-care data and advanced analytics, while protecting privacy; and (5) modernizing rules to increase access to E-care.

Rehabilitation was specifically mentioned as one application in the national broadband plan that would allow consumers to "receive rehabilitation therapy in remote and rural areas" [9] and was cited as an aspect of relevance in terms of adoption and utilization for greater broadband deployment [10].

2.3.7.2   Electronic Health Records

Another spur to greater deployment of health information technology is the new health information technology initiative to support health-care reform. For instance, already 4,000 health-care providers have registered for the EHR incentives program. These would be the records developed and maintained by providers, rather than by consumers. The Centers for Medicare and Medicaid Services said that they expect that number to increase because eligible health-care professionals have the opportunity to receive incentive payments of up to $44,000 from Medicare or $63,750 from Medicaid. Hospitals that are eligible for the incentives can receive millions from both Medicare and Medicaid [14].

While we see the beginnings of greater generalized use of health information technology in this EHR program, the edges are becoming clearer where telerehabilitation could intersect with the health-care services delivery system. For instance, people with disabilities might be expected to utilize their health-care provider's EHRs not only for hospital services but perhaps also as they engage with rehabilitation service providers.

2.3.7.3   Personal Health Records

Use of personal health records (PHRs) by people with disabilities is as nascent as it is for other members of the population, but will surely expand as health-care systems are forced to become more automated for cost savings and effectiveness. PHRs are generally understood to be those health-care records that the consumer maintains and keeps.

A recent preliminary study reported that people with disabilities would find value in PHR use in medical care coordination, but remained cautious about the utilization of that information by government agencies [17]. The study also found a "relatively low rate of interest in the use of a PHR to provide medical records and information to federal agencies" [17]. The study concluded that there is a need for increasing awareness among those with disabilities as to the range of benefits PHRs can provide, especially in longer-term complex situations. These conclusions point the way to how connection with PHRs owned by people with disabilities could deploy: rehabilitation services providers, who are not perceived as "federal agencies" or other government authority figures, could find themselves among the professionals that consumers with disabilities "allow" to use their PHR records.

2.3.7.4 Health Information Exchanges

By 2014, states are expected to have set up technology systems to support other new health-care reform requirements to assure that everyone has health insurance. This effort includes states setting up HIEs that will start helping small business and people—including people with disabilities—select and pay for health plans. Typically, these will be websites with information on tax credits, cost sharing, Medicaid eligibility, children's health care, and available health-care insurers.

There is every reason to believe that HIEs and rehabilitation service provision could intersect via these HIE efforts. People with disabilities go online like everyone else to find out about health-care information, and these sites have the potential to facilitate and provide links to all kinds of services.

2.3.7.5 Accessible and Usable Health-Care Systems

While health information technology generally has not yet become ubiquitous, there is movement in the direction to ensure accessibility and usability for people with disabilities, which may support telerehabilitation efforts. For instance, in November 2010, the U.S. Health and Human Services (HHS) agency provided guidance to the states that included affirming that standards for accessibility by people with disabilities in new health-care delivery information technology systems were part of the technical standards [27].

While this is targeted to Medicaid information systems, purchase of such systems will ensure fewer barriers to access and can drive greater accessibility to more systems. This effort will affect both consumers with disabilities using such health-care systems and employees of entities who have disabilities. Such standards—if properly implemented—could ensure retention of jobs, more jobs available for people with disabilities, and ease of use for all consumers and will likely affect many state-level efforts in regard to provision of health care, a companion service to rehabilitation.

Specifically, the HHS guidance (Section "5.1.3 Standards for Accessibility") clearly states that "enrollment and eligibility systems should be designed to meet the diverse needs of users (e.g., consumers, state personnel, others) ... Systems shall include usability features or functions that accommodate the needs of persons with disabilities, including those who use assistive technology..." This standard invokes Sections 504 and 508 of the Rehabilitation Act for compliance purposes and cites to WCAG 2.0 website accessibility guidelines. *Note*: This HHS guidance also addresses security and privacy standards, including the HIPAA requirement for protection of personal health information, all of which are essential components of a system that users can trust.

The new guidance is a significant step forward in ensuring that states address accessibility needs and could go a long way to make sure that concurrent rehabilitation efforts are not stymied by electronic barriers to access.

2.3.8 Rehabilitation Worldwide to Expand

In the larger global view, the worldwide demand for rehabilitation services and professionals will be growing, and this should influence the growth of telerehabilitation as there will be rising numbers of people across the world expecting, and needing, such services. This will occur as a result of the rising expectations of people with disabilities worldwide, as they come to understand how their civil rights will be enhanced by the international policy driver, the United Nations Convention on the Rights of People with Disabilities (UNCRPD).

There are several provisions, both direct and indirect, in the UNCRPD that address rehabilitation. For instance, "Article 26, Habilitation and rehabilitation" asserts that states or countries "shall organize, strengthen and extend comprehensive habilitation and rehabilitation services and programmes, particularly in the areas of health, employment, education and social services, in such a way that these services and programmes...begin at the earliest possible stage, and are based on the multidisciplinary assessment of individual needs and strengths..." This same UNCRPD article encourages the development of training for professionals and staff working in habilitation and rehabilitation services, and the use of assistive devices and technologies [28].

Likewise, indirectly, the UNCRPD provisions for education; health; work and employment; standard of living; participation in political, public life, and cultural life; recreation; and leisure and sport (Articles 24–30) [30] will raise, and are raising, the expectation of millions of people with disabilities and their families worldwide to participate in every area of social and civic life in a greater way.

Now with over 147 countries as signatories to the UNCRPD [29], there is a clear trend worldwide toward advancement of the civil rights of people with disabilities and which, through rising expectations by people with disabilities, will require rehabilitative effort. There is little doubt that this will drive change, even if not fast enough for some, at the state and local levels. Part of this change will be the establishment of rehabilitation programming. To meet these needs, there will have to be developed systems of telerehabilitation that will bring services to even the most remote locations, through wireless broadband or related technologies.

2.4 General Policy Outlook

The policy challenges are many for telerehabilitation if these trends continue, and will impact the constituency of people with disabilities directly and in a negative way if they are not resolved. Teleassessment and teletherapy must be seen as more equivalent to clinical "on-site" encounters and thus reimbursable. If payment for remote monitoring, certain diagnostic procedures, some forms of counseling, and assessment and management also become part of the health-care technology ecosystem, then telerehabilitation can grow concurrently. Privacy and security concerns and the ability to trust entities to handle very personal information will be critical for consumers. More research on awareness and more education will be necessary to ensure that consumers find relevance and want to participate in telerehabilitation practices.

Similarly important, however, is the overall technology policy environment, with an active technology policy agenda expected in the next 2 years as the U.S. Congress grapples with issues such as Internet taxes, Internet traffic management, digital ownership, Universal Service Fund reform, web tracking, and privacy and related issues. Often, for technology, however, the issues are likely to be framed within economic policy and seen as part of "getting the economy back on track" and to create jobs. This will help ensure that technology policies do not become too mired in partisan gridlock [15]. Also, as health information technology becomes more ubiquitous, due to the drive for cost savings and efficiencies, there is little doubt that solution of those policy problems will also assist telerehabilitation.

Summary

- Rehabilitation of people with disabilities encompasses the programmatic efforts aimed at maintaining and improving their lives, with a focus on their employment.
- Telerehabilitation is where rehabilitation for people with disabilities intersects with broadband technologies.
- Rehabilitation activities such as assessment, evaluation, review, training, cueing, reminding, etc. are surely candidates for transfer to information technology processes. However, less usage and lower rates of adoption to broadband or Internet by people with disabilities are a challenge for telerehabilitation practitioners.
- Implementation of national policies with specific targets for health information technology initiatives will spur other efforts to ensure more broadband-based health-care services delivery, which can partner with rehabilitation efforts.
- The worldwide demand for rehabilitation services and professionals is expected to grow, which should influence the growth of telerehabilitation as well.

Abbreviations/Acronyms

EHR	Electronic health record
GPII	Global inclusive information infrastructure
HHS	Health and Human Services
HIE	Health information exchange

HIPAA   Health Insurance Portability and Accountability Act of 1996
NHIS   National Health Interview Survey
PHR   Personal health record
UNCRPD   United Nations Convention on the Rights of People with Disabilities

References

1. Allen E, Seaman J. Online Education in the United States. Sloan-C Report on Online Education Enrollment. Sloan Foundation. 2010. Available at: http://www.usdla.org/assets/pdf_files/2010%20Sloan-C%20Report%20on%20Online%20Education%20Enrollment.pdf.
2. Blumberg SJ, Luke JV. Wireless substitution: early release of estimates from the National Health Interview Survey, July–December 2008. National Center for Health Statistics. 2011. Available at: http://www.cdc.gov/nchs/data/nhis/earlyrelease/wireless200905.htm. Accessed 1 Nov 2011.
3. Bureau of Labor Statistics. Employment status of the civilian population by sex, age, and disability status, not seasonally adjusted. Available at: http://www.bls.gov/news.release/empsit.t06.htm. Accessed 1 Nov 2011.
4. Business Wire. Research and markets: mobile broadband in North America: forecasts and analysis 2010–2015. 2011. Available at: http://www.businesswire.com/news/home/20110131006962/en/Research-Markets-Mobile-Broadband-North-America-Forecasts. Accessed 31 Jan 2011.
5. Cisco Visual Networking Index. Global mobile data traffic forecast update, 2010–2015. 2011. Available at: http://www.cisco.com/en/US/solutions/collateral/ns341/ns525/ns537/ns705/ns827/white_paper_c11-520862.html. Accessed 1 Nov 2011.
6. Comscore Press Release. ComScore Releases March 2010 U.S. online video rankings. 2010. Available at: http://www.comscore.com/Press_Events/Press_Releases/2010/4/comScore_Releases_March_2010_U.S._Online_Video_Rankings. Accessed 1 Nov 2011.
7. Evans D. Top 25 technology predictions, IBSG innovations practice. Cisco Internet Business Solutions Group (IBSG). 2009. Available at: http://www.cisco.com/web/about/ac79/docs/Top_25_Predictions_121409rev.pdf.
8. Federal Communications Commission. Broadband and health care. In: National broadband plan: connecting America, Chapter 10, p. 197. 2010. Available at: http://www.broadband.gov/issues/healthcare.html. Accessed 24 Jan 2011.
9. Federal Communications Commission. National broadband plan: connecting America, Chapter 1. 2010. Available at: http://www.broadband.gov/plan/1-introduction/?search=rehabilitation.
10. Federal Communications Commission. National broadband plan: connecting America, Chapter 9. 2010. Available at: http://www.broadband.gov/plan/9-adoption-and-utilization/?search=rehabilitation. Accessed 1 Nov 2011.
11. Fox S. Americans living with disability and their technology profile. 2011. Available at: http://www.pewinternet.org/Reports/2011/Disability.aspx. Accessed 24 Jan 2011.
12. Global Public Inclusive Infrastructure, GPII.Org. GPII and NPII discussion. Available at: http://npii.org/index.html.
13. Google. Adding and editing automatic captions in YouTube. Available at: http://www.google.com/support/youtube/bin/answer.py?answer=100077.
14. Government Health IT. CMS counts 4,000 providers initially registering for EHR incentives. 2011. Available at: http://govhealthit.com/newsitem.aspx?nid=75862. Accessed 7 Jan 2011.
15. Gross G. Congress may be able to tackle tech issues in 2011, in Computer World. 2011. Available at: http://www.computerworld.com/s/article/9204458/Congress_may_be_able_to_tackle_tech_issues_in_2011. Accessed 1 Nov 2011.
16. Horrigan JB. Broadband adoption and use in America. OBI Working Paper Series No. 1. Available at: http://hraunfoss.fcc.gov/edocs_public/attachmatch/DOC-296442A1.pdf. Accessed 1 Nov 2011.

17. Lytle N, Simpson J, Horan T, et al. AAPD. Uncovering interests and concerns about personal health record use by individuals with disabilities: results of a preliminary survey. 2010. Available at: http://www.aapd.com/site/c.pvI1IkNWJqE/b.6422581/k.6DAC/Uncovering_Interests_and_Concerns_About_Personal_Health_Record_Use_By_Individuals_with_Disabilities_Results_of_a_Preliminary_Survey.htm.
18. National Center for Educational Statistics. Adult literacy in America. 3rd ed. 2002. Available at: http://nces.ed.gov/pubs93/93275.pdf. Accessed 1 Feb 2012.
19. National Council on Disability. The impact of the Americans with disabilities Act: assessing the progress toward achieving the goals of the ADA. Washington, D.C.: John R. Vaughn; 2007.
20. Perry MJ. Computers just keep getting cheaper and better. 2010. Available at: http://www.britannica.com/blogs/2010/04/computers-just-keep-getting-cheaper-and-better-and-we-should-eagerly-await-the-days-ahead/. Accessed 1 Nov 2011.
21. Pleis JR, Lucas JW. Provisional report: summary health statistics for U.S. adults: National Health Interview Survey; 2008. National Center for Health Statistics. Vital Health Stat 10(242), p 36. Available at: http://www.cdc.gov/nchs/data/series/sr_10/sr10_242.pdf. Accessed 1 Nov 2011.
22. Posny A. Live webcast. 2010. Available at: http://jfactivist.typepad.com/jfactivist/un_convention_on_the_rights_of_persons_with_disabilities/. Accessed 6 Dec 2010.
23. Rehabilitation Research and Training Center on Disability Statistics and Demographics. A NIDRR-Funded Center. 2011 Annual disability statistics compendium, Table 12.1 vocational rehabilitation—applicants: federal fiscal year 2008. Available at: http://disabilitycompendium.org/pdf/Compendium2011.pdf. Accessed 1 Nov 2011.
24. The United States Access Board. Section 508 facts: understanding Section 508 and the Access Board's standards. Available at: http://www.access-board.gov/sec508/brochure.htm. Accessed 1 Nov 2011.
25. U.S. Census Bureau. American community survey. 2008. Available at: http://www.census.gov/acs/www/index.html. Accessed 20 Jan 2011.
26. U.S. Commerce Department's Economics and Statistics Administration. Exploring the digital nation: home broadband Internet adoption in the United States. 2010. Available at: http://www.esa.doc.gov/Reports/exploring-digital-nation-home-broadband-internet-adoption-united-states. Accessed 1 Nov 2011.
27. U.S. Department of Health and Human Services. Guidance for exchange and Medicaid information technology (IT) systems, p. 5. Available at: http://www.hhs.gov/ociio/regulations/joint_cms_ociio_guidance.pdf. Accessed 1 Nov 2011.
28. UNCRPD. Article 26. Available at: http://www.un.org/disabilities/default.asp?id=286. Accessed 1 Nov 2011.
29. UNCRPD. Historic progress of signatories. Available at: http://www.un.org/disabilities/countries.asp?navid=12&pid=166. Accessed 1 Nov 2011.
30. United Nations Convention on the Rights of People with Disabilities. Available at: http://www.un.org/disabilities/default.asp?id=259. Accessed 1 Nov 2011.
31. Wikipedia. Definition of cloud computing. Available at: http://en.wikipedia.org/wiki/Cloud_computing.

Chapter 3
Telerehabilitation in the Military

Katie Ambrose Stout, Philip Girard, and Kristina Martinez

Abstract Traditional rehabilitation was born out of the military's need to treat injured soldiers after World War II. The number of military personnel incurring disabilities in recent conflicts is larger than that has been seen in the United States in over three decades. Rehabilitation trajectories for the improvement of physical function, cognition, psychosocial adjustment, and integration into society depend on the military's ability to detect problems and treat service members early after injury. Telerehabilitation is increasingly accepted within the military as a flexible alternative for providing critical access to specialty care for the growing number of service members returning with traumatic injuries.

3.1 Background

The Military Health System (MHS) is a global medical network within the Department of Defense (DoD) that provides cutting-edge health care to U.S. military personnel worldwide. The 59 hospitals and 364 health clinics within the MHS

K.A. Stout, PT, DPT, MS CBIS (✉)
Department of Tele-Health, Tele-Rehabilitation Chief,
Kimbrough Ambulatory Care Center,
Fort Meade, MD/Rosslyn, VA, USA
e-mail: katharine.c.ambrose.ctr@health.mil

P. Girard
Department of Clinical Initiatives, Defense and Veterans Brain Injury Center,
Walter Reed Army Medical Center, Washington, DC, USA

Manchester VA Medical Center, Manchester, NH, USA

K. Martinez
Tele-Rehabilitation Services, Henry M. Jackson Foundation CTR for Defense and Veterans
Brain Injury Center, James A. Haley Veterans' Hospital,
13000 Bruce B. Downs, PMRS, Tampa, FL 33612, USA
e-mail: kristina.martinez1@va.gov

S. Kumar, E.R. Cohn (eds.), *Telerehabilitation*, Health Informatics,
DOI 10.1007/978-1-4471-4198-3_3, © Springer-Verlag London 2013

deliver high-quality care to a beneficiary population of 9.6 million service members, veterans, and family members [16]. Clinicians at these military treatment facilities (MTFs) are committed to saving the lives and caring for service members and their beneficiaries having illnesses such as cancer, heart disease, and diabetes. The MHS is best known for its emergency life-saving procedures for combat-wounded troops on the battlefield and for the coordination of care for all soldiers, sailors, airmen, and Marines in times of war and peace. Once medical services are rendered, the goal of the MHS is to help injured service members rebuild their lives physically, socially, and emotionally. Efforts by the MHS to promote restorative healing of service members in remote and isolated areas may involve the use of advanced communication technology. These programs may take many forms and are collectively known as telerehabilitation. An understanding of the development of both "rehabilitation" and "telemedicine" within the military is helpful to understand the intersection of these two fields.

3.2   Evolution of Rehabilitation in the Military

The history of rehabilitation in the military goes back to World War II when restorative aides cared for and rehabilitated injured service members [2]. Since the middle of the twentieth century, physical therapists and occupational therapists have been billeted officer positions in the U.S. military. Additionally, the military provides specialized training in physical therapy (PT) and occupational therapy (OT) for qualified enlisted members to assist in therapy clinics [3]. Speech-language pathology (SLP) services within the MHS are provided solely by civilian and contract providers [9]. Officers, enlisted members, DoD civilians, and contract rehabilitation providers work collectively to care for injured service members and beneficiaries throughout the MHS.

Psychological distress often accompanies combat injury as service members simultaneously cope with adjustment to disability, separation from their unit, and the emotional burden of combat [5]. Thus, the rehabilitation team also includes combat-injured peer mentors who work to ease medical transitions for wounded warriors and their families. Individual family members are encouraged to join their loved ones during the rehabilitative process because they motivate the service member and contribute to their emotional healing.

The rapid growth of rehabilitation services within the DoD has led to the creation of high-tech, state-of-the-art rehabilitation programs, such as the Military Advanced Training Center (MATC) at Walter Reed Army Medical Center (WRAMC) and the Center for the Intrepid at Brooke Army Medical Center. Both facilities have the very latest in rehabilitation technology, including the Computer-Assisted Rehabilitation Environment (CAREN) system. CAREN is an immersive environment simulator that allows recovering warriors to perform virtual activities, simultaneously challenging cognitive, neurologic, and musculoskeletal functions [13]. This system, and others similar to it, provides unique opportunities for therapeutic breakthrough, which is crucial throughout the rehabilitative process. Most often, the rehabilitation process may continue for many years depending on the severity of injury and the resilience of the service member. Thus, exporting the capabilities of these advanced systems and developing methods to continue needed therapy in places where service members can receive care closer to home becomes the priority.

3.3 Telehealth in the Military

Prior to high-tech computer rehabilitation systems, the military developed a comprehensive electronic medical record (EMR) that provides a platform for all health operations worldwide. Designed for multidisciplinary and transcontinental use, the EMR ensures communication of patient health status during deployments, following injury, and throughout any medical transition or change of duty station. Clinicians at multiple military facilities can view the patient's medical information and work together to provide the best care for the patient, regardless of geographical distances. The EMR allows information sharing for direct patient care anywhere within the MHS, thereby making networking via telemedicine technology possible [14].

Telehealth applications were initiated by the U.S. military to meet the medical needs of service members in remote and isolated areas. The unique nature of military operations makes expanding and maintaining robust treatment options imperative. Telemedicine initiatives for direct patient care in the military were first described more than two decades ago. In 1988, disaster-support telehealth services were provided by military and civilian facilities to victims of the Armenian earthquake. In 1990, the Alabama National Guard was able to deploy teleradiology services to help victims of Hurricane Hugo living in the Virgin Islands. Telemedicine services were also deployed to augment care to service members involved in the first Gulf War Conflict, as well as for humanitarian missions in Haiti and Somalia [6, 14].

Most recently, telemedicine has been used to connect providers at MTFs and thereby leverage resources and streamline care within the MHS. In 2002, a pilot project to provide ear, nose, and throat (ENT), behavioral health, and sleep assessments began to take shape at MTFs around the world [12]. The outcomes included improved access to care, improved utilization of clinicians already working within the MHS, and improved continuity of care for patients who had a change in duty station while receiving medical care.

In 1998, the Telemedicine and Advanced Technology Research Center (TATRC) was established as part of the U.S. Army Medical Research and Materiel Command (USAMRMC) to address critical gaps in DoD medical programs and foster research on telemedicine, mobile health, and hundreds of other key scientific portfolios [1, 6]. The use of advanced technologies to support deployed forces had been a common theme as far back as 1993, when Lt. Col. (Dr.) Ronald Poropatich was deployed to Somalia during Operation Restore Hope. Today, TATRC continues to support partnerships between the military, the Veterans Administration (VA), universities, and community health systems to improve services for patients in remote and medically underserved areas and especially in response to the need for technological solutions that can expedite the care of service members currently deployed and returning from duty.

At present, the military utilizes a robust communications infrastructure to deliver familiar technological applications for operational purposes, including teleconsultation, distance learning, assistive technology, mobile health, and a variety of web-enabled applications. These systems are often readily used by the military medical system to treat effectively the service personnel who are more transient by the nature of their obligation to move with their unit or change duty stations as needed. In addition, the urgent need for clinical interventions on the battlefield and at all levels of care fosters innovation that helps shape the future of medical technology. Ultimately, the goal of telerehabilitation in the military is to support the alliance between military medical professionals, patients, families, and peers to maximize therapy and provide optimal health and wellness.

3.4   Patient–Provider Health-Care Alliance

Like any medical intervention, the success of a telerehabilitation program relies on a strong patient–provider relationship. If the patient is unable to perceive the effectiveness of the activity or doubts the credibility of the provider, the patient will demonstrate little motivation and poor compliance [7]. The military's technology systems and EMR allow for successful collaboration between providers and patients, creating strong patient–provider relationships and instilling confidence in patients about the telerehabilitation programs. A reliable connection to the patient is as important as good rapport in ensuring trust and motivation, which will, in turn, increase consistency and compliance of the patient, resulting in successful treatment outcomes. Considering this need for effective communication, interactive video is typically used for most types of telerehabilitation. Store-and-forward applications and web-based technologies may also be used independently for patient follow-up or in addition to interactive video.

While the technical approaches to telerehabilitation in the military are the same as in the civilian world, there exist many challenges unique to providing care to the military: nature of the injury, environment of care, military unit demands, and deployments. In addition, service members have to evaluate both short- and long-term goals following injury and the changes that may take place in their career. Navigating the complex military medical system can be particularly challenging for those in transition who have symptoms that affect cognition and behavior.

Additionally, delays in treatment can reduce health outcomes. Although service members may receive immediate treatment for injuries while being deployed, they may not begin needed therapy until later (unless they are severally injured, in which case they are medically evacuated). There are many reasons for this, including limited access to therapists in forward locations or the denial of symptoms that stems from a desire to remain actively engaged with their unit in theater. The stigma associated with revealing mental health and emotional symptoms also prevents many service members with comorbid conditions from seeking treatment early. For these reasons, there is an increased need for rehabilitation services when troops return home. Military health-care providers must have an understanding of these issues and an appreciation for the commitment that each service member has to his or her comrades and country, in order to gain the trust of the service member and thereby increase his or her overall motivation and chances for success.

Orders to change duty stations can have a significant effect on the rehabilitation processes. Rehabilitation services may not be available at the new location, which complicates the transfer as service members attempt to initiate services through a new provider after they are enrolled at the new duty station. These challenges are particularly disruptive to the consistency of rehabilitation care for the patient, which can adversely affect their compliance.

Telerehabilitation technology can help smooth the continuum of care by facilitating provider handoff or continued treatment from the initial provider. Education may be offered for the new provider through the telehealth device, or even a discussion on the patient's progress throughout the treatment and where the treatment was left off. If such rehabilitative services are unavailable at the service member's new location, their current provider may be able to continue treatment through telerehabilitation. A similar model is used in the care of patients with traumatic injuries during transition from the military to the VA system. Interactive video teleconferencing (VTC) allows all members of the clinical team at a military medical center to meet with the receiving rehabilitation team at the VA medical center, to plan important medical transitions. These meetings usually include the individual patient and patient's family who are able to meet the VA team for the first time, ask questions, and discuss elements of the care plan. Later on, VTC may be used again to allow the military medical team to follow up with the patient from a distance.

Telehealth technology can also be used to provide clinical and therapeutic services to the service member when they move closer to home. Telerehabilitation may alleviate stressors and allow for a smooth introduction to a civilian health-care professional by providing real-time assistance through video or telephone. Although it is not possible to complete all types of therapy using telerehabilitation or telemonitoring, the added connection to a health-care provider or therapist can have a positive effect on motivation. Telehealth methods can also be used to support patient care in the home and help deter negative behaviors, reduce depression, and otherwise provide an important safety system. The DoD is introducing mobile health technologies designed to allow providers the ability to track changes in a patient's health status that can be input daily in response to simple questions. Similarly, web-based "self-help" applications allow service members and family members to track personal health goals. Access to counselors is also available through the web as needed to augment continued therapy. Together these technologies are supporting the patient–provider alliance by improving communication and follow-up.

3.5   Access to Rehabilitation Specialists

The U.S. military has bases on all continents, which may, in some cases, be a long distance away from rehabilitation services. The rehabilitation model in the military is similar to that of the civilian world: physical therapists and occupational therapists perform evaluations and reevaluations; active duty technicians with specialty training in PT or OT then carry out the exercise treatment plans, similar to the civilian PT or OT assistant. However, some of the smaller military facilities may employ a staff, with only a few full-time clinicians. A specially trained military technician may work full time at one remote facility while a therapist covers three or four remote sites with monthly site visits. Small military sites do not usually have OT or SLP services due to the lack of a continuous demand. Moreover, the remote nature of smaller sites makes it more difficult to recruit and maintain qualified staff. Depending on the region (or state within the United States), access to clinical rehabilitative services may be limited.

By contrast, larger military bases have ample access to specialty care, including PT, OT, and SLP. However, as troops return from deployment in large numbers, even well-staffed, high-volume centers may be challenged to meet sudden temporary demands for immediate evaluation and treatment. Thus, troop surges create another unique challenge for which telemedicine provides a possible solution.

3.6   Traumatic Brain Injury

Conflicts in Iraq and Afghanistan have left a large number of soldiers in need of specialized assessment and treatment for traumatic brain injury (TBI). TBI has been identified as the signature injury of the wars in the Middle East. More than 195,000 service members have sustained a TBI as a result of current conflicts, including 5,400 with severe or penetrating brain injuries that required medical evacuation from theater [15]. Severely injured service members receive prompt and comprehensive care within the MHS, which typically includes a multidisciplinary, long-term plan for rehabilitation when indicated. However, non-medically evacuated service members who return with their unit may deny symptoms or may have a variety of subtle symptoms related to a TBI that are difficult to detect early. Rehabilitation can play an important role in restoring physical, cognitive, and emotional health for those with TBI of any severity.

Lack of neurologists, neuropsychologists, physiatrists, and other specialists within the military leaves some commands in need of assistance. Prior to the huge influx in military members in need of TBI care, patients were referred to the civilian community where TBI treatment models had been developed and used for decades. Although the rehabilitative care provided in the civilian community can be very good, disruption in care still occurs when a military member changes duty stations to locations where no rehabilitation services, whether civilian or otherwise, exist. In the continental United States, high-quality civilian rehabilitation programs are found primarily in the most densely populated areas of the country and are usually not available in remote areas that are often home to military personnel.

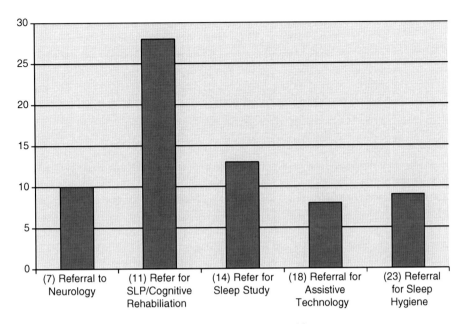

Fig. 3.1 Recommendation prevalence from remote neurocognitive assessments

In 2008, the U.S. Army Medical Command established a tele-TBI network to address the need for greater access to specialty care and rehabilitation services to its geographically dispersed military population. Five regional medical commands spanning 14 time zones (from American Samoa to Germany) were organized with personnel and telehealth equipment procured, based on the clinical needs identified in each region [4]. Initially, the U.S. Army's Northern Regional Medical Command, in partnership with the Defense and Veterans Brain Injury Center (DVBIC) Office of Telemedicine, set up a program to provide remote neuropsychological assessment of service members with cognitive or behavioral problems following a TBI. In 2010, three neuropsychologists had completed 78 comprehensive neuropsychological assessments of service members in remote locations. Of the top five referral recommendations, three included therapy services: SLP/cognitive rehabilitation, assistive technology, and sleep hygiene counseling. All the top five referral recommendations are services that can be successfully implemented through telemedicine modalities (see Fig. 3.1).

Experience with this program to date has helped identify the need for specific treatments that could also be offered via telehealth. Specifically PT, OT, and SLP services were all identified as possible areas where provider access could be augmented remotely within the MHS.

In 2008, DVBIC began to develop a multidisciplinary team that would be staffed like a traditional TBI clinic, but with clinicians who would work entirely remotely. This model allows clinical services to be easily redirected in response to demand fluctuations at distant sites.

Working together with the dental clinic at Ft. Lee Virginia, DVBIC developed a remote temporomandibular joint (TMJ) dysfunction clinic. Ft. Lee dental clinic identified an influx of patients returning from combat with TMJ disorders. The dental clinic has the capacity to provide dental splinting and education; however, TMJ dysfunction often has a stress and a cervical spine posture component to the symptom complex. Without behavioral health and PT interventions, the dental clinic has limited capabilities to treat these patients successfully. The DVBIC tele-TBI physical therapist was contacted to assist with this project because many of the service members with TMJ dysfunction had been diagnosed with mild TBI. Using interactive video already in place at Ft. Lee, the tele-TBI physical therapist sees the patients in conjunction with the onsite behavioral health biofeedback therapist. Posture education is completed and service members are coached through a three- to five-item home exercise program. Symptom management and lifestyle changes are also taught during these sessions to decrease the pain associated with TMJ and improve quality of life.

Ft. Sill, Oklahoma, a geographically isolated military facility with limited specialty services, also benefits from telerehabilitation for their TBI population. Like many MTFs, Ft. Sill had a large number of soldiers returning from Iraq and Afghanistan with significant TBI-related symptoms, which were the results of exposure to blasts or other traumatic events. A VTC link to Brooke Army Medical Center in San Antonio, Texas, made it possible for soldiers at Ft. Sill to receive cognitive rehabilitation services from a specially trained speech-language pathologist.

3.7 Tele-Speech Language Pathology

Prior to large demand for telerehabilitation services due to TBI, telerehabilitation in the military began in the late 1990s when the SLP department at Tripler Army Medical Center recognized a need for telerehabilitation services in the Pacific Rim region, which is made up of many small islands with remote military bases [11]. Service members and their families stationed at some small Pacific islands had to travel long distances to the main treatment facility to access SLP treatment. The time and cost of travel often limited the help that those in need of SLP services received. Using telehealth technology, the SLP team at Tripler began to conduct speech and cognitive evaluations with VTC for improved accessibility to the specialized service for those stationed on the remote islands, and this service was proved to be equally effective as face-to-face services.

3.8 Tele-Physical Therapy

Current applications of tele-PT in the military are varied and include services provided within formal teleneurosurgery programs, the tele-TBI programs, and programs within the European Command. Several independent duty stations in Europe are staffed by a PT technician. These duty stations are supported by a remote physical therapist who visits monthly to conduct evaluations and re-evaluations. Because many of the sites are separated by long distances, the therapists are limited in the number of evaluations that can be completed and in their ability to assess the progress of patients already seen. In September 2010, a physical therapist in Europe responsible for four independent duty stations conducted a trial of remote PT. The physical therapist met with the patient and the PT technician over VTC to discuss the progress made since the last visit. The physical therapist also performed a functional evaluation with the hands-on assistance of the PT technician. The physical therapist was then able to make adjustments to the EMR treatment plan in real time with the technician and the patient. This program clearly resulted in considerable cost savings, increased access to care, and supported the continuation and expansion of the tele-PT model in Europe.

3.9 Teleneurosurgery

The military teleneurosurgery service connects WRAMC in Washington DC to several MTFs without neurosurgeons, including Ft. Bragg, North Carolina, and Ft. Knox, Kentucky. A particular focus of the program is low back pain, which is one of the leading causes for musculoskeletal pain syndromes in the military due to the physical demands placed on service members [8]. Service members with back pain require a neurosurgical evaluation to determine the need for medications, PT, and, in rare cases, surgery.

The WRAMC teleneurosurgery clinic uses clinical components from both commands, which consist of a physician assistant (PA), case manager, neurosurgeon, and physical therapist. The neurosurgery PA, located at Ft. Bragg, performs the initial evaluation onsite and orders laboratory work, imaging studies, and other tests depending on the needs of the individual patient. The case manager helps with scheduling and individual case management based on the patient's needs. During a follow-up visit with the PA, there is an interactive video conference with the neurosurgeon, case manager, and physical therapist at WRAMC. Through a military EMR, the team at WRAMC is able to access and review the notes from the initial visit with the PA and any results from the testing that was ordered at Ft. Bragg.

After the interdisciplinary evaluation, patients are referred for surgery or conservative treatment. The conservative treatment plan utilizes the on-site PA and remote physical therapist. The teleneurosurgery physical therapist continues to work with the patient over video, monitoring responses to PT and providing patient education.

Prior to the initiation of the teleneurosurgery clinic, any soldier at Ft. Bragg with back pain was automatically referred to WRAMC for evaluation and treatment planning. This model required the soldier to make multiple trips to and from North Carolina to Washington DC to meet with the neurosurgery team. The teleneurosurgery clinic eliminated much of the previous travel that was often unnecessary while maintaining successful clinical outcomes and patient satisfaction.

3.10 The Future of Telerehabilitation in the Military

As of September 2009, more than 17,000 behavioral telehealth and teleneurosurgery patient encounters have been completed, with an estimated cost savings of over $2 million [10]. Telerehabilitation continues to prove its worth within the MHS through increased access to specialized rehabilitative care, reduced patient and specialist travel, decreased lost work days, and improved unit readiness. Given its vast area of operations, the diverse medical corps, and the constant need for patient care, the growth possibilities for telerehabilitation seem endless. Today's generation of patients and military health-care providers are especially familiar and comfortable with computer technology, including interactive video which is now commonly used in the home. Together with the Veterans Health Administration, the MHS will continue to support innovations in health care to improve the lives of service members.

Summary

- Telerehabilitation is increasingly accepted within the military to provide the service members returning with traumatic injuries with critical access to specialty care and to support the alliance between military medical professionals, patients, and families for optimal health and wellness.
- Rehabilitation in the military was conceptualized during World War II when restorative aides cared for and rehabilitated injured service members. The rapid growth of rehabilitation services within the DoD has created high-tech, state-of-the-art rehabilitation programs.
- Prior to high-tech computer rehabilitation systems, the military developed a comprehensive EMR system to share information anywhere within the MHS for direct patient care.
- Telehealth applications were initiated by the U.S. military to meet the medical needs of service members in remote and isolated areas.
- At present, the military uses a robust communications infrastructure to deliver technological applications such as teleconsultation, distance learning, assistive technology, mobile health, and a variety of web-enabled applications.
- Given its vast area of operations, the diverse medical corps, and the constant need for patient care, the growth possibilities for telerehabilitation seem endless.

Abbreviations/Acronyms

CAREN	Computer-Assisted Rehabilitation Environment
DoD	Department of Defense
DVBIC	Defense and Veterans Brain Injury Center
EMR	Electronic medical record

ENT	Ear, nose, and throat
MATC	Military Advanced Training Center
MHS	Military Health System
MTF	Military treatment facilities
OT	Occupational therapy
PA	Physician assistant
PT	Physical therapy
SLP	Speech-language pathology
TATRC	Telemedicine and Advanced Technology Research Center
TBI	Traumatic brain injury
TMJ	Temporomandibular joint
USAMRMC	U.S. Army Medical Research and Materiel Command
VA	Veterans Administration
VTC	Video teleconferencing
WRAMC	Walter Reed Army Medical Center

Conflicts of Interest The views expressed in this case study are those of the authors and do not necessarily reflect the official policy or position of the Department of the Navy, Department of the Army, Department of Defense, Department of Veterans Affairs, Defense and Veterans Brain Injury Center, or the U.S. Government.

We certify that all individuals who qualify as authors have been listed; that each has participated in the conception and design of this work, the analysis of data (when applicable), the writing of the document, and the approval of the submission of this version; that the document represents valid work; that if we used information derived from another source, we obtained all necessary approvals to use it and made appropriate acknowledgements in the document; and that each takes public responsibility for it.

References

1. A brief history of TATRC. Available at: http://www.tatrc.org/?p=about_history Accessed 23 Dec 2010.
2. APTA history. Available at: http://www.apta.org/AM/Template.cfm?Section=History_and_Information&Template=/TaggedPage/TaggedPageDisplay.cfm&TPLID=48&ContentID=14772. Accessed 15 Oct 2010.
3. Clinical care providers. Available at: http://www.navy.com/navy/careers/healthcare/clinical-care.html. Accessed 15 Oct 2010.
4. Doar CR, McVeigh F, Poropatich R. Innovated new technologies to identify and treat traumatic brain injuries: crossover technologies and approaches between military and civilian applications. Telemed J. 2009;16(3):373–81.
5. Frain MP, Bethel M, Bishop M. A roadmap for rehabilitation counseling to serve military veterans with disabilities. J Orthop Res. 2010;76(1):13–21.
6. Garchnek V, Burkle FM. Applications of telemedicine and telecommunications to disaster medicine. JAMA. 1999;6(1):26–37.
7. Grindley E, Nayspany A, Zizzi S. Use of protection motivation theory, affect, and barriers to understand and predict adherence to outpatient rehabilitation. Phys Ther. 2008;88(12): 1529–40.
8. Hauret KG, Jones BH, Bullock SH, et al. Musculoskeletal injuries; description of an under-recognized injury problem among military personnel. Am J Prev Med. 2010;38(1S):S61–70.

9. Lewis J. Speech pathology jobs in the army. *eHow.* 2010 Available at: http://www.ehow.com/list_6865536_speech-pathology-jobs-army.html. Accessed 16 Dec 2010.
10. Lyness SS, Baynard W. The Walter Reed tele-neurosurgery program. Annual Meeting Presentation, American Telemedicine Association, 2007. Available at: http://www.google.com/url?sa=t&rct=j&q=&esrc=s&frm=1&source=web&cd=2&cad=rja&ved=0CCYQFjAB&url=http%3A%2F%2Fmedia.americantelemed.org%2Fconf%2F2007%2FPresentations%2FTuesday%2FDELTAB%2F1430%2520Lyness%2520DELTAB%2520Tue.ppt&ei=LcxZUL7OO5PC0AGVr4GICA&usg=AFQjCNEnjObmBJOFT3kaqfpJLY-sE2sCVg&sig2=l6UJWk_0SNFMjaSShg0nHg. Accessed 16 Dec 2010.
11. Mashima P, Doarn C. Overview of telehealth activities in speech-language pathology. Telemed J. 2008;14(10):1101–17.
12. Melcer T, Hunsaker D, Crann B, et al. A prospective evaluation of ENT telemedicine in remote military populations seeking specialty care. Telemed J. 2002;83:301–11.
13. Military Advanced Training Center. 2010. Available at: http://www.wramc.army.mil/research/programs/lem/Pages/matc.aspx. Accessed 16 Dec 2010.
14. Morris TJ, Pajak J, Havlik F, et al. Battlefield medical information system – tactical (BMIST): the application of mobile computing technologies to support health surveillance in the Department of Defense. Telemed J. 2006;124:409–16.
15. TBI Categories (2000–2010). Available at: http://www.dvbic.org/images/pdfs/TBI-Numbers/2009-2010Q3-updated-as-of/2000-2010Q3-Updated-as-of-15-NOV-2010.aspx. Accessed 15 Dec 2010.
16. What is the MHS? Available at: http://health.mil/About_MHS/index.aspx. Accessed 20 Dec 2010.

Chapter 4
Nonverbal Communication and Telerehabilitation

Donald B. Egolf

Abstract The purpose of this chapter is to show the importance of nonverbal communication in the telerehabilitation field. Examples showing the relevance of nonverbal communication are provided for a number of nonverbal areas, particularly the monitoring of the patient's vital signs (vitalics), the physical appearance of the patient (organismics, cosmetics, and costuming), touch (haptics), body movements and postures (kinesics), facial characteristics and expressions (personics), voice (vocalics), time (chronemics), and space (proxemics). Stressed in the chapter is that both verbal and nonverbal messages are important in the therapeutic endeavor. The verbal tells, while the nonverbal shows. The vigilant therapist is always looking for any contradictions between verbal and nonverbal messages during therapy sessions. It is stressed that many off-the-shelf gaming products have made telerehabilitation sessions more visible, more affordable, and more motivating for patients.

4.1 Introduction

The purpose of this chapter is to discuss the relevance of nonverbal communication to telerehabilitation efforts. To begin the chapter some definitions will be given. When giving definitions, particularly in the behavioral sciences, it is often wise to keep in mind the warning of Durant [8], who said that to get involved in issues of definition is to:

> ...let loose the dogs of philosophic war. For nothing is so difficult as definition, Nor anything so severe a test and exercise of mental clarity and skill.

D.B. Egolf
Department of Communication, 1117 Cathedral of Learning, University of Pittsburgh,
4200 Fifth Avenue, Pittsburgh, PA 15260, USA
e-mail: ratchet@pitt.edu

S. Kumar, E.R. Cohn (eds.), *Telerehabilitation*, Health Informatics,
DOI 10.1007/978-1-4471-4198-3_4, © Springer-Verlag London 2013

The Durant caveat is given because the definitions presented below may not be agreed upon by all readers and researchers, and may even provoke some quibbles among them. Four key terms that need to be defined are *nonverbal communication, verbal communication, rehabilitation, and telerehabilitation.*

4.2 Definitions

The definitions given below are derived from Egolf and Chester [11].

By *nonverbal communication* is meant that form of communication wherein messages are sent by virtue of an agent's internal bodily activity (vitalics), physical characteristics (organismics), adornment (cosmetics and costuming), touching behavior (haptics), body movements and postures (kinesics), facial expressions (personics), eye behavior (oculesics), vocal behavior (vocalics), utilization of time (chronemics), and utilization and design of spaces (proxemics).

Verbal communication is communication using language: speaking, writing, or signing [e.g., American Sign Language (ASL)]. A language is a system of symbols known by at least two individuals.

Rehabilitation refers to the activity wherein a therapist or clinician works with a patient or client to *restore, gain,* or *maintain* some physical, cognitive, social, or vocational function. An athlete with an anterior cruciate ligament (ACL) tear is often treated first with surgery, then with physical therapy, and then returned to the playing field 9–12 months post injury. The athlete's physical function is *restored.* On the other hand, the soldier who suffers a thigh-level traumatic amputation of a leg will be treated by compensatory procedures in order to *gain* bipedal functioning. In particular, the soldier will be fitted with a prosthetic leg and then be given physical therapy to use the prosthetic device. Finally, alterations might be made to a senior citizen's house or residence to help the occupant *maintain* independence.

Telerehabilitation refers to offering rehabilitation services at a distance. The distance could be from a major urban hospital to a rural hospital, for instance, or, and most frequently, between a hospital or clinic and a patient's home. Telerehabilitation relies on technology and thus a caveat must be given. In the aviation industry, the common saying is that if it flies it is obsolete. Therefore, many techniques reported in this chapter may already be obsolete or significantly altered before the pages fall from the press.

4.3 Comparing and Contrasting Verbal and Nonverbal Communication

Although the boundaries separating verbal communication and nonverbal communication are not always clearly defined, several features can be discerned. Verbal communication and nonverbal communication are similar in that both communication modalities can communicate symbolically. In language, think of the symbolic nature of proverbs; for instance, "don't put all your eggs in one basket" is seldom about eggs and egg baskets. Instead, the phrase is used symbolically in a variety of situations. In the nonverbal realm, the color red can be symbolic of many things: danger, passion, part of the field in football, the devil, and running an engine at too high an rpm rate, for example.

The contrasting factors are greater in number. Nonverbal communication is more primitive both phylogenetically and ontogenetically. Throughout evolutionary development, the vast majority of living organisms communicated nonverbally. And at any instant today, the vast majority of the messages communicated in the world are nonverbal. In spite of the attention given to experiments purporting to show that certain higher-level mammals communicate verbally, no two mammals and no human–mammal pair has ever been observed communicating verbally in nature. Ontogenetic development refers to the development from birth onward. No baby is born speaking, but virtually all babies communicate nonverbally from the moment of birth. The communication modalities are touch, smell, voice, and vision. Early development theorists [2, 19] made note of this communication and its importance for development throughout life.

Nonverbal communication is continuous whereas verbal communication is not. A communicator can always stop talking, writing, or signing (as in ASL), but that same communicator cannot stop communicating nonverbally. This fact has led to the expression of a number of double-negative expressions, for example, you cannot not communicate; nonverbally you can say the right thing or the wrong thing; you cannot say nothing; and nonverbally nothing never happens.

Nonverbal communication is the primary expresser of emotion, while verbal communication is the primary communicator of information. A TV reporter giving the details of a horrific event may become emotionally overwhelmed by the event as evidenced by a hesitant voice, a saddened facial expression, and quivering lips, for instance. So prominent is the emotional impact of the nonverbal message that Mehrabian [21] estimated that only 7% of the effect of a message is transmitted verbally. Even the role of emotion in logical decision making cannot be discounted. The neuroscientist Damasio [7] concluded that you cannot make a decision in the absence of emotion.

Finally, there seems to be a neurological division in the brain that correlates with the verbal–nonverbal dichotomy. In general, for 97% of the people in the world the left hemisphere is dominant for speech, language, and analytic thought and the right hemisphere is dominant for nonverbal processing (including perceiving others and their facial expressions; perceiving time, melodies, and prosody; perceiving emotion and self-awareness, for example). Evidence supporting this neurological division comes from brain trauma cases (stroke, gunshot wounds, head injuries, and so on) and from various brain scans. It is important to note that the division of labor in the brain is a general observation. The two hemispheres of the brain are connected at various points; the largest connector, often referred to as the 300 million lane expressway between the two hemispheres, is the corpus callosum.

4.4   Contradictory and Complementary Aspects of Verbal and Nonverbal Messages

In some cases, the verbal message and the nonverbal messages are contradictory. The person who says "very funny" after hearing a joke, but says it with a dull voice and a bland facial expression, is contradicting the verbal message with the nonverbal messages. In like manner, the person who says "I'm not nervous," but the person's hands are shaking again, is in a contradictory state. Psychologists and psychiatrists often question their clients on these contradictions, and ask their clients, when the clients are the recipients of contradictory messages, "which message do you believe?" In short, which message is more credible? Clients are often told to trust their guts. The contradictory condition is, in fact, a key component in many activities. In polygraph tests, for example, the examiner looks for contradictions between the verbal and the nonverbal. The interviewee answers the examiner's questions; this is the verbal component. At the same time, the examiner is tracking the interviewee's galvanic skin response, blood pressure, and respiration rate via the polygraph; this is the nonverbal component. Telerehabilitation therapists often look for contradictions between the verbal and the nonverbal. There is often a comparison between what the remote patient says, with what the patient shows, wittingly or unwittingly.

In most cases, the relationship between the verbal and the nonverbal messages is complementary. When talking about general physical dimensions, for example, when a speaker mentions "high," the hands and arms will go up; if "low" is mentioned, the arms and hands will go down; and for "wide," the arms and hands will spread. Ask someone to describe a spiral staircase and you most likely will find the person tracing a spiral with the hand. Warm greetings are often a combination of words, smiles, and embracing arms, for instance. On the opposite side of the coin, a person who is upset can express verbally the felt emotion and at the same time show facial expressions that complement the words.

4.5   Sample Nonverbal Messages of Relevance to Telerehabilitation

4.5.1   Vitalic Messages

One area that uses vitalic messages is cardiology. Johnson and Bendixen [18] have extensively reviewed the technology in this area. After a person has had a heart attack and is sent home, the cardiac rehabilitation process can continue remotely. Blood pressure management, blood lipid control, heart rates, arrhythmias, blood pressure, blood glucose, respiration rates, expiratory reserve volumes (amount of air that can be expelled at the end of a normal expiration), and vital capacity (volume of air that can be expelled after a maximum inhalation) can be monitored remotely.

Both electrocardiograms (ECGs) and echocardiogram data can be transmitted from the patient's home to the remote physician.

During the rehabilitation process, the patient is often asked to keep a journal logging activities engaged in while the heart is/was being monitored. Here is an opportunity to compare the verbal with the nonverbal to look for contradictions. For example, if a recovering heart attack patient is planning her daughter's wedding and is under great stress because the groom's mother is upset about the invitation list, there is a good likelihood the patient's heart will reflect the stress. If the patient does not report the stress, there will most likely be a contradiction between the patient's journal entry (the verbal) and the performance of the patient's heart (the nonverbal).

Exercise is also a part of many cardiac rehabilitation programs. A therapist may ask a patient about his/her exercise routine, and the patient may say, "…every day I'm on that treadmill at 8:00 AM." But that statement may stand in contradiction to the nonverbal messages delivered by the heart monitors. In addition, now with Wii, X-Box Kinect, and webcams, it is possible for therapists to not only monitor the heart parameters, but with webcams to actually watch the patient exercise from a distance.

4.5.2 Organismic Messages

Organismic nonverbal messages that can be transmitted remotely would include weight measures and skin scans. Weight is implicated in a number of pathologies, diabetes, and heart disease, for example. Rehabilitating patients with these pathologies involves managing weight issues. Messages from a scale can be transmitted from a patient's home to a therapeutic setting in a number of ways: telephone, Internet, and so on [4]. Dermatology is, in fact, a visually based branch of medicine. Patients can scan their bodies at home with their smart phones and e-mail their scans to their dermatologists. The transmitted scans can provide both diagnostic and/or treatment recovery information to their dermatologists. One study has shown that teledermatologists and face-to-face dermatologists had 100% agreement in their evaluations of the same patients [28].

The perceptual aspects of organismics cannot be ignored. Moore [23] reported that patients were more willing to disclose and discuss personal symptoms to a physician of higher physical attractiveness than one of lower attractiveness. On the other side of the dyad, it was found that a patient's physical attractiveness or at least the patient's physical appearance influenced a physician's interaction with the patient. Although generalization to other nonphysician therapists and their patients has not been documented, the physician–patient studies cited by Moore would suggest that the same perceptual dynamics may be operating in other therapeutic arenas as well.

In 1989, some residents of San Francisco expressed outrage when a spa erected a billboard showing the arrival of aliens. The billboard's message was:

When they come they'll eat the fat ones first.

The billboard caption encapsulated the many aspersions that are often cast at over-weight people. Asher (2000), for example, reported research that found that, in a job interview, the overweight person is out of the running. The discrimination against women was most severe. Some people investigating the discrimination against the overweight have compared the reactions to them as they entered a number of social situations compared to the reactions to them when they were wearing a "fat suit." Lampert [20], for instance, compared the reactions to her when she was wearing a fat suit, which appeared to increase her weight to 250 lb, with the reactions to her at half that weight. In outside the home social situations, Lampert was interpersonally ignored and was negatively looked at; often people would shake their heads in disbe-lief. The most negative looks were given to her at the supermarket when people looked in her shopping cart. They did not know she was buying for a family of five.

With age, there are, of course, physical changes: the muscles weaken, the joints stiffen, the gait slows, and the memory clouds, for example. Moore [23], a 26-year-old designer whose specialty was designing environments for the elderly, did an experiment similar to that done by Lampert. Instead of varying her weight, however, Moore with the help of latex make-up varied her age. She was shocked to find the reactions she received. As an 80-year-old woman she was consistently short changed by the shopkeepers she interacted with every day, was pushed and shoved, and was mugged. What is important to remember in both the Lampert and Moore cases is that personality characteristics were controlled for since it was the same person being reacted to with and without the respective disguises.

4.5.3   Cosmetics and Costuming

Patients in critical-care facilities and even at-home patients are often unable to apply their cosmetics as they do in everyday life. This can often be mortifying when visi-tors drop by and see them as they have never seen them before. The therapists, of course, are not deprived of their cosmetics. This magnifies the asymmetrical power relationship between therapist and client. Teletherapists should always remember that when people look better (often through cosmetics and costuming or dress) they feel better. If a client is being visually monitored at home, therapists should be sen-sitive to the patient's appearance. A poor appearance can be a sign of poor care-taking, decreasing motivation, depression, or a combination of these. Amy Jones-Barlock, a psychotherapist working with depressed individuals, was inter-viewed by Sauer [27]. Jones-Barlock found that dress was a key indicator of how a person was feeling. As concern with dress deteriorated, so did mood.

Therapists are also aware of factors like "White-Coat Hypertension." White-Coat Hypertension (see Fackelmann, [12]) is a spike in blood pressure when that blood pressure is measured by a high-status healer dressed in a white medical coat. For example, a patient visits a cardiologist's office and takes one look at the cardiologist in a white coat, and the patient's blood pressure spikes. The cardiologist records the elevated blood pressure. Later an office staff member in street clothes takes the blood pressure and it is markedly diminished. The conclusion is that the white coat generated anxiety in the patient, which became manifest in the patient's spiked blood pressure. Many therapists have abandoned the white coat and/or have blood pressures taken multiple times by more than one person in a single visit. Acknowledging the possibility of white-coat hypertension shows that therapists are sensitive to patients' emotional states.

4.5.4 Haptics

Haptics or touch poses a problem for the telerehabilitation therapist. Touch can be therapeutic beyond the therapeutic value of the presence of another caring person. It is known that touch and massage can trigger the release of at least one hormone, oxytocin, and at least one opiate, endorphins (see Cozolino, [6, p. 103]). What do most people do reflexively when they bump their elbows in that sensitive spot? They begin to rub the elbow. This rubbing triggers the release of endorphins. This release has therapeutic value. Endorphins mimic the effects of morphine without the addictive side effect. But self-massage is often difficult operationally. One cannot massage one's back. It is most likely less effective as well. While there is no established experimental evidence here, a reasonable assumption would be that self-massage therapeutic effects are less effective than massage administered by a therapist. Perhaps the second best solution is to have a caring caregiver armed with good home instructions do the massage for telerehabilitation clients.

4.5.5 Kinesics

Carignan and Krebs [5] expressed their belief that a strong market for home-based rehabilitation existed, but noted the high cost of that endeavor. Unless the cost of telerehabilitation could be reduced, telerehabilitation will remain aloof. The only solution for these authors was the possibility of off-the-shelf devices becoming available. The devices have become available. The beneficiaries of this availability are of course the patients but physical and occupational therapists as well. This is particularly true in the nonverbal area of kinesics. A number of therapists have successfully used off-the-shelf commodity items in telerehabilitation activities.

Huber et al. [17] from the Tele-Rehabilitation Institute, a joint venture between Rutgers and Indiana Universities, showed how home video games could be adapted for improving hand function in teens with cerebral palsy. Rutgers engineers adapted a Play-Station 3 system so that the researchers could observe the three cerebral palsied participants. After 3 months of therapy conducted remotely by occupational and physical therapists, two participants progressed from being unable to lift heavy objects to being able to do so. All three participants showed varying improvement in tooth brushing, shampooing, dressing, and using eating utensils.

Burke et al. [3] used common webcams to track arm movements in stroke rehabilitation. The webcams presented a dynamic stimulus (e.g., a running rabbit) that the patient had to track and click on when the rabbit stuck its head out of one of four holes. The authors developed games for both unilateral and bilateral rehabilitation. The webcams were programmed so that the patient received immediate feedback and points for correct hits. The therapists received feedback remotely over the Internet. Moreover, webcams have been instrumental in a unique program sponsored by Armed Forces Insurance [29]. In this program, combat-wounded military personnel exercise with the New Orleans Saints via web cams. The wounded were located in Leavenworth, Kansas while the Saints were in New Orleans, Louisiana. Each group could see the other on large wall-mounted flat-screen televisions.

Wii-Gaming has been used extensively in telerehabilitation efforts. The use has been so extensive that people often refer to the process as "Wii-hab." Saposnik [26] reported that in stroke telerehabilitation, Wii-Gaming therapeutic strategies produced results that surpassed more standard strategies. The therapeutic task for the stroke patients involved in the study was to use arm movements required in tennis and to mimic arm movements needed to peel onions and potatoes, slice meat, and shred cheese. The Wii group showed a 30% better improvement than the traditional therapy group in the tasks being taught.

Fitzpatrick and Harding [13] reported their findings in using the Wii in vestibular rehabilitation. Patients engage in a number of activities that have been found to improve their motor performances. For example, patients would walk a tightrope or jump over objects while experiencing visual distraction, do weight shifts, make fine motor movements while shifting their weight, or walk with their eyes closed. Improvement was assessed by computing dizziness scores, duration of one-leg standing, and the number of steps possible with eyes closed. The authors noted that the inexpensive Wii provided patients with visual and balance challenges in a safe and fun environment.

Halton [15] has noted the rapid growth in the use of the Wii in rehabilitation settings. For example, in Halton's rehabilitation facility, the Wii has been used to help patients improve upper arm strength and balance skills. Use of the Wii has influenced participation and overall effort in therapy, according to Halton. However, because of its newness therapists will have to rely heavily on anecdotal reports of its efficacy in therapeutic endeavors. Wii activities can be monitored remotely by the simple use of webcams or with sophisticated electronic modifications.

The most recent entry in the gaming product area is the Xbox Kinect. Niehaus [24] has noted the applications of this product in the health-care arena. Xbox Kinect is similar to the Wii in that it detects the motions of the players, but it distinguishes itself from the Wii in that no controllers (glove-like garments the players must wear) are needed, speech recognition is enabled, and face recognition is possible. As an example of using Xbox Kinect, Niehaus discussed a fitness program where doctors separated from patients could nonetheless connect with the patients through the Xbox's social network capacity. Xbox's appropriately programmed could prescribe patient-specific therapeutic protocols, make assessments, and give feedback to patients.

4.5.6 Personics

Does it make a difference if a radiologist sees a patient's face when computerized CAT scans are reviewed? A study in personics suggests that it does. Helliker [16] reported on a study that found that including photographs of patients in their files enhanced radiologists' performances. Fifteen radiologists reviewed computed CT images along with a photograph of the patient. Months later they reviewed the same CT scans without a photograph. Three hundred CT scans were read. The results showed that when no photograph was present, there was an 80% drop in incidental findings, such as when a search for a kidney stone turns up a tumor.

4.5.7 Vocalics

There are some vocalizations that fall into the nonverbal category without question. Screams and cries would be examples, and few, if any, of these examples would be found in the therapeutic arena. More pertinent would be the vocal tones that accompany speech. Two classic studies would seem to have relevance to the telerehabilitation therapist. Milmoe [22] studied the effects of the physician's voice on patients' compliance. The physicians were making recommendations to detoxed alcoholics, recommending that the alcoholics undergo further treatment. Judgments were made of the emotions expressed in the physicians' voices when they were making their recommendations. Compliance was assessed by whether or not the alcoholic followed the physician's advice and participated in follow-up treatment. Milmoe found least compliance when there was anger in the physician's voice, and the most compliance when there was anxiety in the physician's voice. Vocal anger seemed to communicate chastisement triggering the "I'll show you response" from the patient. Anxiety, on the other hand, seemed to communicate worry. Specifically, the patients seemed to feel that the physicians were worried about them.

Another classic study in vocalics was conducted by Rosenthal [25]. College students participating in a study were greeted by a receptionist who said the same words in all cases. However, in half the cases the greetings and instructions were said in a monotonic, matter-of-fact voice. In the other half, the greeting and instructions were given a friendly voice. Results showed that those participants greeted in a friendly voice gave a superior performance on the tasks presented to them. Rosenthal's study gave credence to the old aphorism, "It is not what the person said but how the person said it."

4.5.8 Chronemics

Time communicates is the message of chronemics, the effects of time on communication. One area in which the telerehabilitation therapist can provide benefit to patients who require an augmentative device to communicate, is to help them increase their rate of message production. Conversation has a rhythm, and to communicate laboriously slow is to break that rhythm. The consequence of this rupture is that communicators often lose their conversational partners. Much effort is expended by researchers to enable augmentative communication device users to increase their speech (natural or synthesized) rates. One approach is to store lists of common utterances into the augmentative device's memories. Using this strategy, an utterance can be retrieved and uttered by a device in a fraction of a second using just a few keystrokes. This approach is not useful, however, when a novel utterance is appropriate. In spite of the impression that many human communication messages are stereotyped, the fact of the matter is that most conversational utterances are novel. Egolf [9] discussed many of these issues. A number of strategies (e.g., word prediction strategies) can be used by the augmented communicator to increase communication rates. A telespeech therapist can remotely receive each keystroke that an augmentative user makes, check on the rate of production, and determine whether or not the augmentative user is using the strategy that would best maximize the rate of production.

4.5.9   Proxemics

In the area of proxemics, a growing telerehabilitation area is telecaregiving. In telecaregiving the living environments of disabled individuals, particularly the elderly, are wired so as to permit monitoring by people in remote locations, most often relatives and friends. For instance, National Public Radio in August of 2010 in the United States featured a piece on an elderly couple in the United States who was receiving telecare. The couple had cameras installed throughout their home that were controlled by a remotely located caregiving provider. The telecaregiver was even able to join the couple through interactive television. The telecaregiver controlled the ceiling-installed cameras in the couple's home remotely. No cameras were installed in the couple's bedroom or bathroom. However, if someone stayed in the bathroom too long, the telecaregiver called the couple's home. The remotely controlled cameras gave the telecaregiver the opportunity to scan a room to look for any signs of possible danger, for example, a stove left on after dinner. A daughter of the couple praised the telecaregiving service and said of the service, "They're diligent, they're on the ball, and I like it."

Some telecaregiving services are based on RFID technology. Most people rely on this technology to some degree and are not aware of it. People who use fobs instead of keys are using RFIDs. Drivers who cruise through toll booths without stopping have their windshield-mounted RFIDs identification information read when they enter a toll booth area and when they depart at their destination point for billing purposes. Egolf [10] described how RFIDs are used in assisted-living communities. The RFIDs are mounted in patients' lanyards and the lanyards can communicate to a central computer all the residents' movements, locations, and activities in a given day. Egolf reported the experience of how a daughter living far away from her mother would call her mother, who lived in a smart assisted-living community, and ask her mother about her day; her mother often could not remember. But with the mother wearing the lanyard, the daughter could check her computer to see exactly what her mother had done even when the daughter was away and at work. Often, knowing what the mother had done facilitated the mother–daughter conversation because the daughter was able to jog her mother's memory on the day's activities.

Egolf [10] also recounted the experience of a reporter who became a "patient" in a high-tech nursing home. RFID tags dotted the walls, cameras marked boundaries, beds were wired to detect patients' movements, and the reporter/patient wore a lanyard around her neck that served as a room key, alarm, and location monitor. The reporter's brother was her "caregiver" 2,300 miles away, and he was able to tell her about her every move even when she was sleeping. Did all the monitors bother the reporter? No. She said that she quickly forgot about them and that she gladly tolerated them because they gave her freedom of movement.

4.6 Conclusions

This chapter has sampled a number of situations showing the use or the potential importance of nonverbal factors in telerehabilitation. Some of the technology has been around for years, for example, the transmitting of heart performance data by telephone or heart monitor. Other efforts are new, particularly those using game technology and sensors (RFIDs, for instance). If telerehabilitation therapists can use off-the-shelf technology (e.g., webcams, Wii, and X-box Kinect) the cost of telerehabilitation will be significantly reduced and the technology will be less threatening to the patient. The field will be somewhat chaotic since the manufacturers of off-the-shelf technology shy away from making any medical claims for their products. Making such claims would probably require them to do clinical trials and apply for FDA approval. Standardization will be difficult if not impossible. It may not even be advisable since any standard will probably be obsolete by the time the standards are established.

In this chapter, the therapist–patient relationship is not addressed in a substantial way. One researcher who has studied that extensively is Zia Agha, MD, MS (zia.agha@va.gov), Veterans Administration San Diego Healthcare System, San Diego, California. In general, when studying physician–patient interactions in telemedicine, Agha finds the physicians to be domineering. He notes, however, that much more research needs to be done. TherapyTimes.com is another valuable resource for those interested in new approaches in telerehabilitation. This Internet site publishes many new and innovative approaches to telerehabilitation before they appear in traditional journals.

While the therapist–patient relationship can be seen as primarily a verbal dialogue, there are many nonverbal exchanges in the dyad. What generates trust, or what causes one therapist to be excellent in motivating a patient while another equally trained not so? A number of studies have shown that patients can tolerate some rough times in their therapies if they trust their therapists. The motivation factor is more of a mystery. Jerome Frank [14], the author of *Persuasion and Healing*, said, "In concluding this section on the therapist's personal attributes we must add that probably the most important one has escaped systematic study. This attribute is healing power or charisma." Frank was talking about psychotherapists, but generalizations to therapists in general are not unwarranted.

In most cases, telerehabilitation services are provided in the patient's home. The therapeutic agent should know about this space. Is the environment physically conducive to telerehabilitation efforts? Does the patient have good social support? Social support has repeatedly been shown to promote not only psychological health but physical health as well. Again there are nonverbal components in each of these areas. Recent literature has shown that many family caregivers are extremely stressed. Take the parent of a severely disabled cerebral palsied child, for example. It may take as many as 4 h for the parent to bath, dress, feed, and then mount the child's augmentative communication device. Then the child says, "I must go to the bathroom." The whole process begins all over again. More hours are spent just getting the day started. It is very stressful.

Summary

- Both verbal and nonverbal messages are important in the therapeutic endeavor: the verbal tells whereas the nonverbal shows.
- Nonverbal communications such as patient's vital signs, physical appearance of the patient, touch, body movements and postures, facial characteristics and expressions, voice, time, and space are of potential importance in the telerehabilitation field.
- In some cases, the verbal and the nonverbal messages are contradictory. Telerehabilitation therapists often look for contradictions between the two expressions; there is often a comparison between what the remote patient says and what the patient shows.
- In any therapy, the patient–therapist relationship is very important. If the patients trust their therapists, they can even tolerate some rough times in their therapies.
- Many off-the-shelf gaming products have made telerehabilitation sessions more visible, affordable, and motivating for patients.

Abbreviations/Acronyms

ACL   Anterior cruciate ligament
ASL   American Sign Language
CAT   Computerized axial tomography

CT   Computerized tomography
ECG   Electrocardiogram
FDA   Food and Drug Administration
RFID   Radio frequency identification

References

1. Asher D. Discrimination: a weighty matter. Psychol Today, May/June 2000;24.
2. Bowlby J. Attachment: attachment and loss. 2nd ed. New York: Basic Books; 1999.
3. Burke J, Morrow P, McNeil J, et al. Vision based games for upper limb stroke rehabilitation. 2008. Available at: www.burkazoid.com/files/documents/burkeej-visiongamesrehabilitation. pdf. Accessed 14 Feb 2011.
4. Cardiocom. 2011. Available at: http://www.cardiocom.com/telescale.html. Accessed 3 Feb 2011.
5. Carignan C, Krebs H. Telerehabilitation robotics: bright lights, big future? J Rehabil Res Dev. 2006;43(5):695–710.
6. Cozolino L. The neuroscience of human relationships. New York: WW Norton; 2006.
7. Damasio A. Descartes' error: emotion, reason, and the human brain. New York: HarperCollins; 1994.
8. Durant W. The story of philosophy. New York: Pocket Books; 1974.
9. Egolf D. Improving the interaction rates of users of assistive communication devices. In: Proceedings of annual California State University conference on technology and persons with disabilities, Northridge, 1998.
10. Egolf D. Assisting the elderly with RFID technology. In: Proceedings of the annual California State University conference on technology and persons with disabilities, Los Angeles, 2007.
11. Egolf D, Chester S. The nonverbal factor. 2nd ed. New York: iUniverse; 2007.
12. Fackelmann K. White-coat hypertension: high risk or harmless to the heart? Sci News. 1998; 154:380–1.
13. Fitzpatrick M, Harding L. Using the Wii for vestibular rehabilitation. Veda Publication No. C-7; 2009. Available at: http://vestibular.org/sites/default/files/page_files/Using%20the%20 Wii%20for%20Vestibular%20Rehabilitation_2.pdf. Accessed 19 Sep 2012.
14. Frank J. Persuasion and healing. New York: Schocken Books; 1974.
15. Halton J. Rehabilitation with the Nintendo Wii: experiences at a rehabilitation hospital. Occupation Therapy Now, May/June 2010.
16. Hellliker K. Face time: the benefits of seeing patients as people. The Wall Street Journal, Tuesday, 3 Dec 2008, p. B9.
17. Huber M, Rabin B, Docan C, et al. Feasibility of modified remotely monitored in-home gaming technology for improving hand function in adolescents with cerebral palsy. IEEE Trans Inf Technol Boimed. 2010;14(2):526–34.
18. Johnson J, Bendixen R. Chapter 5: Telehealth. In: Mann W, editor. Smart technology for aging, disability, and independence. New York: Wiley; 2005.
19. Klaus M, Kennell J. Maternal attachment: importance of the first postpartum days. N Engl J Med. 1972;286(9):460–3.
20. Lampert L. Fat like me. Ladies Home Journal, May 1993.
21. Mehrabian A. Communication without words. Psychol Today. 1968;2:52–5.
22. Milmoe S. The doctor's voice: postdictor of successful referral of alcoholic patients. In: Weitz S, editor. Nonverbal communication: readings with commentary. New York: Oxford University Press; 1979. p. 268–76.
23. Moore P. Disguised. Waco: Word Books; 1985.
24. Niehaus C. Xbox Kinect applications to health and medicine. 2010. Available at: http://sector-public.com2010/11/xbox-connect-applications-to-health-and-medicine. Accessed 2 Feb 2011.

25. Rosenthal R. Self-fulfilling prophecy. Psychol Today. 1968;2:47–51.
26. Saposnik G. Stroke rehab with Wii games. Paper presented at the American Stroke Association's annual conference, San Antonio, 2010.
27. Sauer G. If "you look mahvelous" you probably feel good too. The Pittsburgh Post Gazette, The Magazine Section, 5 Sept 1993, p. 14–15.
28. Shapiro M, et al. Comparison of skin biopsy triage decisions in 49 patients with pigmented lesions and skin neoplasms. Arch Dermatol. 2004;140:525–8.
29. Simmons L. JR Martinez: new face of wounded warriors "virtual rehab" program. A press release from Armed Forces Insurance headquartered in Leavenworth, Kansas, 10 Aug 2010.

Chapter 5
Telerehabilitation Interface Strategies for Enhancing Access to Health Services for Persons with Diverse Abilities and Preferences

Jack M. Winters

Abstract This chapter extends a prior classification scheme for tele-encounters, with the purpose of applying it to human factors and accessibility analysis of electronic and information technology interfaces that are commonly used for telerehabilitation applications. A novel framework is proposed for developing technical guidelines for teleinterfaces that would lead to more equitable access to telerehabilitation (and more generally, telehealth) services for persons with diverse abilities and preferences.

5.1 Introduction

This chapter proposes strategies for designing more effective interfaces that could help the telerehabilitation field reach its full potential for providing both remote and equitable access to persons with the full spectrum of diverse abilities. It is based on a synthesis of concepts derived from three experiences of the author. One involved experiences with the original Rehabilitation Engineering Research Center (RERC) on Telerehabilitation (from 1998 to 2003), including insights from its state-of-the-science conference in 2002 that brought together most of the groups engaged at that time in telerehabilitation research and service delivery activities within the United States [34]. This experience was especially captured in a review of telerehabilitation research [52], with an evolving perspective captured by Feng and Winters [15]. The second experience involved managing the RERC on Accessible Medical Instrumentation (RERC-AMI,

J.M. Winters
Department of Biomedical Engineering, Marquette University,
Cramer Hall, 160 C, Milwaukee, WI 53233, USA
e-mail: jack.winters@marquette.edu

S. Kumar, E.R. Cohn (eds.), *Telerehabilitation*, Health Informatics,
DOI 10.1007/978-1-4471-4198-3_5, © Springer-Verlag London 2013

2002–2008; see www.rerc-ami.org), including synthesizing results from its state-of-the-science workshop [56]. This is especially captured in a review of interfaces that can enhance universal access to health care [53], as well as in a section on "accessibility considerations" (Section 16, pp 229–242) within a new national standard entitled "Human Factors Engineering: Medical Device Considerations" (called AAMI HE 75, under the umbrella of the American Association of Medical Instrumentation; see http://www.aami.org/he75/). Section 16 is the only part of this comprehensive voluntary standard that is freely available to the general public. This is because it is used as a national resource for the development of new technical regulatory standards that will be added to the Rehabilitation Act of 1973 (as Section 510) for medical diagnostic equipment by the U.S. Access Board in consultation with the Food and Drug Administration (FDA), in response to a charge within the Patient Protection and Affordable Care Act of 2010 that was signed by President Obama. The third experience involves serving as a contracting consultant for the FDA, in part to provide assistance to the FDA in addressing this charge for technical accessibility guidelines for certain classes of medical products, along with plans to enhance its in-house human factors capacity related to this initiative.

The Telerehabilitation Special Interest Group (Telerehab-SIG) of the American Telemedicine Association (ATA) has recently developed a blueprint for telerehabilitation guidelines, producing a working document with numbered lists classified under four areas: administration, clinical, technical, and ethical [4]. The six numbered statements under the "technical" category are very general, mostly relating to equipment reliability and clinical quality control. Item 5 addresses "environmental elements of care" and mentions the importance of physical accessibility of the treatment space and usability of equipment, without giving any specifics. Accessibility of the electronic and information technology telerehabilitation interface (telerehab-EIT) is not mentioned (this author views accessibility and usability as different constructs; see Ref. [53]). By nature, many (perhaps most) persons who could benefit from telerehabilitation services have disabilities, in many cases with multiple functional limitations that affect their functional capacity to participate in a tele-encounter. Furthermore, such functional limitations may change over time as tissues remodel, for instance, due to secondary consequences or the aging process. Here, we implicitly assume that the "fault" for any lack of equitable access resides not with the person and their abilities, but rather with the lack of available telerehab-EIT that has a truly accessible interface. The irony is that because of existing accessibility guidelines in the area of EIT and the finite number of types of tele-encounters, producing such guidelines is feasible. They could then serve as a resource to interface designers, clinicians, researchers, policymakers, and other stakeholders, and augment the more general work of the Telerehab-SIG and of the current RERC on Telerehabilitation that is based at the University of Pittsburgh.

This chapter provides a conceptual foundation for classifying tele-encounters and telerehab-EIT interfaces, and then proposes a novel framework for implementing telerehabilitation-specific accessibility guidelines. If gradually implemented, such guidelines can perhaps help overcome some of the existing access barriers to large-scale telerehabilitative service delivery.

5.1.1 *"Systems" Analysis of Telerehabilitation in the Context of the Continuum of Care*

In a review of the state of telerehabilitation research about a decade ago, this author suggested that an underlying principle behind much of the rehabilitation field is that tissues and systems of cells can "remodel" as long as there is access to an adequate internal support infrastructure such as blood supply [59], and that this adaptive process can be influenced by the augmented "use history" of rehabilitative interventions [52]. It was noted that all of the applied health professions view their professions in the context of using timely assessments and strategic interventions to maximize outcomes [9]; indeed, outcomes are central to rehabilitation research [17, 18]. This was tied to the concept that the tools of telerehabilitation can help minimize this barrier, both of patients to rehabilitative services and of researchers to subject populations, and that such enhanced access can open up new possibilities for discovering and implementing optimized intervention strategies across the continuum of care [52].

This previous review also identified a number of possible processes for delivering rehabilitative services [52]: teleconsultation, telediagnosis, teleassessment, telementoring, telesupport, telesupervision, telemonitoring, telecoaching, and teletherapy. Associated services were conceptualized within the context of a "continuum of care" and ranged from pressure ulcer management [11, 48] to provision of assistive technology [6] to approaches for telehomecare [51]. Because of the slow nature of enabling–disabling processes [1], the plan of care is typically implemented over a few weeks to months, with tele-encounters used for only parts of the process. From a "systems" perspective, assessments of health status and functional capabilities can be viewed as "snapshots" in time, and the rehabilitative continuum of care as delivering a finite series of bolus interventions. In such a model, telerehabilitation tends to fit into the plan of care in two ways:

1. Access to remote expertise, especially as related to expert assessments related to diagnosis, prognosis, treatment planning, and outcomes assessment.
2. Delivery of assessments and interventions via telerehab-EIT. These events can replace or coordinate with conventional outpatient/home therapy and health management, and thus fit into the plan for optimal rehabilitative service delivery. Norms of outpatient/homecare practice will typically involve 2–4 visits per week for a given therapeutic modality (e.g., nursing visit or physical therapy session). For many enabling-disabling processes, it turns out that about three interventions per week are sufficient, with additional interventions providing diminishing return on investment (e.g., most types of musculoskeletal and cardiovascular rehabilitation, management of secondary conditions such as loss of muscle strength and joint contractures by physical therapists, and general health management by nurses).

A third way has been emerging: novel approaches for providing larger amounts of rehabilitative intervention, especially as related to neurorehabilitation. This is motivated by research that makes it clear that the current norms of practice (and reimbursement) are inadequate in terms of available time and resources for optimal service delivery. For instance, the evidence demonstrates that intensive movement therapy intervention protocols often can result in significant improvements, even years after the initial injury onset [31, 45]. This has led to considerable research activity, and to research studies that target rehabilitation robotics [8, 25], virtual environments [22, 24, 27, 32], and various gaming technology that includes a telerehabilitation component [16, 26, 55].

5.1.2 Human Factors Analysis Applied to Telerehabilitation Interfaces

It was also recognized by 2002 that telerehabilitation involves, at its core, new ways for humans to work interactively together to achieve certain aims. These aims involve completing tasks, usually cooperatively between sites. Much of the previous review focused on a telerehabilitative process from what could be viewed as a "human factors engineering" perspective. The field of *human factors/ergonomics* focuses on designing system interfaces to optimize the ability of users to accomplish tasks successfully within a satisfactory time period while minimizing the risk of use error [7, 36]. A related concept is *usability*—the extent to which a product can be used by specified users to achieve specified goals in an effective and efficient manner, to the satisfaction of these users [29]. Another important concept that has been deemed as being critical to product acceptance is the *reliability* of the interface. Practitioners, in particular, have little patience for new products that are not reliable, and view this as a major reason for abandonment. Recently, the importance of human factors/ergonomics and usability analysis as related to telerehabilitation have been better developed [2, 30], which is helpful.

5.1.3 Progress over the Past Decade

Although there have certainly been progress and some success stories (e.g., see reviews by Theodoros and Russell [46], Brennan et al. [3], McCue et al. [28]), for the most part the past decade has not been particularly successful in terms of widespread adoption of telerehabilitation-mediated health services. This is despite remarkable technological advances over this past decade, especially with cell phones becoming multimedia devices, Internet protocol (IP) videoconferencing becoming ubiquitous on personal computers, and e-mail and social networking becoming pervasive across the full spectrum of age groups. This suggests that the primary barrier is not the technological capabilities, but rather the classic challenges that have been well recognized for over a decade [33], such as lack of large-scale clinical trials that address outcomes and cost effectiveness, challenges with reimbursement for clinical services, clinician reluctance (and lack of relevant training programs), patient–consumer reluctance, and the continuing lack of sufficient federal research investment in this area as addressed by Seelman [38].

Surmounting such challenges requires various approaches, including large-scale federally funded projects to document effectiveness of various types of telerehabilitation-mediated services. But one of the challenges in implementing such projects is that available technology is always changing, and often multi-year projects cannot change to improved technologies during an ongoing study, which has been viewed as a disadvantage [10]. This common concern implicitly suggests that technology can have an impact on the findings of a given study. Indeed, a case can be made that without attempting to optimize the technological interface for a particular type of tele-encounter that is the focus for a given project, clinical research studies may not be giving telerehabilitation services a fair shot at success [52, 58].

A problem with these conceptual arguments is the implicit assumption that interfaces can be used by persons with diverse abilities, (i.e., that they are accessible). We will see that this is not a good assumption, and, additionally, the telerehabilitation field could benefit tremendously by taking leadership in the area of accessible design (AD) of interfaces for persons with diverse abilities and preferences.

This rest of this chapter considers roles for telerehabilitation for enhancing universal access to health-care services, where universal access goes beyond the classic considerations of the barriers of distance and cost, to also consider the accessibility of the interface.

5.2 Insights from a Greater Focus on the Accessibility of Health-Care Interfaces

How is telerehab-EIT selected? The reality is that most telerehabilitation applications use *off-the-shelf mainstream technology* for implementing tele-encounters, usually selected by clinicians with no formal training in human factors/ergonomics/usability engineering as related to human–technology interfaces. In doing so, they are implicitly depending on any human factors analysis that went into designing the interface. Typically the primary market for such devices is mainstream users, with products designed primarily with able-bodied users in mind. Consider, for instance, the features of most advanced cell phones: the trend has been toward smaller keys (some only available via a touchscreen), small screens containing images with very small fonts and icons, and small touchcreens for navigation and pointing controls. Furthermore, they tend not to be designed to be operated with only one hand, at least for many tasks.

5.2.1 Limitations of Conventional Usability Testing and Human Factors Approaches

These limitations make sense when one considers how conventional usability testing protocols are designed, where the standard of practice consists of user testing on 6–12 participants who are considered to be "typical" users; among these participants, 0–2 can be expected to have disabilities. This is true even for interfaces for medical devices (e.g., usability section of the AAMI HE 75 consensus standard). Indeed, for medical equipment and devices it is the manufacturer who defines the "intended users" of their product during the regulatory approval process involving the FDA. Most often, the "intended users" are able-bodied clinical professionals, even for technologies such as infusion pumps that are now routinely used by persons with disabilities within the home environment. There has been considerable indirect evidence that inaccessible interfaces can lead to unsafe events and injury (although disability data cannot be collected as part of "adverse event" reporting to the FDA). The RERC-AMI's national surveys and focus groups also documented that individuals with disabilities would often take risks to get access to essential medical services [57]. The multi-site RERC-AMI had to confront this challenge.

5.2.2 RERC-AMI Strategies for Addressing Accessibility Considerations

One of our strategies was to engage in considerable testing of classes of medical equipment/devices by developing a technology that we called the Mobile Usability and Accessibility Lab [57]. This included a formalized pre- and postactivity interview process [based largely on the principles of universal design (UD)] plus a video-based systematic analysis that focused on identifying events associated with accessibility difficulties and use errors [43]. Unique in our approach was our proactive effort to *recruit persons with diverse abilities as subjects*. Used for about eight IRB-approved human subject's studies, one of our insights was the *clear distinction between usability analysis and accessibility analysis*. This is formally addressed in Ref. [53], but a summary is that maximizing usability for most persons can often decrease accessibility for some people. This is true even when the principles of UD are considered (which basically represent "best practices" for inclusive usability). UD principles have been reviewed extensively [40, 42], including in the context of telerehab-EIT interfaces [30], and this will not be repeated here except to note that they are often articulated as seven principles:

1. Equitable use
2. Flexibility in use
3. Simple and intuitive use
4. Perceptible information
5. Tolerance for error

6. Low physical effort
7. Size and space for approach and use

Addressing all these principles does not imply that an interface is accessible; for example, improving "simple and intuitive use" for most people can cause lack of access for others. UD is not intended to be inclusive of all persons, or to address accessibility directly.

The distinctions between UD and AD are formally addressed in Ref. [13], where UD is viewed as a principle to consider and AD relates primarily to meeting applicable accessibility regulations and guidelines. But of note is that this distinction is especially dramatic for EIT, where federal accessibility guidelines allow two approaches for achieving AD: *direct access* (often based in part on UD principles) and *indirect access*. Indirect access involves a very different approach: the manufacturer provides and supports a "hook" interface, often standardized, that provides access via the user's assistive technology (AT) or user agent. Relevant ATs include (see also Ref [48]): text telephone (TTY), screen readers, Braille, voice recognition/activation, assistive listening systems, physical magnifiers, operating system accessibility features (e.g., sticky keys, magnifiers, and alternative keys), and mobility aids for access to facilities (e.g., wheelchairs, scooters, lifts, and crutches). Generally, direct access is preferred, when possible. But for telerehab-EIT of the future, a possible advantage of indirect access is that it could enable the user to obtain access through a *personalized interface* that is more fully matched to their abilities and preferences [15].

In the context of telerehab-EIT, it is useful to mention the six "...abilities" described by Winters [53]:

- Accessibility (ability to access)
- Usability (ability to use)
- Reliability (ability to depend on)
- Interoperability and cooperability (ability to work with other entities)
- Learnability (ability to learn the effective use the interface)
- Safeability (ability to safely access the intended use)

Historically, telerehab-EIT tends to focus on three of these: usability, reliability, and interoperability. But an alternative strategy, especially relevant for telerehab-EIT, is personalized design (PD) of interfaces based on a given user's abilities and preferences. An example is the universal remote console (URC) standard that was lead by a team from the RERC on Information Access and resulted in ISO 24752 (e.g., see Ref. [60]), which the RERC-AMI helped develop as part of an INCITS (InterNational Committee for Information Technology Standard) working group [23]. In this standard, a "user agent" (a type of AT) creates an alternative interface, based on information about the target device plus user abilities and preferences, as described by XML files. The RERC-AMI created simulated products such as vital sign and exercise monitors, used the standard to create "on-the-fly" alternative interfaces based on UD and PD principles, and then evaluated user performance for persons with diverse abilities [12, 15]. We found that performance improved the most for PD interfaces, both for able-bodied and for diverse-ability populations, including when personalized for PDAs [37] and exercise monitors [19]. For telerehab-EIT, the key concept is that because teleinterfaces naturally tend to be inherently multimodal, and it is not a stretch to recognize that for certain applications, PD interfaces could be customized based on the abilities and preferences of the end user.

Another strategy of the RERC-AMI was our participation in the AAMI Human Factors Committee that was involved in a multiyear process to establish what became the ANSI-AAMI HE 75 Design of Medical Devices: Human Factors Considerations standard in 2009. This large committee of expert stakeholders was charged with promulgating human factors best practices as related to designing medical device interfaces. Consideration of accessibility was not part of the original agenda, but through our participation; eventually Section 16 (Accessibility Considerations) was included as part of this national standard for the medical device industry. This content was based on two primary sources: (1) our own research on various types of medical interfaces for various classes of medical equipment used by persons with diverse abilities; and (2) language motivated by existing federal accessibility standards, especially the "Functional Performance Criteria" (Subpart C) of Section 508 amendments to the Rehab Act that relate mostly to EIT (http://www.access-board.gov/sec508/standards.htm), and certain parts of the ADA accessibility guidelines (http://www.access-board.gov/ada/index.htm). Interestingly, before our participation, most members of the committee—experts in human factors—had clearly never heard of these laws, or of the Web Content Accessibility Guidelines (WCAG) (http://www.w3.org/WAI/intro/wcag.php, see also Ref. [5] for how these relate to health care). In addition to the content in Section 16, a summary of this work is available [41] and more detailed guidelines are maintained at an online archive (http://rerc-ami.org/ami/projects/d/4/1/index.aspx).

5.2.3   Relevance to Telerehabilitation

In telerehabilitation, the consequence of use error, or access difficulties, commonly appears to be abandonment rather than injury. With no "essential" health service requiring telerehab-EIT as part of the standard norm of clinical practice, it becomes easy for access barriers to be hidden from collective view. Perhaps this explains why there appears to be little research on whether difficult or hard-to-use interfaces prevent access to teleservices. However, a case could be made that there likely are many applications where persons with disabilities, participating in the role of a patient or consumer (or even a telepractitioner), are not even being considered because of obvious cases of lack of accessible teleinterfaces. Addressing this interface challenge is actually quite complex, and thus it makes some sense that neither the original RERC on Telerehabilitation nor the current one based at the University of Pittsburgh has had a specific research focus on the use of telerehab-EIT by persons with diverse abilities and preferences.

But standards-based guidelines for telerehab-EIT might be a good strategy for impacting on need, even with the rapidly changing technology landscape. The basic types of tele-encounters, and of human–technology interface modes, will still apply.

Section 3 proposes a framework for addressing this challenge: accessibility of telerehab-EIT interfaces for persons who come to a tele-encounter with diverse abilities and preferences.

5.3 Proposed Framework for Telerehab-EIT: Tele-Encounters, Interface Features, Guidelines

5.3.1 Framework for Tele-Encounters

We assume that telerehab-EIT interfaces matter only in the context of how they are used during a tele-encounter and that, from a human factors task analysis perspective, there are different classes of tele-encounters. In Fig. 5.1, we use an idealized

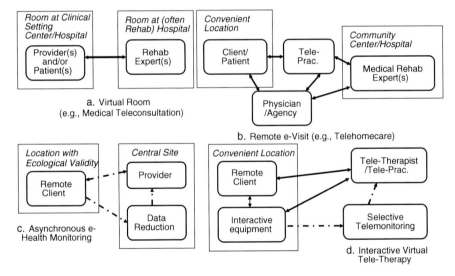

Fig. 5.1 Four conceptual models for classes of tele-encounters that use telerehab-EIT interfaces. (**a**) "Virtual room" uses interactive videoconferencing, typically with high bandwidth between clinical sites for a "teleconsultation" to get access to specialty expertise. In this setting, all participants should have equitable access to all information that is transmitted, with multimodal flexibility. The virtual room can be extended to additional sites. (**b**) This is the classic "access anywhere" concept for interactive televisits (e.g., telesupport, telecare), typically involving moderate bandwidth. It should be fully accessible for the client and provider, with at minimum universally designed interfaces and support for indirect access via a person's AT or user agent, and in some cases with a personally designed interface. (**c**) Setup for minimally intrusive, asynchronous telemonitoring, designed with full asynchronous access to information for which there is benefit, and with accessible interfaces related to maintenance of reliable data collection; often this type of tele-encounter is supported by (**b**), or embedded as part of (**d**). (**d**) Model for interactive virtual teletherapy in which a client "plays" or "exercises" or receives an interactive service (e.g., worksite accommodation) at home. This should include the ability of the teletherapist/practitioner to interactively participate in telecoaching, to access performance measures, and to change certain strategic interventional settings remotely during the interactive session

extension of the four process-oriented types of telerehabilitation processes that were described by Winters [52]: teleconsultation (now called virtual room), telehomecare (now called remote televisit), telemonitoring/teleassessment (now called asynchronous e-health monitoring), and teletherapy (now called interactive virtual teletherapy). Note that these four processes were recently used by Parmanto and Saptono [29] to classify the state-of-the-art telerehabilitation research from an informatics perspective, with between 36 and 61 citations found for each of these four categories, plus 45 falling under an "other" category of telerehabilitation services; this suggests that this classification encompasses about 80 % of all studies, and with the augmentations of Fig. 5.1 probably even a larger percentage. Furthermore, this classification does not include e-health resources, which could be considered a fifth area; however, we do not consider informational e-health here because there does not really exist a unique "teleprocess" to evaluate, and furthermore, there are existing WCAG and Section 508 guidelines that are available and applicable. Related to this, electronic health records (see Ref. [49, Chapter 9]), most of which should already fully comply with the aforementioned accessibility guidelines, are not addressed here.

From a human factors perspective, a tele-encounter involves task demands. To break down task demands, we start with the following statement motivated by Health Level Seven (HL7) [20] international ad hoc standard that is widely used by for interoperable medical communications and billing, as developed by Winters [53]:

> ...an *entity* in a *role participates* in an *act*

Here an *entity* is defined as the physical objects in health care, which are nouns that can represent a person, place, or thing (e.g., device); the *role* ascertains the part that entities play as they partake in health-care acts; the *act* (a verb) refers to the health-care sequence of task actions; and to *participate* requires an "entity in a role" performing an act (task sequence).

In our context, the "act" is the tele-encounter, and entities include both persons in a role (e.g., clinician, patient, consumer, and technician) and technologies in a role (e.g., interfaces for synchronous or asynchronous telecommunication of information to/from persons and/or storage media). Task demands such as time constraints can affect the quality of the tele-encounter—but so can the capabilities of the participating entities, including both persons (e.g., abilities and experience) and interfaces (e.g., controls, display quality, and bandwidth). Performance depends on matching capabilities and demands; here we assume that persons who are trained to participate in the role of user are likely to have a diversity of abilities. Thus, the scope of the intended users is large.

5.3.2 Classification of Interface Features and Design Strategies

We assume that five types of human–technology EIT interface modes can participate in a tele-encounter, as outlined in Fig. 5.2, from the human perspective: text/

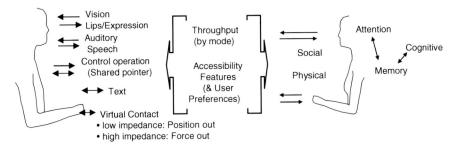

Fig. 5.2 Overview of information transmission modalities from a human factors perspective, with human–technology teleinterfaces emphasized on the *left* and human information processing on the *right*. *Left* (five core modes): *Vision* is a unicausal sensor system, although accomplished through an active eye–head gaze system (including fast voluntary saccadic eye movements, smooth pursuit eye tracking movements, and the vestibulo-ocular reflex for eye stabilization during head and body movement), and with certain indirect motor feedback (e.g., facial expressions). *Hearing* is also a unicausal information transfer interface, although involving elaborate signal-noise extraction capabilities; when coupled with speech, a near-synchronous bidirectional information exchange is created. *Text*, while language specific, can readily be used as an alternative mode to vision or hearing, and even simple contact switches, and assumes language skills. *Control operations* are commonly used for text entry and operating controls; however, most controls can be accomplished through any of these modes (including, in the near future, through noncontact gestures), and frequently there are shared pointers. *Virtual contact* interfaces, in contrast, are inherently bicausal, transferring both forces and position, enabling power transfer (force × velocity) when the human–environment impedances are fairly matched, and a unidirectional signal with impedance mismatch. One-way contact interfaces (e.g., force reflection without position) can be useful, but do not replicate natural contact. *Right*: For interaction, the perceptual to working memory to cognitive flow has a limited attentional capacity, and if overloaded, performance degrades. Similarly, multiple motoric tasks require skill development, especially for contact tasks. It is well documented that transmission time delays degrade performance, especially when delays differ between modes during multimodal operation

language (including within shared files), vision (used for conferencing, images, and shared files), hearing/speech, control operations (including shared pointers), and virtual contact (usually manual). The first four models have telecommunications technical standards behind them, with those associated with traditional videoconferencing previously reviewed [52]. The anticipated trend of pervasive IP-based multimedia has emerged, with vision now routinely being part of IP instant messaging programs and shared data now being ubiquitous with e-mail and many messaging systems. As a society we are transitioning toward fully integrated multimedia, with cell phones and web-enabled video games being the most remarkable examples. A shared pointer goes back as far as Netmeeting (Microsoft) in the 1990s. Virtual contact is more of a challenge, but is technically feasible, including at low cost [14, 15, 44]. Each type of channel may be uni- or bidirectional, and in some cases multidirectional.

One common challenge of EIT progress is that new technological innovation *can also cause steps backward in accessibility*. For instance, the trend has been toward smaller displays with smaller fonts, smaller manual keys, less tactile support, and more manual coordination (e.g., iPods and iPhones provide an innovative interactive environment for those with manual dexterity, good motor coordination, good vision, and disposable income).

Interfaces are now less constrained by the *throughput* of the communication link, that is, the amount of information that can be exchanged per unit time. This especially applies to video, which demands greater throughput than the other modes. The wireless 3G (third-generation) cell phone/PDA infrastructure that was anticipated to become pervasive in 2002 now is, and the 4G networks that are now emerging provide the final step. Additionally, 3G capacity is reaching more and more rural areas. It is notable that cell phones (and basic computers with build-in accessibility features) are gradually becoming ubiquitous across racial and economic landscapes, with prices now in a range that could be covered by health providers when cost is a barrier. The distinction between metropolitan area networks (MAN; e.g., cell phone coverage areas) and local area networks (LAN; e.g., WiFi areas) is blurring, while a rich variety of lower-power personal area networks (PAN; e.g., Bluetooth) devices are now available in the market. Perhaps it is clearer now that MAN/LAN connectivity provides access across distance for modes than can now include video, while PAN can be used to provide personalized AT (e.g., hands-free use and speech recognition).

5.3.3 Proposed Framework for Guidelines for Accessible Telerehab-EIT

What follows is a *brief* collection of examples of *telerehab-EIT accessibility guidelines*, organized under the four classes of tele-encounters of Section 3.1, while considering the five modes of interfaces of Section 3.2, and the simple list of functional impairments in the left column of Table 5.1.

1. *Virtual room.* This approach is most often identified with telerehabilitation. Although important, it is not and cannot be the pillar of telerehabilitation, in part because access to virtual rooms tends to be limited to clinical sites with restricted access. We can assume two types of acts for which entities can participate:
   (a) *Management of meeting set-up.* It is reasonable to assume that persons in this role have a basic ability to access and evaluate all five types of interface modes, although there may be minor sensory and manual deficit. Tasks involve turning on equipment and then using a remote control to operate controls that are within windows on the display.
      (i) The remote control should be universally designed, including all control buttons, and should preferably support shared remote/mouse control so that there can be multiple operators.
      (ii) The display windows should support accessibility features of the operating system or, if not, at minimum, should have an option for adjustable font size of the menu.

Table 5.1 Summary of mapping of well-recognized categories of functional limitations to federal guidance statements within Section 508 of Rehab Act and Section 255 of Telecommunications Act[a]

Class of functional impairment	Section 508 of Rehab Act (§ 1194.31a–f)	Section 255 of TAAG (§ 1193.41a–i)
Vision—blind	Extracted from part (a)	Similar to part (a)

"*At least one mode of operation and information retrieval that does not require user vision should be provided, or support for assistive technology used by people who are blind or visually impaired should be provided, unless the abilities of all intended users of the interface explicitly demand the requirement of vision.*"

Vision—partially sighted	First part from part (b)	Second part from part (c)

"*a. At least one mode of operation and information retrieval that does not require visual acuity greater than 20/70 should be provided in audio and enlarged print output working together or independently, or support for assistive technology used by people who are visually impaired should be provided, unless the abilities of all intended users (of this interface) explicitly demand the requirement of visual acuity above this level.*

b. At least one mode of operation and information retrieval that does not require color vision should be provided, in all cases. ..."

Hearing—deaf	Extracted from part (c)	Similar to part (d)
Hearing—limitations	Extracted from part (d)	
Tactile	Wording motivated by 508	
Speech	Extracted from part (e)	Similar to part (h)
Fine motor	Extracted from part of part (f)	Similar to part (e)

"*At least one mode of operation and information retrieval that does not require fine motor control or simultaneous actions should be provided.*"

Gross motor	Extracted from part of part (f)	Similar to part (f)
Positioning/orienting), reflects physical nature of many devices	Wording motivated by 508	
Cognitive	Wording motivated by 508	Extracted from part (i)
Time-independent use (applies to subset of interfaces)	Wording motivated by 508	Extracted from part (g)

[a]These helped motivate the original form of proposed accessibility guidance to the AAMI Human Factors Committee charged with developing HE 75. For each of the functional limitations to the left, there was a statement, which is given here for three cases: vision bind, vision partial, and fine motor. The first two represent examples where direct *or* indirect access is possible, while also providing a qualifier to acknowledge that a given mode may be essential for a trained profession. The third provides an example where there is no such qualifier.

(iii) Both local and remote interactive zoom-pan control should be available, with the control rate being scalable and available in at least two modes (manual and voice activated).

(b) *Interactive meeting.* Here it should be assumed that persons participating in the tele-encounter may have very diverse abilities, and may also be bringing an AT (or user agent) to the tele-encounter (e.g., magnifier, wheelchair, and assistive listening device) that can be used to help them attain equitable access. Accessibility guidelines should go well beyond UD principles and include at least the following:

(i) Large size display or displays for direct access (preferably two displays, one dedicated to data sharing), plus support for an external jack or wireless interface that enables each person to project onto their own device.

(ii) A clear line of sight to all displays for all participants.

(iii) Audio with *redundant methods of volume control* for direct access (up to at least 65 dB, which should also be the default volume), while also supporting *indirect access* via an external jack or wireless interface that supports personal listening devices, and/or closed captioning (e.g., if there is a captioner).

(iv) Noise-canceling microphones designed for human voice, and used by default.

(v) A room environment that is ADA compliant (e.g., wheelchair accessible), including accommodations to reach seats located closest to the primary display.

(vi) Remote control of any zoom-pan camera should be multi-modal, operated by means of manual operation of a remote or voice commands by certain participants.

(vii) If the type of tele-encounter includes physiotherapy or similar encounters where physical touch has value, the room should support a basic level of simple virtual touch (e.g., one bicausal channel).

(viii) Support for use of the "least common denominator" of modes, that is, video, audio, and text, should be able to be simply and *selectively deactivated* during a session at any time. This relates to the UD principles of equitable access (as it is very easy for participants to accidentally communicate through a mode that is unavailable to some participants), flexibility in use, and perceptible information (for all participants).

(ix) Use of multiple (redundant) *modes for essential information*, with text or data highlighted (e.g., larger or bold font—note that color cannot be used as the only method).

(x) If the room is using IP conferencing, control and display interfaces should meet at least the WCAG specified by the most current version of Section 508 of the Rehab Act. (Note that this acknowledges that this is not usually readily achievable for dedicated ISDN videoconferencing using the ITU 320 collection of conferencing standards.)

2. *Televisit.* This is assumed to be a goal-directed, interactive virtual visit that minimizes the barrier of distance, while also having the benefit of being timely. It is also assumed that the primary purpose is *synchronous* communication (Item 3 addresses asynchronous tele-encounters) that does not require physical

contact or a formal therapy session (Item 4 addresses teletherapy tele-encounters). Unlike for virtual rooms, these visits (which can be brief) occur at *convenient locations* for the 1–2 participants on either side of the connection, and may occur within settings where there are *environmental challenges* (e.g., poor lighting and background noise). We divide visits into two types: ad hoc and preplanned (where environmental factors can be better controlled):

(a) *Ad hoc visits.* These are usually brief, with the key aim of the tele-encounter to interactively communicate health information.

   (i) Many mass-market technologies are available, with reliability and ease of use being critical. Phones (landline or cell) tend to be the mode of choice if audio communication is possible and the user can operate the interface, with an important alternative being interactive text messaging via a computer with accessibility features.

   (ii) Any proprietary software should support a user's preferred AT for audio and/or text modes, including handwriting, voice recognition software, and/ or closed captioning.

(b) *Preplanned televisits.* These virtual visits are assumed to be facilitated by teleinterfaces that are set up within the client/patient's home (or school/ workplace) and the practitioner's office (e.g., at a clinic setting or within their home).

   (i) Unless there are bandwidth limitations, the preferred approach is IP-based multimedia conferencing using desktop/laptop computers running software on standard operating systems. Any proprietary software should fully support the accessibility features that are provided with popular operating systems, as well as meet WCAG as outlined in Section 508.

   (ii) During the preparation/planning phase, site accommodations should be made by a clinical staff person, such as a rehabilitation engineer. Often this can mean assuring that the client's personal AT works with the interface, and in some cases providing the client with appropriate AT (and training).

   (iii) Accessibility features, including for controls and/or displays, should be personalized to the abilities and preferences of the client. Note that the entire suite of control and display interface should be viable options, including voice control, and options are expanding. In particular, newer noncontact control operations (e.g., using the Microsoft Kinect system) hold great promise for remote-free operation of controls during virtual visits, when this is a preference.

   (iv) Multichannel data transfer modes should be supported by the system (e.g., for transmitting vital signs and performance data), with the interfaces for operating these modes fully accessible. Additionally, accessible file sharing should be supported, using interfaces meeting WCAG standards.

3. *Asynchronous e-health telemonitoring.* In the context of rehabilitative services, this can include reasonably unobtrusive monitoring of health-related metrics (e.g., vital signs and body weight), self-performed intervention sessions (e.g., assessment metrics related to performance), and/or daily activity events (e.g., environmental switches and motion sensors within a kitchen; wearable kinematic sensors for postural tilt, location, or contact force; or pressure sensors within the shoes or gloves). In the context of a tele-encounter, the operative word is asynchronous; synchronous tele-encounters would fall under Item 2 (televisit) or Item 4 (teletherapy). There are two types of acts with roles for participants: (1) timely data collection of the person in the role of client/patient being monitored and (2) periodic data monitoring, usually in the form of a person reviewing data collected over time and/or already in a summary form. Both have accessibility concerns.

(a) *Data collection.*

   (i) An individual being telemonitored must have been informed about the protocol, and their participation must be voluntary at all times. The interface should have the option (potentially disabled for a given clinical application) for turning off data collection, and furthermore to be able to do so via multiple modes of operation (e.g., a button on equipment, a remote, text entry on a computer, and a certain voice command).

   (ii) The telemonitoring system must provide quality data, reliably, and be able to identify and process adverse events as appropriate for the health and rehabilitative aims. When loss of quality data collection is determined, the appropriate entity (person) should be informed by means of a context-appropriate message in an accessible format, and preferably telecommunicated in a timely manner that minimizes the response time. Since the abilities (and perhaps preferences) of the person being monitored are known, the accessibility modes should include those that are accessible for the user, and ideally, also support their personal preferences. This lowers the risk of use error, as well as the possibility of personal inconvenience.

   (iii) Support for a mobile connection (e.g., cell phone) and call to a person in the role of an evaluator should be timely, and should also include both text and voice messaging capability.

(b) *Periodic data monitoring.* Data may be collected in continuous and/or sampled modes, with the data available for monitoring in an accessible format, intended for evaluation by users who may have diverse abilities.

   (i) There is considerable advantage in having the data interface use a standard operating system platform such as Windows, as the user can then take advantage of built-in accessibility features and/or their personal AT software.

   (ii) Any web-based interface should at least follow the version of WCAG that is part of current Section 508 guidelines.

(iii) There is advantage to support for a mobile interface, at least for scanning data. Note that the client will often participate at different times in different roles, including the role of an evaluator.

4. *Interactive virtual teletherapy*. Here we assume that the aim is interactive therapy that is similar in terms of quality to a physical face-to-face encounter, and indeed may even improve on such an encounter through "virtual environment" interfaces and/or storage of data from teleinterfaces. As was true a decade ago [51, 52], this still remains the greatest challenge for telerehab-EIT; progress has been mostly in the areas of rehabilitation where physical contact is not a necessary part of the intervention (e.g., psychological and speech–language sessions), which according to our schema really falls under televisits. Here we target intervention sessions that fall under physical/occupational therapy (e.g., see Refs. [35, 50] for possibilities), plus assessment/interventions such as remote worksite accommodations that could benefit from a physical contact mode. Physical contact is fundamentally bicausal [54]: human performance depends on the dynamic properties of the contacted environment. Two variables are passed during the period of contact: force and position (velocity), the product of which is mechanical power. Bicausal interfaces with a low time delay provide a natural "feel" that, through practice, can make a device appear like an extension of the body (e.g., the extended physiological proprioception concept in prosthetics [39]). Design of contact interfaces can broadly be classified by their mechanical impedance [21]. We include both bidirectional (e.g., with force-reflecting client interface, with "resist" and "assist" modes) and unidirectional contact interfaces (for evaluation or training, including of virtual environments on the client side that include the graphics workstation and software, plus the sensors that measure real-time position/orientation of certain body segments). A related concept is telepresence—the use of telecommunications to allow a remote operator to be "present" (e.g., to manipulate objects for a remote client). All accessibility guidance from Item 2 (televisits) also apply here, along with these additional ones:

(a) Selected therapeutic gaming and virtual reality technologies, both hardware and software, should support the standardized human interface device (HID) ports for interoperable mouse/joystick/gaming devices that connect via USB or wireless ports. This facilitates (1) rehabilitation software development for selective data collection of performance measures and (2) use of alternative interface devices (e.g., a different brand of joystick, mouse–joystick signal conversion, and voice-activated control of a switch channel).

(b) Ranges of motion of device degrees of freedom, and force application levels, should be able to be scaled based on the abilities (or preferences) of the user [14, 15].

(c) Usually, there should be two display monitors for the telepractitioner (one for multimodal conferencing and the other related to the therapeutic gaming environment), and perhaps for the client.

5.3.4 Use of Proposed Framework

It is important to note that guidance associated with more than one of the four types of tele-encounters will be relevant for many telerehabilitation programs. As an example, consider the types of tele-supported home rehab therapy programs that are reviewed by Johnson et al. [25]. These involve the use of tools such as rehabilitation robotics, force-reflecting joysticks, and other gaming technology (see also Refs. [14, 15, 26]) often placed in the home. While interactive teletherapy sessions are an important type of tele-encounter, there is no question that telemonitoring must also be integrated into the plan, as it relates to adherence and assessments that are critical for timely adjustments to the intervention proposal (e.g., as performance changes and/or tissues remodel). Furthermore, conventional televisits can be expected, for instance, to integrate in professionals from other aspects of health intervention. Thus, different telerehab-EIT technical guidelines apply to different components of the intervention protocol. Other examples include speech therapy telepractice (involving televisits and telemonitoring, see Towey, Chap. 8) and telerehabilitation for occupational therapy (see Cason, Chap. 10).

It could be argued that some of these guidelines may be too strong. Not really – there are no technological barriers to implementation. Actual telerehab-EIT technical guidelines would, of course, need to *go through a consensus process*, involving representative stakeholders, but the proposed guidelines of Section 3.3 might provide a useful starting point. Perhaps an entity such as the RERC on Telerehabilitation could help facilitate the process. With broad consensus, such guidelines can serve as a *resource* for:

- product developers (who would have specifications to consider during the design process);
- procurers of telerehab-EIT (who could use this guidance and specifications as a resource for identifying desirable features for the types of tele-encounters of interest);
- policy-makers (who would have "enabling" guidance for addressing access policies; see Seelman [38]);
- rehabilitation, disability, and telehealth researchers;
- most importantly, persons with a diversity of abilities who would be better informed about what is theoretically possible in terms of their ability to equitably participate in the types of tele-encounters from which they feel that they could benefit from having better access.

As telerehabilitation is most closely associated with expertise in disability research and human–technology interfaces, any telerehab-EIT accessibility guidelines could *easily become more general telehealth-EIT accessibility guidelines*. This could expand the scope of application and, in turn, expand the magnitude of impact on the lives of persons with disabilities.

Finally, because rehabilitation researchers are generally not experts in either accessibility or modern EIT, such guidelines might help spark a recommendation of

Winters [51, 52] that has been not yet been realized: enabling rehabilitation research-ers to have more timely and frequent access to subjects operating in their natural, more ecologically valid environments.

5.4 Future Directions

As noted by Winters [51, 52], the ultimate challenge in telerehabilitation is to achieve location-independent, integrated therapeutic intervention at a distance. This chapter addresses a component that has seemed to be missing: formalized consideration of the diverse abilities and preferences of our most important entities—the end users who can benefit from more accessible telerehab-EIT. Specifically, it suggests that the time is right to start seriously considering technical guidance for accessible telerehab-EIT.

Perhaps such telerehab-EIT accessibility guidelines could set the stage for a product accessibility certification process that could be of great benefit to this emerging field. A good example of how this process can work and be effective is the Inclusive Fitness Initiative's accreditation mark for fitness equipment in England (see http://www.efds. co.uk/page.asp?section=1595&sectionTitle=Inclusive+Fitness+Initiative+%28IF I%29). The focus is on accessibility of the interface(s), with accessible equipment then classified by core types of functional use. Health facilities in England now tend to be full of equipment that meets their core accessibility guidelines, and a few years ago the RERC on Recreational Technologies helped found the Inclusive Fitness Coalition (IFC; see http://www.incfit.org/node/69/) to help replicate some of these successes in the United States. For telerehabilitation, the starting point, probably, would be to gather a collection of stakeholders and a few EIT and web-accessibility experts to see if there is sufficient momentum for launching and maintaining such an effort.

The good news is that many existing standards are available for use as resources, and that, even as technology continues to evolve, it would be relatively straightfor-ward to update such telerehab-EIT accessibility guidelines because a mature collec-tion of the types of tele-encounters and classes of teleinterfaces can already be developed. Mainstream developers of hardware and software products with teleinter-faces would likely benefit from having these guidelines available as a resource, which in turn would benefit the field and, mostly importantly, the quality of life of persons with diverse abilities and preferences—who deserve better teleaccess to health care.

Summary

- Telerehabilitation is aimed at achieving location-independent, integrated thera-peutic intervention at a distance.
- The Telerehabilitation Special Interest Group (Telerehab-SIG) of the American Telemedicine Association (ATA) has recently developed a blueprint for telereha-bilitation guidelines.

- By 2002, it was recognized that telerehabilitation involves new ways for humans to work interactively together to achieve certain aims such as completing tasks, usually cooperatively between sites.
- Despite remarkable technological advances over this past decade, widespread adoption of telerehabilitation-mediated health services did not happen. This suggests that the primary barrier is not the core technological capabilities, but rather the classic challenges such as lack of federal investment in large-scale clinical trials on outcomes and cost effectiveness and patient–consumer and clinician reluctance. More focus on access to effective use of telerehabilitation interfaces by persons with diverse abilities could help tip the scale in overcoming such challenges.
- In telerehabilitation, the limited documentation of use errors and access difficulties are likely more a result of abandonment by persons with disability, or even lack of initial access.
- More effective interfaces need to be designed to help the telerehabilitation field reach its full potential for providing both remote and equitable access to persons with the full spectrum of diverse abilities. A framework for guidelines that could lead to more accessible telerehabilitation interfaces is proposed.

Abbreviations/Acronyms

AD	Accessible design
ADA	Americans with Disabilities Act
AT	Assistive technology
ATA	American Telemedicine Association
EIT	Electronic and information technology
FDA	Food and Drug Administration
HID	Human interface device
HL7	Health Level Seven
IFC	Inclusive fitness coalition
INCITS	InterNational Committee for Information Technology Standard
IP	Internet protocol
IRB	Institutional review board
ISDN	Integrated services digital network
LAN	Local area network
MAN	Metropolitan area network
PAN	Personal area network
PD	Personalized design
PDA	Personal digital assistant
RERC	Rehabilitation Engineering Research Center
RERC-AMI	RERC on Accessible Medical Instrumentation
SIG	Special Interest Group
Telerehab-SIG	Telerehabilitation Special Interest Group

TTY   Text telephone
UD   Universal design
URC   Universal remote console
USB   Universal Serial Bus
WCAG   Web Content Accessibility Guidelines

Conflicts of Interest This work does not reflect the viewpoints of Marquette University or of the FDA.

References

1. Brandt EN, Pope AM, editors. Enabling America, assessing the role of rehabilitation science and engineering. Washington, D.C.: National Academy Press; 1997.
2. Brennan DM, Barkder L. Human factors in the development and implementation of telerehabilitation systems. J Telemed Telecare. 2008;14:55–8.
3. Brennan DM, Mawson S, Brownsell S. Telerehabilitation: enabling the remote delivery of healthcare, rehabilitation, and self management. Stud Health Technol Inf. 2009;145:231–48.
4. Brennan D, Tindall L, Theodoros D, et al. A blueprint for telerehabilitation guidelines. Int J Telerehabil. 2010;2:31–4.
5. Brewer J. Access to medical instrumentation: the role of web accessibility. In: Winters JM, Story MF, editors. Medical instrumentation: accessibility and usability considerations. Boca Raton: CRC Press; 2007. p. 297–303, Chapter 23.
6. Burns RB, Crislip D, Daviou P, et al. Using telerehabilitation to support assistive technology. Assist Technol. 1998;10:126–33.
7. Card S, Moran T, Newell A. The model human processor. In: Boff K, Kaufman L, Thomas J, editors. Handbook of perception and human performance, vol. 2. New York: Wiley; 1986.
8. Carignan CR, Krebs HI. Telerehabilitation robotics: bright lights, big future? J Rehabil Res Dev. 2006;43:695–710.
9. Carr JH, Shepherd RB. Neurological rehabilitation: optimizing motor performance. Oxford: Butterworth-Heinemann; 1998.
10. Chumbler NR, Quigley P, Sanford J, et al. Implementing telerehabilitation research for stroke rehabilitation with community dwelling veterans: lessons learned. Int J Telerehabil. 2010;2:15–21.
11. Dang T, Rosen MJ, Halstead L. Remote evaluation of pressure ulcers for wound care management of individuals with spinal cord injury: a preliminary report. In: Proceedings of the IEEE/ EMBS, Atlanta, 1999.
12. Danturthi RS, Shroff P, Winters JM. Progress in using the universal remote console standard to create user-customized interfaces for future medical devices. In: Winters JM, Story MF, editors. Medical instrumentation: accessibility and usability consideration. Boca Raton, FL: CRC Press; 2007. p. 373–92. chapter 28.
13. Erlandson RF, Enderle JD, Winters JM. Educating engineers in universal and accessible design. In: Winters JM, Story MF, editors. Medical instrumentation: accessibility and usability considerations. Boca Raton: CRC Press; 2007. p. 101–18.
14. Feng X, Winters JM. An interactive framework for personalized computer-assisted neurorehabilitation. IEEE Trans Inf Technol Biomed. 2007;11:518–26.
15. Feng X, Winters JM. Emerging personalized home rehabilitation: integrating service with interface. In: Winters JM, Story MF, editors. Medical instrumentation: accessibility and usability considerations. Boca Raton: CRC Press; 2007. p. 355–72, Chapter 27.
16. Feng X, Winters JM. A pilot study evaluating use of a computer-assisted neurorehabilitation platform for upper-extremity stroke assessment. J Neuroeng Rehabil. 2009;6:15.

17. Fuhrer MJ, editor. Assessing medical rehabilitation practices. The promise of outcomes research. Baltimore: Paul H Brookes Publ. Co.; 1997.
18. Granger CV, Brownscheidle CM. Outcome measurement in medical rehabilitation. Int J Technol Assess Health Care. 1995;11:262–8.
19. Haines J, Winters JM. Evaluating automatically generated personalized interfaces on an ergometer for people with disabilities. In: Proceedings of the EMBC, Vancouver, 2008.
20. HL7. Health Level Seven (HL7) International, see standards, Version 3.0. 2010. Available at: http://www.hl7.org.
21. Hogan N. Adaptive control of mechanical impedance by coactivation of antagonist muscles. IEEE Trans Automatic Control. 1984;AC-29:681–90.
22. Holden MK, Dyar TA, Dayan-Cimadoro L. Telerehabilitation using a virtual environment improves upper extremity function in patients with stroke. IEEE Trans Neural Syst Rehabil Eng. 2007;15(1):36–42.
23. INCITS. InterNational Committee for Information Technology Standard, V2 – IT access interfaces. 2008. Available at: http://zing.ncsl.nist.gov/incits/v2/. National: ANSI/INCITS 389–393:2005. International: ISO/IEC 24752:2008.
24. Jack D, Boian R, Merians A, et al. Virtual reality-enhanced stroke rehabilitation. IEEE Trans Neural Syst Rehabil Eng. 2001;9:308–18.
25. Johnson MJ, Feng X, Johnson LM, et al. Potential of a suite of robot/computer-assisted motivating systems for personalized, home-based, stroke rehabilitation. J Neuroeng Rehabil. 2007;4:6. doi:10.1186/1743-0003-4-6.
26. Lange B, Flynn SM, Rizzo AA. Game-based telerehabilitation. Eur J Phys Rehabil Med. 2009;45(1):143–51.
27. Lewis JA, Deutsch JE, Burdea G. Usability of the remote console for virtual reality telerehabilitation: formative evaluation. Cyberpsychol Behav. 2006;9(2):142–7.
28. McCue M, Fairman A, Pramuka M. Enhancing quality of life through telerehabilitation. Phys Med Rehabil Clin N Am. 2010;21:195–205.
29. Parmanto B, Saptono A. Telerehabilitation: state-of-the-art from an informatics perspective. Int J Telerehabil. 2009;1:73–84.
30. Pramuka M, Roosmalen L. Telerehabilitation technologies: accessibility and usability. Int J Telerehabil. 2009;1:85–98.
31. Reinkensmeyer D, Lum P, Winters JM. Emerging technologies for improving access to movement therapy following neurologic injury. In: Winters JM, Robinson C, Simpson R, et al., editors. Emerging and accessible telecommunications, information and healthcare technologies. Arlington: RESNA Press; 2002. p. 136–50.
32. Rizzo AA, Strickland D, Bouchard S. The challenge of using virtual reality in telerehabilitation. Telemed J E Health. 2004;10:184–95.
33. Rosen MJ. Telerehabilitation. NeuroRehabilitation. 1999;3:3–18.
34. Rosen MJ, Winters JM, Lauderdale D. Summary of the state of the science conference on telerehabilitation. In: Winters JM, Robinson C, Simpson R, et al., editors. Emerging and accessible telecommunications, information and health technologies. Arlington: RESNA Press; 2002. p. 220–45.
35. Russell TG. Physical rehabilitation using telemedicine. J Telemed Telecare. 2007;13(5):217–20.
36. Sanders MS, McCormick EJ. Human factors in engineering design. New York: McGraw-Hill; 1993.
37. Scroff P, Winters JM. Generation of multi-modal interfaces for hand-held devices based on user preferences and abilities. In: Transdisciplinary conference on distributed diagnosis and home healthcare, Arlington, 2006. p. 5.
38. Seelman KD. Technology for full citizenship: challenges for the research community. In: Winters JM, Story MF, editors. Medical instrumentation: accessibility and usability considerations. Boca Raton: CRC Press; 2007. p. 307–20. chapter 24.

39. Simpson DC. The choice of control system for the multimovement prosthesis: extended physiological proprioception (E.P.P.). In: Herberts P et al., editors. The control of upper extremity prostheses and orthoses. New York: Charles C Thomas; 1974. p. 146–50.
40. Story MF. Applying the principles of universal design to medical devices. In: Winters JM, Story MF, editors. Medical instrumentation: accessibility and usability considerations. Boca Raton: CRC Press; 2007. p. 83–92, Chapter 6.
41. Story MF, Lemke MF, MacDonald C, et al. Guidelines for designing and selecting accessible medical equipment. In: Proceedings of the RESNA 31st international conference, Arlington, 2008.
42. Story MF, Mueller JL. Universal design performance measures for products. A tool for assessing universal usability. In: Winters JM, Robinson C, Simpson R, et al., editors. Emerging and accessible telecommunications, information and health technologies. Arlington: RESNA Press; 2002.
43. Story MF, Winters JM, Lemke MR, et al. Development of a method for evaluating accessibility of medical equipment for patients with disabilities. Appl Ergon. 2010;42(1):178–83. Epub 2010 Aug 17.
44. Sugarman H, Dayan E, Weisel-Eichler A, et al. The Jerusalem telerehabilitation system, a new low-cost, haptic rehabilitation approach. Cyberpsychol Behav. 2006;9(2):178.
45. Taub E, Uswatte G, Pidikiti R. Constraint-induced movement therapy: a new family of techniques with broad application to physical rehabilitation – a clinical review. J Rehabil Res Dev. 1999;6:237–51.
46. Theodoros D, Russell T. Telerehabilitation: current perspectives. Stud Health Technol Inform. 2008;131:191–209.
47. Vanderheiden GC, Zimmermann G. State-of-the-science chapter: access to information technologies. In: Winters JM, Robinson CJ, Simpson RC, et al., editors. Emerging and accessible telecommunication, information and healthcare technologies. Arlington: RESNA Press; 2002. p. 95–111, Chapter 16.
48. Vesmarovich SH, Walker T, Hauber RP, et al. Extending the continuum of care: the use of telerehabilitation for the treatment of pressure ulcers in persons with spinal cord injuries or multiple sclerosis. Adv Wound Care. 1999;12:264–9.
49. Watzlaf V, Moeini S, Firouzan P. VOIP for telerehabilitation: a risk analysis for privacy, security and HIPAA compliance. Int J Telerehabil. 2010;2:3–9. doi:10.5195/ijt.2010.6056.
50. Winters JM. Motion analysis and telerehabilitation: healthcare delivery standards and strategies for the new millennium. In: Gerald F, Smith PA, editors. Pediatric gait: a new millennium in clinical care and motion analysis technology. Piscataway: IEEE Press; 2000. p. 16–22.
51. Winters JM. Emerging rehabilitative healthcare anywhere: was the homecare technologies workshop visionary. In: Winters JM, Robinson CJ, Simpson RC, et al., editors. Emerging and accessible telecommunication, information and healthcare technologies. Arlington: RESNA Press; 2002. p. 152–84, Chapter 16.
52. Winters JM. Telerehabilitation research: emerging opportunities. Annu Rev Biomed Eng. 2002;4:287–320.
53. Winters JM. Future possibilities for interface technologies that enhance universal access to healthcare devices and services. In: Winters JM, Story MF, editors. Medical instrumentation: accessibility and usability considerations. Boca Raton: CRC Press; 2007. p. 321–40, Chapter 25.
54. Winters JM, Lathan C, Sukthankar S, et al. Human performance and rehabilitation technologies. In: Winters JM, Crago PE, editors. Biomechanics and neural control of movement. New York: Springer; 2000. p. 493–551, Chapter 37.
55. Winters JM, Feng X, Wang Y, et al. Progress toward universal interface technologies for telerehabilitation. Conf Proc IEEE Eng Med Biol Soc. 2004;7:4777–80.
56. Winters JM, Story MF. Results of the workshop on interfaces for accessible medical instrumentation. In: Winters JM, Story MF, editors. Medical instrumentation: accessibility and usability considerations. Boca Raton: CRC Press; 2007. p. 419–44. chapter 31.
57. Winters JMW, Story MF, Barnekow K, et al. Results of a national survey on accessibility of medical instrumentation for consumers. In: Winters JM, Story MF, editors. Medical instru-

mentation: accessibility and usability considerations. Boca Raton: CRC Press; 2007. p. 13–28, Chapter 2.

58. Winters JM, Wang Y, Winters JMW. Wearable sensors and telerehabilitation: integrating intelligent telerehabilitation assistants with a model for optimizing home therapy. IEEE/EMBS Mag Spec Issue Wearable Med Technol. 2003;22:56–65.

59. Woo SL-Y, Debski RE, Zeminski J, et al. Injury and repair of ligaments and tendons. Annu Rev Biomed Eng. 2000;2:83–118.

60. Zimmermann G, Vanderheiden G. A dream. The universal remote console. 2010. ISO Focus+, p. 11–3.

Chapter 6
Telerehabilitation as a Means of Health-Care Delivery

Alan Chong W. Lee and Nancy D. Harada

Abstract Telehealth is defined by the American Physical Therapy Association as the use of electronic communications to provide and deliver a host of health-related information and health-care services, including, but not limited to, physical therapy-related content and services over large and small distances. Telehealth encompasses a variety of health-care and health promotion activities, including, but not limited to, education, advice, reminders, interventions, and monitoring of interventions. Telerehabilitation is a form of telemedicine and involves the delivery of therapeutic rehabilitation interventions using telecommunication technologies. This chapter will discuss the current telerehabilitation literature related to physical therapy. In addition, novice telehealth PT practitioners will learn of telerehabilitation resources available from national and international professional associations. By looking at the current evidence and guidelines related to telerehabilitation, we hope to glean future opportunities for practice, research, and education for physical therapy practitioners.

6.1 Introduction

Telehealth is defined by American Physical Therapy Association (APTA) as the use of electronic communications to provide and deliver a host of health-related information and health-care services, including, but not limited to, physical therapy-related content

A.C.W. Lee (✉)
Physical Therapy Program, Mount St. Mary's College,
10 Chester Place, Los Angeles, CA 90007, USA
e-mail: allee@msmc.la.edu

N.D. Harada
Department of Health Services, Fielding School of Public Health,
650 Charles Young Dr. S., 31-269 CHS, Box 951772, 90095-1772 Los Angeles, CA, USA
e-mail: nhrada@ucla.edu

S. Kumar, E.R. Cohn (eds.), *Telerehabilitation*, Health Informatics,
DOI 10.1007/978-1-4471-4198-3_6, © Springer-Verlag London 2013

and services over large and small distances. Telehealth encompasses a variety of health-care and health promotion activities, such as education, advice, reminders, monitoring, and intervention delivery [3]. As discussed in this book, telerehabilitation for occupational therapists as well as telepractice for speech-language pathologists have been developing in recent years. The purpose of this chapter is to describe evidence-based telehealth practice in physical therapy and the potential implications for clinical practice. We will discuss the current telerehabilitation literature related to physical therapy as well as resources available from national and international professional telerehabilitation associations. By looking at the current evidence and guidelines related to telerehabilitation, we hope to glean future opportunities for practice, research, and education for physical therapy practitioners.

Telerehabilitation is a form of telemedicine and involves the delivery of therapeutic rehabilitation interventions using telecommunication technologies [12, 25]. Patients undergoing rehabilitation may benefit from telerehabilitation programs that offer more convenient and efficient service choices [18]. For example, older adults often have access barriers such as functional limitations and fewer transportation options, which may interfere with their ability to visit a rehabilitation provider regularly for ongoing treatment. Indeed, the use of telemedicine has grown in rural areas where patients often have to travel long distances to see their health-care providers.

An early application of telerehabilitation was reported in 1984 by Fletcher and colleagues, who found that the use of transtelephonic electrocardiographic monitoring in patients with coronary artery disease who exercised at home was efficacious and safe [21]. Patients who benefited the most were located in rural areas where distance posed a barrier to traveling to a hospital-based program. In another early study, Sparks and colleagues randomized patients to either a 12-week home exercise program using transtelephonic exercise monitoring (TEM) or a 12-week hospital-based exercise program [22]. They found significant improvement in cardiac function for both the groups. No medical emergencies arose in either group, and only two patients in the TEM group developed new arrhythmias while exercising that required medication changes. The researchers concluded that TEM was an effective alternative for the rehabilitation of patients who were unable to return to a hospital-based exercise program.

More recently, telehealth technology has been applied to monitor and deliver health care in the patient's home [9, 14, 17]. These programs have demonstrated promising results with respect to clinical outcomes and cost savings. Kaiser Permanente evaluated the effectiveness of a remote video system (PTS 100 home video system, American Telecare, Minneapolis, Minnesota) that allowed patients and nurses to interact in real time [14]. Patients who used this system had chronic diseases (i.e., congestive heart failure, chronic obstructive pulmonary disease, cerebrovascular accident, cancer, diabetes, anxiety, or need for wound care). Although no differences were found in quality indicators (i.e., medication regimen compliance, knowledge about their disease, and ability to move toward self-care), investigators found similar patient satisfaction and lower mean costs of care for the video-monitoring group compared to the control (usual care) group. This study demonstrated that despite fewer in-home visits made by a nurse (but more video contact), patients continued to report satisfaction and lower costs.

At the Physical Therapy and Society Summit in 2009, Dr. Joseph C. Kvedar [16], an expert telemedicine practitioner, stated that telehealth in physical therapy may provide exercise monitoring, pain management monitoring, and telerehabilitation opportunities to address the adherence rates to exercise.

In the U.S. Department of Veterans Affairs (VA), telehome health programs have been developed and targeted toward frail older veterans with complex chronic disease conditions, who are high-cost, high-risk, and high-resource users [9, 17]. These programs monitor specific disease conditions such as stroke, chronic obstructive pulmonary disease, congestive heart failure, and diabetes, with the aims of improving health status, increasing the efficiency of health-care delivery, decreasing resource utilization, and maintaining veterans in their own homes. Early evaluation of these programs utilized quasi-experimental designs and demonstrated reductions in emergency room visits, hospital admissions, hospital bed days of care, VA nursing home admissions, and VA nursing home bed days of care [9, 17]. The patient dropout rates in these early programs were low, and survey results reported excellent patient, family/caretaker, and provider satisfaction. Moreover, patient quality of life and functional status showed significant improvements, representing a positive therapeutic response for the frail older adult population [17]. Randomized controlled trials are now being conducted to determine the effectiveness of telerehabilitation interventions utilizing more rigorous study designs [10].

A recent systematic review of clinical outcomes, clinical process, health-care utilization, and costs associated with telerehabilitation by Kairy and colleagues found unclear conclusions from 28 studies due to methodological limitations [15]. They recommended more methodologically robust studies that investigate resource allocation and costs with patient focus and clinical process measurements to address sustainability of telerehabilitation.

The use of telerehabilitation by physical therapists is promising. However, much work needs to be done to advance the science of telerehabilitation within the PT profession. As a basis for this work, we conducted a literature review to describe the state of telerehabilitation delivery in physical therapy, as documented in the literature over the past 10 years.

6.2 Methods

We reviewed the PubMed database for the period January 2000 through October 2010 to identify all the published studies related to physical therapy telerehabilitation. The keywords used to search PubMed were "telerehabilitation" followed by "telerehabilitation physical therapy." The search yielded a total of 117 articles. Each of the article abstracts was independently reviewed by both authors and classified according to the following framework:

1. *Conceptual or descriptive*: The article describes conceptual issues related to telehealth or potential clinical applications, but no data have been reviewed.
2. *Financial or resource use*: The article describes issues related to reimbursement, legislative, licensure or professional standards, or resource utilization (e.g., number of outpatient visits or number of hospitalizations).
3. *Screening, evaluation, and assessment*: The article discusses measurement issues including reliability, validity, evaluation, and examination.
4. *Monitoring*: The article discusses the use of telerehabilitation for the purpose of monitoring a patient over time. This category may include pilot studies of monitoring interventions.
5. *Intervention efficacy or effectiveness*: The article describes studies that test the efficacy or effectiveness of a telehealth intervention. Results are reported for specific outcome measures.

6.3   Results

The interrater reliability was 95% on classification of the abstracts using the above framework. Differences in classification between the authors were resolved by discussion until an agreement was reached.

Of the 117 articles, 44% ($n=53$) were conceptual or descriptive, followed by 21% ($n=24$) relating to screening, 21% ($n=24$) to monitoring, 7% ($n=8$) to financial, and 7% ($n=8$) to efficacy/effectiveness. Eighteen percent of the articles ($n=21$) were directly related to physical therapy practice. The majority of the studies (59%, $n=69$) were conducted in the United States, followed by 19% ($n=22$) in Europe, 14% ($n=16$) in Australia, and 8% ($n=9$) in other countries such as Japan and Canada.

Articles classified as conceptual or descriptive provided overviews of telehealth technologies with a clinical perspective for applying these technologies to physical therapy practice. Many of these articles were case studies describing the application of telerehabilitation to a patient with a specific diagnosis. As an example, Hermann and colleagues [13] described the efficacy of an Internet-based exercise regimen to enhance activities of daily living and functional task performance for a post stroke patient with the implication for further development of this type of application.

The majority of articles classified as screening focused on reliability and validity of the telerehabilitation application compared to an in-person or a clinic-based screening method. These studies typically showed moderate-to-high reliability of the telerehabilitation method compared to the in-person method. For example, Cabana and colleagues [8] found interrater reliability coefficients of >0.80 for outcome measures of range of motion and functioning when assessed through videoconferencing compared to face-to-face assessment for patients with total knee arthroplasty.

Articles classified into the monitoring category typically described the use of telerehabilitation technology to follow a patient over time. As an example, Harada and colleagues [11] evaluated the feasibility of monitoring home exercise for physically inactive older adults using a text-messaging device.

The fewest number of articles were related to financial or resource use, which essentially described utilization, reimbursement, legislative, licensure, or professional standards. Many of these articles described the impact of telerehabilitation on resource use, such as clinic visits, hospital, and nursing home stays, with mixed results. Bendixen and colleagues [6] evaluated the use of a system to monitor self-care and safety within the home and found no significant different in costs compared to patients receiving standard care. While clinic visits increased following this intervention, there were decreases in hospital and nursing home stays.

Finally, there were few studies describing intervention effectiveness or efficacy utilizing randomized controlled trials. The US Department of Veterans Affairs is a leader in this respect because it has conducted several randomized controlled trials of home telehealth. For example, Chumbler and colleagues [10] have recently conducted a randomized controlled trial of home telehealth for stroke patients, with outcome measures being physical function, disability, falls-related self-efficacy, and patient satisfaction.

6.4   Discussion

Our review found that the majority of articles published in the literature over the past 10 years were conceptual or descriptive, thus identifying numerous potential clinical applications of telehealth in physical therapy. There were fewer studies investigating reliability and/or validity, and the fewest number of studies were conducted in the financial/resource use or effectiveness categories. For a newly emerging technology in physical therapy, we would expect to see this pattern of literature as clinicians and researchers first identify potential applications, investigate the reliability and validity of technology use, and then begin to explore reimbursement/policy issues and intervention effectiveness.

The current body of literature highlights the opportunities for future advances in telehealth practice for physical therapy practitioners. The promotion of telehealth and telerehabilitation is strongly supported by both national and international professional associations. The American Telemedicine Association (ATA) published a blueprint for telerehabilitation guidelines in 2010 [2]. This document provides valuable insight to administrative, clinical, ethical, and technical standards for practitioners to implement telerehabilitation services.

The states of Alaska and Washington implemented regulations for telehealth practice in 2009 and 2010, respectively [1, 24]. Within Alaska, telerehabilitation is used to provide physical therapy to patients who are located at distant sites that are not in close proximity of a physical therapist [1]. Five Alaskan standards for practice require that the clinician: (1) must physically be present in the state while performing telerehabilitation; (2) must interact with the patient maintaining the same ethical conduct and integrity; (3) must comply with the requirements of licensed physical therapist assistant supervision; (4) may conduct one-on-one consultation, including initial evaluation; and (5) must provide and ensure appropriate client confidentiality and HIPAA compliance, establish secure connection, activate firewalls, and encrypt confidential information [1]. Within the state of Washington, telehealth is defined as providing physical therapy via electronic communication wherein the physical therapist or physical therapist assistant and the patient are not at the same location [24]. In addition, electronic communication is defined as the use of interactive, secure multimedia equipment that includes, at a minimum, audio and video equipment permitting two-way, real-time interactive communication between the physical therapist or physical therapist assistant and the patient. When physical therapy is practiced via telehealth within the state of Washington, the clinical record must include a statement that the physical therapy encounter occurred via telehealth technology.

Australian physical therapy researcher Dr. Trevor G. Russell, Clinical Informatics Committee Chair of the Australian Physiotherapy Association (APA), recommended that the PT profession adopt and integrate telerehabilitation into routine clinical practice, as empirical research emerges demonstrating its efficacy. In an editorial on telerehabilitation, Russell concluded by stating that a failure to do so would constitute a grave disservice to clients [19]. Furthermore, the APA published a position statement on telerehabilitation in 2009. This position statement included the definition, benefits, limitations, and barriers to telerehabilitation. The APA position concluded that care must be taken to ensure client safety and appropriateness of treatment when choosing to deliver physiotherapy services through telerehabilitation while adhering to the APA Code of Conduct at all times [5]. Finally, Australian physiotherapists gained national licensure to practice across jurisdictions and published a reimbursement policy for physiotherapy telerehabilitation services in 2011 (Russell, September 2010, personal communication).

6.5 Implications

Recently, great strides have been made to integrate telerehabilitation for physical therapy practice. To continue along this path, the following issues must be addressed:

1. As a hands-on profession, future research must address the effectiveness and efficacy of telerehabilitation compared to face-to-face physical therapy practice to mitigate the potential risks. Seelman and colleagues [20] reported the following benefits of telerehabilitation: greater access to services in rural areas, improved timing intensity and sequencing of interventions, and enhanced motivation for end users within their own social and vocational environments. However, potential challenges for telerehabilitation include professional license portability and the training required to replicate hands-on, face-to-face practice.

2. Physical therapists should investigate the financial reimbursement issues in the public and private sectors, with the implications for cost-effective care. For example, use of telerehabilitation in Alaska could avoid travel to a regional hospital in Dillingham, Alaska, thus saving a round trip airfare of $448 plus costs of food, housing, and local transportation for follow-up physical therapy services to patients [7]. In Washington, fifth visit re-evaluation via telehealth between a physical therapist located at a distant site (Oregon) and a physical therapist assistant located in the home site (Washington) may save between $12,000 and $18,000, as found in a recent financial analysis carried out by Infinity Rehab, Inc. [7]. In an economic evaluation of interactive teledermatology practice compared with conventional care, Armstrong and colleagues [4] noted that the hourly cost of operating a teledermatology practice was lower than that of a conventional clinic ($274 versus $346). The cost savings found in this study were due to less office space use and lower cost of technology. However, this saving was dissolved if a physician's compensation rose to $197. Therefore, cost savings in telehealth should not be shifted to other resources or personnel. For system-wide adoption of telerehabilitation, direct and indirect savings must be reinvested toward consumers of health care.

3. Practitioners must address ethical and legal regulation including malpractice risk management.

4. Future education must include how to best inform all stakeholders on the value of telehealth practice in physical therapy.

5. Physical therapy telepractitioners should check the proper regulatory standards in his or her licensed jurisdiction.

6. Physical therapy telepractitioners must be responsive to the needs of individual patients.

7. Physical therapy practitioners should collaborate with other telemedicine providers to progress the practice, research, and education of telerehabilitation.

A questionnaire is provided in Table 6.1 to assist physical therapy practitioners who might offer telerehabilitation services appreciate the general issues related to telehealth practice. Furthermore, physical therapy practitioners are urged to both seek out current recommendations and replicate best practices (and lessons learned) from telehealth and telemedicine practitioners. Table 6.2 lists national and international organizations where a practitioner may locate such information. For example, the California Telemedicine and eHealth Center (CTEC) published the seven steps to successful program development for a novice practitioner to assess, develop, and implement a new program in telemedicine [23].

6.6 Conclusions

Telerehabilitation in the physical therapy profession is gaining momentum for practice, research, and education in the global health-care arena, with the promotion of telehealth and telerehabilitation strongly supported by both national

Table 6.1 Essential questions for PT telepractitioners

Professional Guidelines

- What are the state licensure requirements for telehealth (telemedicine credentialing, interstate licensure) for the states within which I intend to telepractice?
- What are the professional standards (fees, reimbursement, licensure/continuing education, and legislative agenda) for the states within which I intend to telepractice?
- How do these requirements compare to those for other telerehabilitation professions? (e.g., speech-language pathology; occupational therapy)

Professional Association Guidelines

- What telehealth guidelines are provided by physical therapy (APTA) and other professional associations? (AOTA, ASHA, ATA, and APA)

Malpractice Coverage

- Does my malpractice insurance cover telehealth practice?

Technical Standards

- What are the technical standards for telepractice in physical therapy (technology use including setup costs and maintenance of equipment, consultants/technical assistance)?

Ethical Standards

- What are the ethical standards (informed consent, quality assurance, and consumer protection)?

Outcome Measures

- What are the outcome measurements (patient satisfaction, functional outcomes, cost/benefit ratio, and health-care economics/outputs) for physical therapy telepractice?

Table 6.2 Association telepractice resources

- American Physical Therapy Association—1111 North Fairfax Street, Alexandria, VA 22314-1488. Phone: 703-706-3252. www.apta.org. (Internet search terms—APTA: definition and guidelines on telehealth; technology in physical therapy, special interest group in health policy and administration)
- Australian Physiotherapy Association—Level 1, 1175 Toorak Road, Camberwell VIC 3124 Australia, PO Box 437, Hawthorn, BC VIC 3122, Australia. Phone: +61-3-9092-0888. http://www.physiotherapy.asn.au. (Internet search terms—APA: position statement on telerehabilitation)
- Federation of State Boards of Physical Therapy—124 West South Street, 3rd floor, Alexandria, VA 22314. Phone: 703-299-3100. www.fsbpt.org. (Internet search terms—FSBPT: 2010 Regulation of Telehealth—best practices)
- American Telemedicine Association—1100 Connecticut Avenue, NW, Suite 540, Washington, DC 20036. Phone: 217-398-1792. www.americantelemed.org. (Internet search terms—ATA: a blueprint for telerehabilitation guidelines)
- California Telemedicine & eHealth Center—1215 K Street, Suite 2020, Sacramento, CA 95814. Phone: 877-590-8144. http://www.CTEConline.org. (Internet search terms—CTEC: telehealth program developer)
- American Speech-Language-Hearing Association—2200 Research Boulevard #220, Rockville, MD 20850-3289. Phone: 301-296-5666. www.asha.org. (Internet search terms—ASHA: 2004 telepractice position statement and model regulation)
- The American Occupational Therapy Association, Inc.—4720 Montgomery Lane, PO Box 31220, Bethesda, MD 20824-1220. Phone: 301-652-2682. www.aota.org. (Internet search terms—AOTA: 2010 telerehabilitation position paper)

and international professional associations. Benefits of telerehabilitation include greater access to services in rural areas, improved timing intensity and sequencing of interventions, and enhanced motivation for end users within their own social and vocational environments.

The current body of literature highlights the opportunities for future advances in telehealth practice for physical therapy practitioners. Our review of literature found more descriptive studies compared to financial, screening, monitoring, and intervention trials.

In conclusion, this chapter has examined the current evidence on telerehabilitation and physical therapy to progress the future practice, research, and education of telehealth for physical therapy practitioners.

Summary

- Telehealth is the use of electronic communications to provide health-related information and health-care services, such as education, advice, reminders, monitoring, and intervention delivery, over large and small distances.
- Telerehabilitation is a form of telemedicine that involves the delivery of therapeutic rehabilitation interventions using telecommunication technologies. Telerehabilitation in the physical therapy profession is gaining momentum in the global health-care arena.
- Telehome health programs have been developed to provide health-care services to frail older veterans in their own homes, with the aims of improving their health status, increasing the efficiency of health-care delivery, and decreasing resource utilization.
- Benefits of telerehabilitation include greater access to services in rural areas, improved timing intensity and sequencing of interventions, and enhanced motivation for end users within their own social and vocational environments.
- The current body of literature highlights the opportunities for future advances in telehealth practice for physical therapy practitioners. The promotion of telehealth and telerehabilitation is strongly supported by both national and international professional associations.
- Physical therapy practitioners should collaborate with other telemedicine providers to progress the practice, research, and education of telerehabilitation.

Abbreviations/Acronyms

APA   Australian Physiotherapy Association
APTA   American Physical Therapy Association

AOTA   American Occupational Therapy Association, Inc.
ASHA   American Speech-Language-Hearing Association
ATA   American Telemedicine Association
CTEC   California Telemedicine and eHealth Center
HIPAA   Health Insurance Portability and Accountability Act of 1996
TEM   Transtelephonic exercise monitoring
VA   U.S. Department of Veterans Affairs

References

1. AK Department of Commerce, Community and Economic Development website. Statues and regulations physical therapy and occupational therapy June 2010 main page. Available at: http://commerce.state.ak.us/OCC/pub/PT-OTStatutes.pdf. Accessed 3 Jan 2011.
2. American Telemedicine Association website. A blueprint for telerehabilitation guidelines resource page. Telemedicine standards & guidelines. Available at: http://www.american-telemed.org/i4a/pages/index.cfm?pageid=3311. Accessed 3 Jan 2011.
3. APTA telehealth website. Telehealth – definition and guidelines main page. Available at: http://www.apta.org/AM/Template.cfm?Section=Home&CONTENTID=67435&TEMPLATE=/CM/ContentDisplay.cfm. Accessed 21 Dec 2010.
4. Armstrong AW, Dorer DJ, Lugn NE, et al. Economic evaluation of interactive teledermatology compared with conventional care. Telemed J E Health. 2007;13:92–100.
5. Australian Physiotherapy Association website. Telerehabilitation and physiotherapy position statements page. Available at: http://www.physiotherapy.asn.au/images/Document_Library/Position_Statements/2012%20telerehabilitation.pdf. Accessed 3 Jan 2011.
6. Bendixen RM, Levy CE, Olive ES, et al. Cost effectiveness of a telerehabilitation program to support chronically ill and disabled elders in their homes. Telemed J E Health. 2009;15(1):31–8.
7. Brannon JA, Brown CA, Esau TD, et al. Regulation of telehealth – best practices part I. Paper presented at the Federations of State Boards of physical therapy, Denver, 16 Oct 2010.
8. Cabana F, Boissy P, Tousignant M, et al. Interrater agreement between telerehabilitation and face-to-face clinical outcome measurements for total knee arthroplasty. Telemed J E Health. 2010;16(3):293–8.
9. Chumbler NR, Mann WC, Wu S, et al. The association of home-telehealth use and care coordination with improvement of functional and cognitive functioning in frail elderly men. Telemed J E Health. 2004;10(2):129–37.
10. Chumbler NR, Rose DK, Griffiths P, et al. Study protocol: home-based telehealth stroke care: a randomized trial for veterans. Trials. 2010;30:74.
11. Harada ND, Dhanani S, Elrod M, et al. Feasibility study of home telerehabilitation for physically inactive veterans. J Rehabil Res Dev. 2010;47(5):465–76.
12. Hatzakis M, Haselkorn J, Williams R, et al. Telemedicine and the delivery of health services to veterans with multiple sclerosis. J Rehabil Res Dev. 2003;40(3):265–82.
13. Hermann VH, Herzog M, Jordan R, et al. Telerehabilitation and electrical stimulation: an occupation-based, client-centered stroke intervention. Am J Occup Ther. 2010;64(1):73–81.
14. Johnston B, Wheeler L, Deuser J, et al. Outcomes of the Kaiser Permanente Tele-home health research project. Arch Fam Med. 2000;9:40–5.
15. Kairy D, Lehoux P, Vincent C, et al. A systematic review of clinical outcomes, clinical process, healthcare utilization and costs associated with telerehabilitation. Disabil Rehabil. 2009;31:427–47.

16. Kvedar J (2009) Innovative perspectives: technological drivers of change. In: APTA physical therapy and society summit, Leesburg, 27–28 Feb 2009.
17. Meyer M, Kobb R, Ryan P. Virtually healthy: chronic disease management in the home. Dis Manag. 2002;5(2):87–94.
18. Morgan RE. Computer-based technology and caregiving for older adults: exploring the range of possibilities and beyond. Public Policy Aging Rep. 2004;14(1):1–5.
19. Russell TG. Telerehabilitation: a coming of age [editorial]. Aust J Physiother. 2009;55:5–6.
20. Seelman KD, Hartman LM. Telerehabilitation: policy and research tools. Int J Telerehabil. 2009;1:47–58.
21. Shaw DK, Sparks KE, Jennings HS, et al. Cardiac rehabilitation using simultaneous voice and electrocardiographic transtelephonic monitoring. Am J Cardiol. 1995;76:1069–71.
22. Sparks KE, Shaw DK, Eddy D, et al. Alternatives for cardiac rehabilitation patients unable to return to a hospital-based program. Heart Lung. 1993;22:298–303.
23. The California telemedicine and eHealth center website. Program developer page. Available at: http://www.cteconline.org/program-developer.php. Accessed 11 Jan 2011.
24. WA State department of health website. Pre-Proposal (CR-101) Washington State Register main page. Available at: http://apps.leg.wa.gov/documents/laws/wsr/2009/15/09-15-002.htm. Accessed 3 Jan 2011.
25. Winters JM. Telerehabilitation research: emerging opportunities. Annu Rev Biomed Eng. 2002;4:287–320.

Chapter 7
Implementation and Management of a Successful Telerehabilitation Program in Speech Language Pathology

Lyn R. Tindall

Abstract Development of a successful telerehabilitation program involves planning in the initial stages and continuous quality improvement throughout the implementation of such a program. Key elements include choice of telecommunication technology, setting up of the environment, attention to business aspects, staff preparation, and client selection. This chapter offers guidelines for planning and starting a telerehabilitation program that includes essentials to consider during this phase. A general overview of technology is presented. Pointers for preparing an environment conducive to a successful telerehabilitation application are outlined. Preparation and training of staff and clients are components of a thriving program. And finally, a marketing plan is the process for communicating to clients and partners who may benefit from a telerehabilitation program.

7.1 Introduction

Traditional systems of delivery of speech pathology services may be difficult to access for many individuals, yielding results that are inadequate or compromised. To achieve the objective of delivering speech pathology services that meet the needs of all clients, it is incumbent on speech-language pathologists to seek alternative ways to provide effective, less expensive care [5]. The delivery of rehabilitation services at a distance, using telecommunication systems, holds the promise of enhancing and expanding the delivery of speech pathology services by increasing the options available, consequently enabling persons with disabilities to have

L.R. Tindall
Department of Physical Medicine and Rehabilitation,
Veterans Affairs Medical Center,
Lexington, KY 40505, USA
e-mail: lyn.tindall2@gmail.com

S. Kumar, E.R. Cohn (eds.), *Telerehabilitation*, Health Informatics,
DOI 10.1007/978-1-4471-4198-3_7, © Springer-Verlag London 2013

equitable access to treatment. Thus, telerehabilitation technology has the potential to bridge this gap by providing rehabilitation services to distant sites.

The American Speech-Language Hearing Association (ASHA) [2] has adopted the term *telepractice* to describe the delivery of speech pathology services at a distance using telecommunication technology. ASHA recognizes the need for optional delivery of services to clients unable to travel to a hospital or clinic for treatment, while ensuring the quality of those services. According to ASHA guidelines [2], speech-language pathologists must be responsible to deliver evidence-based care that is comparable to traditional face-to-face treatment. Use of telecommunication technology should not be recommended solely on convenience and cost savings. The notion that delivery of speech pathology services using telecommunication technology is "better than nothing" must be avoided [4]. Success of a telepractice program must include thorough and careful planning as well as continued management to provide the best care for clients. Such a program should include *planning and startup, choice of technology, continued management*, and *special consideration for the client encounter.*

7.2   Planning and Startup

Initial stages of program planning provide opportunities to identify and analyze client care issues and develop realistic goals. To accomplish this, the selection of a team of individuals to guide the process is important for the development of a successful telepractice program. Suggestions for members of this team include the following:

- A clinical lead
- A support person from executive leadership
- A representative from information technology (IT)
- Others may be added depending on the setting

If these individuals are not available, as in a small private practice, collaboration may be necessary to assist in the initial planning stages.

A needs assessment should be the first step in developing a telepractice program. This could include collection of data on underserved clients, costs of providing care (including costs of implementing the telepractice program), missed opportunities, etc. This step will provide a clear understanding of the how the program will be expected to meet the needs of clients and the organization, and these data will be a guide for developing quality improvement measures. The development team should then identify resources and barriers relevant to the program within the organization. Monetary barriers such as third-party reimbursement issues, licensure, credentialing and privileging barriers, training of clinicians, scheduling difficulties, and technology problems need to be considered. Identification of barriers and resources at the initial phase of implementation will eliminate or minimize problems that may arise during implementation of a telepractice program. Return on investment analysis will provide information about cost effectiveness of the investment. Finally, continuous quality improvement methods to evaluate the program will help sustain and improve the quality of services.

7.3   Technology and Environment

7.3.1   *Technology*

The dilemma in choosing a technological system is that technology is ever-changing. With the goal of sustainability in mind, technology must be flexible beyond the initial funding stage. Therefore, in choosing a system, decisions must be made about specific equipment, identification of types of services, and client needs before deciding on technology options [3]. Decisions must also be made concerning peripheral accessories. The entire system may be purchased from a single vendor or separately, if it results in a better quality system.

The first consideration in choosing the technology is to determine if a live interaction with a client or a review of clinical data is desired. The two modalities are as follows:

1. *Real-time* (*synchronous*): This encounter is similar to a face-to-face clinic visit. Use of this modality will require scheduling for all parties involved and allocation of space and time for both the client location and the clinician site.
2. *Store-and-forward* (*asynchronous*): Data are recorded and then sent to a supporting site for review. These data may be recorded images (e.g., a modified barium swallow or videostroboscopy) or client files.

After choosing the modality of an encounter, the place of service delivery must be determined. Clients can receive services in their homes, within a clinic, or at distant sites, such as other clinics, hospitals, or offices. Room videoconferencing and/or desktop conferencing systems are available for these applications. These decisions will determine the type of equipment needed and help in setting up the environment. The quality of service of a network is significant. Interrupted video or audio signals are not acceptable in clinical videoconferencing; therefore, input from IT personnel will assist in making informed decisions about technology for each application.

Concerns for security and privacy are of high priority when choosing telecommunication equipment. Manufacturers should be able to discuss available security features to protect client's privacy and comply with regulations.

Bandwidth refers to the data rate supported by a network connection or interface. It represents the capacity of the connection. The greater the capacity, the more the information it can carry. A low-bandwidth connection, such as a dial-up modem, may be best used for store-and-forward applications. High-bandwidth connections are preferred for real-time videoconferencing and are associated with better quality of video and smoothness of motion.

Several telecommunication networks are available. They include the following:

- POTS (plain old telephone service): POTS is synonymous with basic telephone service over the public telephone network. These connections are of low bandwidth and are available through dial-up modems.
- ISDN (integrated services digital network): ISDN Group systems in large-scale settings, such as conference rooms and classrooms, use videoconferencing over integrated services digital network (ISDN), which is an all-digital replacement for POTS. A connection is made by dialing a phone number, and then the switching equipment at the telephone company completes the call.
- IP (Internet protocol): Each device connected to Internet or Intranet has an IP address that enables systems to communicate with each other.

However, all these systems have limitations. The best strategy is to make it certain that a knowledgeable network engineer is consulted during the planning stages of development to determine which telecommunication equipment will best meet the needs identified. Each setting is different and each caseload is unique; therefore, avoid the notion of "one size fits all" while choosing a telecommunication system for telepractice.

7.3.2 Environment

Careful consideration must be given to the environment of both the client's and clinician's space to be used in a telepractice application. The environment should be set up in such a way that client comfort and ease of accessing services are maximized, and should be private and secure. Ease of access to a quiet room that is also convenient to clients with disabilities provides the best setting. This includes doorways that are wide enough for wheelchairs and rooms that are large enough to accommodate telecommunication equipment and additional staff if needed. Keep in mind the type of clients served when choosing furniture. Tables and chairs should be at comfortable levels for both children and adults.

In addition to telecommunication equipment required for transmission of the speech therapy application, other equipment should minimally include a telephone and fax machine. A computer may also be necessary during a speech therapy session. A telephone is essential if problems arise during the therapy session. A fax machine can be used to transmit therapy materials, letters, etc. A light or sign placed outside the treatment room will indicate that the room is in use and will protect the privacy of clients.

Lighting and décor are important factors to consider when planning a room designed for telepractice. Lighting on the face of clients and clinicians should be adjustable to minimize shadows on their faces. If the room has exterior windows, they should be covered with room-darkening blinds or draperies. Objects such as mirrors, artwork, plants, fans, and wallpaper with patterns should be eliminated as they may cause reduced video quality of the signal. A neutral non-white color such as light grey, blue, or beige is best for the walls.

Audio quality is another important factor to consider. If possible, room reverberation and echo should be eliminated. A IT or audio–visual (AV) person can provide advice on optimal placement of microphones to achieve the best audio quality and eliminate feedback. Camera placement is crucial for the best video image of the client and clinician. The camera image ought to display the head and shoulders of a client and clinician, and should also include the capability to zoom in and out so that others in the room can be identified or to zoom in on therapy materials.

7.4 Successful Management of a Telerehabilitation Program

7.4.1 Business Plan

Development of an appropriate business infrastructure will enhance technical and clinical aspects of a telepractice program. Goals and timelines are components of a business plan that should be developed and modified as necessary. Evaluation of progress and outcomes are critical components of a successful program. Establishment of measureable goals and timelines will allow tracking of accomplishments and identification of obstacles to success. Communication concerning performance to leadership, providers, and clients will encourage their support and participation. Therefore, an effective business plan should include:

- policies, procedures, and standards of practice (SOP);
- a memorandum of understanding (MOU) with sister facilities;
- financial goals to maximize resources;
- quality indicators;
- a marketing plan;
- a backup plan for technical difficulties.

7.4.2 Staff Preparation

Competent staff is essential and may present a challenge to the development and maintenance of a program. Clinicians must obtain education and training on all aspects of a telepractice endeavor. They must also complete credentialing and privileging when required. Licensure in the state where a client is located is required and supported by the ASHA guidelines. According to the ASHA position statement, "The use of telepractice does not remove any existing responsibilities in delivering services, including adherence to the Code of Ethics, Scope of Practice, state and federal laws (e.g., licensure, HIPAA, etc.), and ASHA policy documents on professional practices." Therefore, the quality of services delivered through telepractice must be consistent with the quality of services delivered face to face.

Organizations such as ASHA and the American Telemedicine Association (ATA) provide workshops, short courses, etc. during their annual conferences. Additionally, the ASHA Special Interest Group (SIG) #18 offers opportunities to obtain training via its continuing education publication. Local and statewide professional organizations may also offer training programs in telepractice.

Staff preparation may also include rehabilitation technicians, such as speech-language pathology aids (SLP-A), or family members to assist in the presentation of stimulus items or pictures. Staffing issues must be paired with the abilities of clients to assure a successful encounter. Thus, careful assessment must be made of a client, and identification and training of support staff as needed.

7.4.3 Marketing

Marketing is the activity, set of institutions, and processes for creating, communicating, delivering, and exchanging offerings that have value for customers, clients, partners, and society at large [1]. Marketing strategies are used to convince a clientele to use particular services or products. To do this, the first step is to identify a particular client base, and then to direct marketing strategies toward them.

A telepractice marketing plan should include the following:

- Description of telepractice services
- Identification of clients, physicians, and rehabilitation personnel who might be interested in telepractice services
- Promotion and dissemination of information about the program
- Evaluation of marketing performance

7.5 The Client Encounter

As in all other aspects of telepractice, planning and preparation of the client encounter are critical for the success of a telepractice therapy session. Client-centered care must be the goal, with results being comparable to a traditional face-to-face visit. Awareness of all facets that will affect the outcome of a session ought to be provided prior to the encounter, during the telepractice session, and after the session has ended with preparation for the next encounter.

Planning and preparation include selection of an appropriate candidate for this type of service delivery system. Client selection should include:

- evaluation of sensory deficits of a client such as vision and hearing and if the telecommunication equipment can accommodate these deficits;
- client's cognitive ability to attend and focus on a therapy task;
- client's capability to detect stimulus items presented by clinician;
- client's ability to manipulate objects during a session if appropriate.

Deficits in any of these areas may necessitate recruitment of an aide or a family member to assist in presentation of stimulus items, encouragement of the client to stay on task, or providing information to the distant clinician about the appropriateness of a response. If there is uncertainty about whether a client would be able to summon help in an emergency, then another person should always be present in the therapy room with him or her, or a way should be provided to summon help. Staff roles and responsibilities should be defined and accepted by all persons involved in a telepractice session.

Prior to a telepractice session, a process should be in place to educate and orient a client about the session, technology, and what to expect. Therapy materials may be mailed ahead of time or faxed just before a session begins. Clients should also be given the opportunity to consent to or decline telepractice services. When a client arrives, a staff person should be charged with the responsibility of greeting, checking in the client, and escorting him or her to the therapy room.

During the therapy session, a light or "do not disturb" sign outside of the treatment room door will alert others that speech therapy is in session and protect the privacy of clients. A split screen view that includes the client and clinician will allow a clinician to see what the client sees. This enables a clinician to determine if a stimulus item is in focus and within camera range for the most effective presentation. Everyone in the room at the time of the treatment session must be identified. Clinicians should look into the camera and reduce extraneous movement during a session to avoid pixilation of the image. Slow, deliberate movements work best when switching from one stimulus item to another. At the conclusion of the therapy, the clinician should wait until the client has left the treatment room and is in the company of others before disconnecting equipment.

After the therapy session is completed, a mechanism for assessing satisfaction of both the clinician and client should be used. Outcome measures taken during therapy will be beneficial in determining progress, compared to traditional face-to-face outcomes, and for assessing quality improvement. Information gathered using these methods will help plan the next telepractice session. If technical problems arose during the treatment session, trouble shooting may be necessary by technical support personnel.

7.6   Lessons Learned

The following items are "pearls of wisdom" gleaned from many years of delivering speech-language pathology services to clients at a distance. Telepractice can be a rewarding experience by enabling many individuals to have access to speech pathology services who would otherwise not be able to benefit from speech intervention.

- Planning ahead and anticipation of all possible scenarios cannot be emphasized enough.
- Telepractice should never be undertaken alone. Experts in the field of telecommunication technology and delivery of telerehabilitation services are a valuable asset.

- Cultivate a good relationship with your technical person. Success or failure may hinge on that person.
- Know what your equipment is capable of doing and be an expert on how to use it.
- Have a thorough understanding of your client's abilities and level of acceptance in using telepractice to receive services.
- Accept that there will always be individuals for whom telepractice is not well suited.
- Always have a backup plan for when things do not work.

Summary

- Telepractice describes the delivery of speech pathology services at a distance using telecommunication technology.
- The first step in developing a telepractice program includes collection of data on underserved clients, costs of providing care (including costs of implementing the telepractice program), missed opportunities, etc.
- In choosing a system for telepractice, decisions must be made about specific equipment, identification of types of services, and client needs before deciding on technology options. Concerns for security and privacy are of high priority when choosing the telecommunication equipment.
- The environment of a telepractice application should be set up in such a way that client comfort and ease of accessing services are maximized, and should be private and secure.
- Clinicians must obtain education and training on all aspects of a telepractice endeavor. Prior to a telepractice session, a process should be in place to educate and orient a client about the session, technology, and what to expect.

Abbreviations/Acronyms

ASHA	American Speech Language Hearing Association
ATA	American Telemedicine Association
AV	Audio–visual
CEU	Continuing education unit
HIPAA	Health Insurance Portability and Accountability Act of 1996
IP	Internet protocol
ISDN	Integrated services digital network
IT	Information technology
MOU	Memorandum of understanding
POTS	Plain old telephone service

SIG	Special Interest Group
SLP-A	Speech-language pathology aids
SOP	Standards of practice

References

1. American Marketing Association. Definition of marketing. 2007. Available at: http://www.marketingpower.com/AboutAMA/Pages/DefinitionofMarketing.aspx. Accessed 30 Dec 2010.
2. American Speech Language Hearing Association. Speech-language pathologists providing clinical services via telepractice: position statement. 2005. Available at: http://www.asha.org/practice/telepractice/. Accessed 30 Dec 2010.
3. Bashshur R, Shannon G. History of telemedicine. New Rochelle: Mary Ann Liebert; 2009.
4. Tindall L, Huebner R. The impact of an application telerehabilitation technology on caregiver burden. Int J Telerehabil. 2009;1(1):3–8.
5. Wilson L, Onslow M, Lincoln M. Telehealth adaptation of the lidcombe program of early stuttering intervention: five case studies. Am J Speech Lang Pathol. 2004;13:81–93.

Chapter 8
Speech Therapy Telepractice

Michael Towey

Abstract For more than 30 years, speech therapy telepractice has been recognized as an effective substitute when no therapist was available. This chapter describes a speech therapy telepractice model that can provide treatment better than traditional methods and is not restricted to patients living in areas without qualified professionals. Using web-hosted applications, telepractice can be provided securely and effectively on virtually any computer, smart phone, or tablet at low cost to the therapist and no cost to the patient. This chapter provides the information necessary to develop an effective speech telepractice program, including low-cost/no-cost telepractice video connections and digital treatment materials and use of Web 2.0 approaches to enhance treatment and competencies required for effective speech therapy telepractice.

8.1 Introduction: Our Maine Experience

Speech therapy telepractice is emerging not only as a way to provide service when none is available [2, 3, 4, 16, 21] but also as a delivery system that can produce better results than the traditional model.

What began as an attempt to provide voice therapy to a teacher in a rural area 5 years ago has become a transformative way to provide virtual face-to-face speech therapy at Waldo County General Hospital (WCGH), a 25-bed critical access hospital in Belfast, Maine. The Speech Pathology Department at WCGH includes the

M. Towey
Voice and Swallowing Center of Maine,
Waldo County General Hospital, Belfast, ME, 04915, USA
e-mail: speech@wcgh.org

S. Kumar, E.R. Cohn (eds.), *Telerehabilitation*, Health Informatics,
DOI 10.1007/978-1-4471-4198-3_8, © Springer-Verlag London 2013

Voice & Swallowing Center of Maine. Eight speech-language pathologists deliver primarily pediatric treatment in preschool and school settings. Specialized voice and swallowing services are provided to patients referred from across the state, with patients often traveling 4 h for the specialized services of the Center.

Following deliberate review, therapists at WCGH recognized that speech therapy telepractice was an opportunity to create an entirely new treatment model, not just a way to videoconference traditional tabletop speech therapy across distances.

As WCGH therapists have developed competencies and approaches using speech therapy telepractice, a new way of providing therapy has evolved using a variety of digital Web 2.0 [30] applications in virtual face-to-face speech telepractice at WCGH.

Speech therapy telepractice continuously evolves, with patients actively helping to create authentic treatment content, using videos, Internet uploads, e-mails, and smart phones, and becoming fully engaged in capturing the power of the computer and Internet as forces of communicative change.

Speech-language pathologists at WCGH organized full-day meetings to critically review treatment techniques, outcomes, and service delivery. A consensus was reached that existing treatment techniques and methods of service delivery fell far short of the expectations and needs of the twenty-first century. While all therapy outcomes and practices at WCGH are considered exemplary and representative of evidence-based practice, therapists knew that they must do much better on behalf of patients and those who pay for therapy services.

Therapists at WCGH confronted the brutal reality that speech therapy service delivery has changed little in the last 40 years. It is true that speech-language pathology had changed professional identity from speech correctionist to speech-language pathologist and benefited from a rapidly increasing knowledge base about communicative function [17]. It is also true that the way speech therapy is provided in clinics and schools is much the same model today as it was 40 years ago. The therapist sits across the table from the patient, and using print materials, attempts to have the patient practice and master speech tasks – somehow hoping the gains in therapy will "stick" and generalize to different settings. Sometimes therapists use computers in therapy, but most applications are digitalized versions of the same drill books and work sheets that are photocopied and printed.

8.1.1 Aligning Speech Therapy Telepractice with the Digital World

Teachers and parents label today's school students as bored and unmotivated. At home however, these same focus intense attention for hours on iPhones, play stations, Twitter, Facebook, and gaming. In reality, today's students do not lack attention or motivation. They are bored and uninspired by instructional materials and approaches used in schools and speech clinics that are unrelated to how they live and learn [32].

Students are instantly connected to more information than ever before in human history. Yet when students go to speech therapy, they have to sign off and power down their devices that allow them to connect to a powerful learning tool that is changing the way people think and learn [26]. When not in school, students are connected to information, entertainment, and social networking around the clock. It is no surprise that therapy patients (children and adults) are bored by the outdated, slow-moving, and dull treatment strategies still being used in speech therapy rooms and clinics across the country.

Telepractice offers the opportunity to transform speech therapy using the power of an interactive, content-rich, and motivating Web 2.0 environment that people are already using every day, in many aspects of their lives [27].

The treatment approach at WCGH captures the power of the Internet and digital capacities that reside, across all age groups, in virtually every school, clinic, and home in the United States [43, 44]. Therapy approaches at WCGH were changed to use these applications to provide the authenticity, intensity, and repetition for learning opportunities necessary to rewire the way speech therapy patients think, create, and communicate.

When utilizing interactive digital application in speech therapy telepractice, treatment is not limited by the knowledge of the speech-language pathologist or the treatment materials in the therapy file cabinet. Speech-language pathologists can help patients access an array of communication experiences and learning with well-designed speech therapy telepractice.

At WCGH, therapists are learning how not to limit patient progress because of therapists' limitations in professional training and knowledge. Therapists are learning how to get patients more connected to produce multiple opportunities for communicative learning, across multiple cycles of interaction throughout the day, using computers, smart phones, virtual learning, and digital therapy treatment.

8.1.1.1 Crossing over the Digital Bridge

There are societal concerns about the thousands of hours spent playing video games; sending/receiving hundreds of thousands of text messages, tweets, and e-mails; and on cell phones by today's digital users, many as young as 3 years old. Personal judgments about these changes should not limit professional understanding of how technological connectivity has changed society and the way speech therapy patients live, learn, and process information when using their digital gadgets [36, 43].

Effective use of technology in speech therapy telepractice allows patients to engage actively in sharing information in multiple formats, communicating through video, text, Facebook, and smart phones.

Five years ago, speech-language pathologists at WCGH learned that they were using techniques and approaches from the last century, and did not understand new technologies or even how to speak the language associated with them.

Speech-language pathologists at WCGH have begun to cross over the digital bridge, understanding that today's patients who are moving at twitch speed are

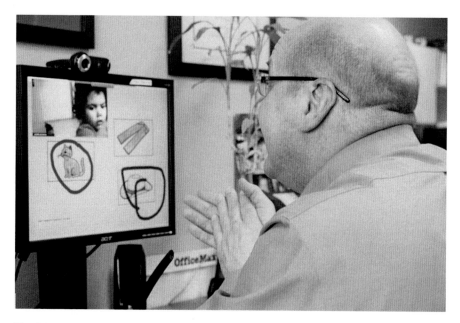

Fig. 8.1 A 4-year-old child engages with the therapist by following directions using an electronic crayon in a speech telepractice session

limited by speech therapy approaches based on how fast picture cards can be flipped in a game of Go-Fish.

Everyone has been challenged trying to program a TiVo or a smart phone and surprised that a digitally literate 10-year-old can do it without even reading the instructions. People today are using a new digital language and interacting in ways barely imagined 10 years ago.

As immigrants to the new digital world, speech-language pathologists are learning a new language and vocabulary that includes avatars, alternate realities, search technologies, supported literacy, 3D modeling, LAN parties, cloud computing, virtual reality, folksonomy, mashups, and Wikis. This new language is all available to be used and applied in speech therapy telepractice.

Speech-language pathologists may not have acquired the new digital language, but increasingly speech therapy patients are using this language in school, at work, and to maintain social relationships. Speech-language pathologists must learn to surf the crest of this digital tsunami to be the initiators of change in delivering speech therapy telepractice [15].

Speech therapy telepractice can provide the tools and skills, enabling patients to go far beyond therapist's clinical skills, knowledge, and drill cards, to succeed in a world that increasingly demands an array of communication and digital literacy skills. When connected on the Internet, patients can talk to friends, socialize, find entertainment, make purchases, and look things up, creating wonderful opportunities for therapists to develop treatment approaches (Fig. 8.1).

It is exciting to think about the power of cell phones, readily available across all ages. These are powerful and inexpensive communication devices integrated with cameras, video, Internet, and easy-to-download content; open to both external and internal input; and perfect for developing speech therapy telepractice applications in a way that makes communicative change inevitable.

What has been holding our profession back? We have been held back by our lack of imagination to use these devices to create new ways to engage speech therapy patients in meaningful activities.

At WCGH, the therapy task has become one of directing patients to multiple learning opportunities throughout their day. Clinicians help patients identify and filter content that targets specific communicative behaviors with varied content and contexts through daily living and learning activities.

Speech therapy telepractice allows therapists to be programmers for therapy patients and to guide patients to create their own content with videos, digital pictures, social interactions, video calling, and blogs in intrinsically motivating activities. Speech therapy telepractice immerses patients into a fully engaged experience and helps create autonomous learners, fully capable of navigating the digital learning world.

The future holds boundless opportunities for communicatively disordered individuals through speech therapy telepractice. It is entirely possible that speech therapy telepractice can improve speech therapy treatment dramatically and have children become literate and even reading before they enter school.

The remainder of this chapter describes the essential tools and vital clinical behaviors necessary to cross over the bridge into the speech therapy telepractice world.

8.2 New Patients—New Methods

Speech therapy telepractice should not be just an extension of traditional speech therapy by a "video conference." Speech therapy telepractice, applied by well-trained clinicians, provides a transformative effect on service delivery and treatment outcomes.

It is unnecessary to seek funding for expensive "telemedicine videoconferencing" systems linking one facility to another over dedicated connections. These systems are expensive, and limit the full array of digital treatments available and where service can be provided. These systems were designed for highly specialized medical or group meeting purposes.

The influence of digital experiences has fundamentally changed the way in which children and adults think and process information more than ever before [31]. Today's patients are no longer the same patients for whom traditional speech therapy was designed.

Speech telepractice is a new way to delivery treatment, requiring training and competencies in digital clinical skills, development of digital treatment materials, deep understanding of today's learners, and preparation for virtual therapy sessions.

The advantages of speech telepractice and associated supportive technology fit well with the continued emergence of computers and the Internet as a powerful force of social change, creating new learning methodology essential for today's new learners [8, 33].

Speech telepractice "costs" people less to get service, in technology expense, and in time spent traveling. Geography or physical limitations are no longer barriers to treatment. For patients who must get services at home, telepractice provides a less intrusive method of service delivery than admitting strangers into the privacy of a home for "home visits."

Speech-language pathologists at WCGH have been providing speech telepractice for almost 5 years.

At WCGH, treatment was first provided for a patient with Parkinson's disease and then expanded by carefully selecting patients for speech therapy telepractice. The present level of speech therapy telepractice service at WCGH includes five telepractice-trained speech-language pathologists providing speech telepractice 6 days a week. The caseload composition is as diverse as expected in any speech clinic: preschool and school-age children and adults with an array of disorders.

A broad array of technological skills, competencies, and digital treatment materials has been developed to support the delivery of speech therapy telepractice. The WCGH telepractice treatment model is now beginning to document outcomes to support speech therapy telepractice as a primary service delivery model that is as good as or better than the traditional "across the table" model [14].

A few patients and caregivers have initially been hesitant about how effective speech telepractice would be. The parent of a 3-year-old child from a remote area near the Canadian border made the following comments after receiving speech therapy telepractice:

> We were waiting a long time to get into face to face speech therapy. In the back of my mind I knew the computer was available. I just didn't think it was going to work. So I tried it and I think my child benefitted more from the computer sessions...It's almost like you're still doing one on one face to face...everything is still the same. I love it!

8.3 Speech Teletherapy Advantages

The obvious advantages of services when none are available have been the primary focus describing the advantages of speech therapy telepractice. According to the American Speech Language Hearing Association, "telepractice *may be used* (emphasis added) to overcome barriers of access to services caused by distance, unavailability of specialists and/or subspecialists, and impaired mobility" [3].

At WCGH, speech therapy telepractice offers an entirely new treatment model approach not available in traditional speech therapy.

Speech therapy telepractice delivers service directly to where patients live and learn, and the digital capacity co-occurring with telepractice allows for the creation of a therapy "cloud" influencing patient progress throughout the day.

Speech therapy telepractice is more immediate and focused than traditional therapy. Treatment takes place in the small, focused space of the video screen.

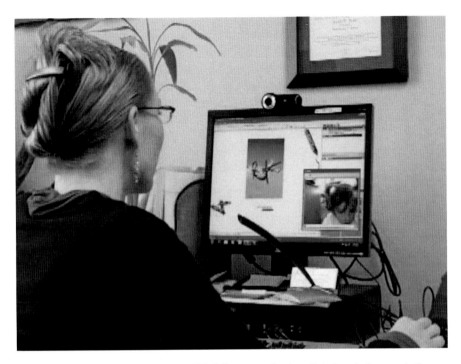

Fig. 8.2 Therapist and a 4-year-old child fully engaged using digital tools in speech therapy telepractice

Speech telepractice is an entirely different experience for both the therapist and the patient.

Communicatively disordered patients live, socialize, learn, and work in a digital age that continues to change society [8]. This increasingly is the experience and expectation patients bring to speech therapy.

Today, therapists at WCGH find it boring to deliver speech therapy using picture cards placed on a table or give photocopied "practice materials" when exciting, interactive digital materials are readily available.

The therapist's role has changed from being the "sage on stage" and main focus of the patient–therapist interaction, to one of directing treatment across a range of different contexts and settings to influence the daily environment and support communicative change [11].

Today's digital age allows for customization of therapy materials to create high interest among patients, personal treatment objectives intrinsically interesting to the patient, and a desirable level of difficulty to assure patient progress and learning [40].

In Fig. 8.2, notice how engaged and focused the 4-year-old child is as she works on comprehension and maneuvers a digital crayon on screen.

Speech telepractice allows for the delivery of services, using an array of easily accessible technologies that can serve as a force multiplier for the speech-language pathologist.

Effective use of available technologies creates opportunities to support speech telepractice in an array of applications. Speech therapy telepractice sessions can be recorded, edited, and stored online, for anytime/anywhere access by patients and caregivers on home computers or smart phones.

The types of therapy delivered by telemedicine are broad, with innovations in technology and competencies allowing for greater service delivery across age groups and disorders. The broader application and use of telepractice make it a legitimate therapy tool just like any other treatment modality [7].

8.3.1 Telepractice Treatment Efficacies

In very early phases of telepractice, use of telephone, filmstrips, and other supplemental materials were reported to be used to reach patients in rural areas. This approach, called "telecommunicology," was delivered through the Birmingham VA Hospital 35 years ago [39].

Continued successful application of speech telepractice was described 15 years ago, using a NASA advanced communications satellite connection between several states. These early results demonstrated reliable evaluation data and good patient satisfaction using telemedicine [18].

Almost a decade later, 11,000 speech "teletherapy" sessions were successfully provided in Oklahoma public schools with very favorable results [19].

Other published articles identify the use of telepractice in management of stroke [9], in delivery of research-based speech therapy to Parkinson's patients [37], in audiology [20, 24], in the reliability of speech telepractice assessment [41, 42], and in gaining reimbursement for speech telepractice [38].

An ongoing 3-year pilot project in Ohio public schools reports that children make equal progress in therapy with telepractice as in the traditional manner, with students and parents being very pleased with telepractice [29].

Overall, parents/caregivers, teachers, and administrators appeared to find telepractice a satisfactory service delivery model for school-based speech-language therapy [13].

8.4 Getting Started in Speech Telepractice

Speech telemedicine can be provided at a very low cost using existing web-based technology and available computers. Early speech therapy telepractice used expensive video conference systems to deliver traditional therapy across a distance. Today, the rapid advancements in web-based technologies, low-cost, high-quality audio/video, and improved broadband have created a whole new service delivery model.

Now, the therapist and patient only require to have a computer with a high-speed Internet connection, a web cam/microphone, speakers, and a secure web telepractice host. Most computers available today are fully capable of supporting effective telepractice service delivery right out of the box.

8.4.1 Technology Requirements

1. Computer: A computer with adequate processing speed is required. Most computers purchased within the last several years are adequate. If a computer can play video and music, there is adequate capacity.

   Tip: Check the computer speed to assure a download speed of 1 Mbps. Generally, if the upload/download speed is 1–1.5 Mbps, there is adequate capacity.

   Hint: To check computer connection speeds, Google search "computer speed check." There are several free sites that give a good evaluation of connection speed.

2. Web camera/microphone: Many models of web camera/microphone are available online and in retail stores. Web cameras (cams) provide high-quality imaging at a very little cost. Many laptops have a web cam built in, most with microphones and speakers.

3. Connecting: A reliable, high-speed Internet connection is required. Most of the currently available high-speed connections in homes, clinics, and schools are adequate. It is also important that the telepractice connection operates across different systems (Mac and PC) and interface with existing network firewalls and other security measures [34].

   Tip: If connecting on a networked computer in a school or hospital, check with the information systems technician about settings and connecting permissions.

4. Connecting therapist to patient: Therapists must find and select an online web host to make the connection between the therapist and the patient possible. Connection is similar to video conferencing, with many critical clinical differences.

   Tip: Online video connecting: A number of low-cost, flexible web-hosting applications are readily available, including Adobe Connect [1], WEBEX [12], and applications that integrate electronic medical records [23]. These systems are web based. This means that the program and connections do not "live" on a local computer. The therapist does not make any investment in expensive hardware or special programs. The telepractice can be done from any computer, smart phone, or tablet from anywhere.

   Tip: Most vendors allow free trials for 2 weeks to 1 month. Insist on a free trial. Be sure to try out technical support and any online tutorials during the trial period. If the system is not easy to use during the trial period, it will not get any easier when you sign the contract.

   Hint: Security/confidentiality: All online vendors are not the same. Make sure that the system you use is encrypted. Ask the vendor for their security standards.

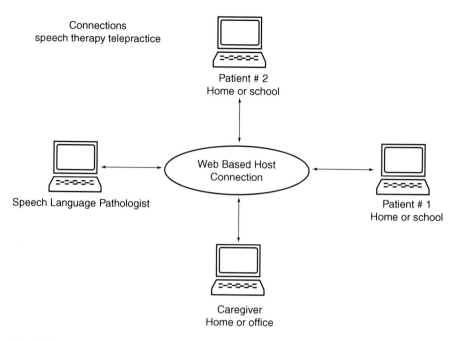

Fig. 8.3 Low-cost, high-quality, web-based speech telepractice connections

This is very important to meet legal and ethical standards for patient confidentiality. When connecting online, the therapist and patient are connecting through a web-based "server." This server encrypts therapy information for security. These connections are safe and secure, and can be password protected.

Hint: Look for a vendor with (a) dedicated security department, including a GIAC-certified forensic analyst; (b) restricted site access (the therapist controls who can access the telepractice site); (c) the ability to require all therapy sessions to have a password; and (d) an encrypted connection using the 128-bit SSL encryption standard.

Hint: HIPAA and FERPA standards would be met if the online web host meets the security features described here. To be sure, check with the compliance person in your work setting.

Hint: Look for WebTrust certification.

Hint: Some vendors offer a price reduction if the account is paid in advance.

Tip: Choose a web host that allows several people to be connected with each other at the same time from different locations for group therapy, teaming, and collaboration. Fig. 8.3 illustrates a schematic of how these multiple connections might look.

Figure 8.3 illustrates a web-based telepractice connection. The therapist e-mails the connection information, and the patient and selected others can connect and join the session. There is no equipment/hardware to buy, no special software to purchase, and no connection cost for the patient.

Hint: Any system selected should cost no more than a few hundred dollars for the vendor to set up and customize the therapists' telepractice page. Monthly fees should be no more than $50–75 per month for unlimited usage.

Hint: Choose voice-over Internet protocol (VOiP) for audio connections. Some systems have separate video and audio connections and allow users to choose audio connection by phone or VOiP. VOiP costs much less than audio by phone, usually a few cents a minute.

Hint: Choose a system capable of easy expansion, so that other therapists can be added at little additional cost. Adding another user to an existing account should be as easy as one phone call to the customer service department of the vendor.

Some additional, must-have requirements for successful telepractice are as follows:

1. Web cam: Web cams provide high-quality imaging for very little money, usually less than $50. Many laptops have web cams built in.

   Tip: Having a separate web cam makes it easier to move the camera. High-definition web cams are now available at very low cost (less than $75), but one should be careful while purchasing one. These require high-speed broadband connections and may slow down connection speeds. Some online vendors already use high-definition connections and a standard good-quality web cam with very good video quality.

2. Store-forward therapy: This allows for recording all or part of any treatment session. The recording is stored on a secure web location. An e-mail or Internet link to the recording is sent to the patient and other caregivers for practice and review. This is a very helpful feature for patients, families, and caregivers to review and practice therapy activities. For patients, this allows access to multiple treatment times during the day in different locations and situations (home, school, rehab setting, etc.).

   Tip: Recording should be in easy-to-use formats and should allow choice of recording formats, such as WMV, FLV, and MP4. Avoid any vendor without a recording function or one that offers recording in difficult-to-manage formats such as ARF or AVI.

   Hint: Recording must be simultaneous for patient, therapist, and the therapy materials being used onscreen. Some systems may record only the onscreen document but do not record audio or video streaming of patient and therapist.

   Hint: Using FLV or MP4 recording formats allows the therapy session to be downloaded onto the patient's smart phone, iTouch, iPad, or similar device for easy access and practice throughout the day. This is very helpful to increase practice opportunities or provide instructions and reminders to patients about managing their communication disorder.

3. Online functionality: The telepractice system selected should have (a) a whiteboard function, allowing therapist and patient choice to write and draw; (b) the ability to have multiple documents/therapy materials available at the same time; (c) the ability to go to full-size screen with materials easily; and (d) the ability to resize video images of therapist and patient.

   Tip: A desirable feature is the function that allows the therapist to give the patient control of the screen (shared host) to allow for independent writing, marking responses, and following directions.

4. Privacy screen: Place a backdrop behind the therapist when providing speech telepractice. This eliminates background distractions, creates privacy, and gives

a much more professional presentation. Privacy screens are commonly found in health-care settings.

Tip: Privacy screens can be bought online or can be easily made with a frame draped with a blue-colored muslin sheet to create a neutral background.

5. Ease of patient connection: Typically, when the therapist schedules a speech tele-therapy session, the patient receives an e-mail, with a link to the session. The patient "clicks" the link and is connected to the speech telepractice session. When con-nected, the patient typically clicks "join session" to start the speech teletherapy.

Tip: Patients connecting for the first time may need a bit of coaching with audio or video settings. Most of the time, connection is very intuitive. The thera-pist must know how to adjust audio and video setting to help the patient.

Hint: To provide clear instructions for patients, make digital instructions. Use screen shots of each part of the connection process. To take a screen shot, select/ print scr/or/print screen/on the keyboard, and then paste into a document or a PowerPoint slide. Label each of the steps and then e-mail the document to the patient. This works very well and patients appreciate the help.

Hint: Schedule a brief practice connection with the patient prior to the date of the therapy session. This only takes a couple of minutes and helps orient the patient and caregivers to the format of the telepractice session.

6. Improving audio quality: For most speech telepractice sessions, the built-in microphone will be adequate. To improve audio quality, open the computer con-trol panel and go to audio or sound settings. The microphone and sound settings can be adjusted for the best audio quality. Have the patient do the same thing. Place the microphone close to the therapist and instruct the patient to place it close to their mouth. In some telepractice systems, when connecting, an auto-matic audio adjustment will "pop up" for step-by-step configuration.

Tip: Desktop computers typically do not have in-built microphones, speakers, or cameras. These must be purchased and added to the computer. Purchase a microphone that connects through a USB port, for ease of connection. Laptop computers, smart phones, and tablets are typically well configured with camera/ microphone and speakers.

Hint: To improve audio quality, add a microphone that connects though a USB. Place it close to the mouth of the therapist and the patient.

Hint: For highest-quality audio, the patient can use a headset with a micro-phone. This is most helpful when speech articulation or voice must be heard clearly. A good-quality headset/microphone can be purchased at most retail stores for less than $10.

Hint: A separate set of external speakers, plugged into the computer, improves sound quality and makes listening easier for both therapist and patient. The increased audio boost from external speakers may be very helpful for patients with hearing impairments.

7. Looking good online: Be sure to have adequate facial lighting during speech telepractice. If the light is behind the therapist, the therapist's image will be washed out and create a distraction, making it difficult for the patient to pay attention.

Tip: Adjust the camera to zoom in to create a "head/shoulder shot." If the zoom is too far out, the therapist will look very distant. Good close-up images of both the therapist and the patient create a real sense of closeness and joint attention.

Hint: Properly applied makeup and lip gloss will help avoid the harsh look the camera and lighting may create.

8.4.1.1 Speech Therapy Telepractice Materials

Speech therapy telepractice requires a high degree of planning, anticipation of materials needed through the entire session, and availability of digital therapy materials.

Clinicians must have very strong clinical skills in identifying the vital behaviors to target therapeutically and how to make those targets memorable and "sticky" for the patient and eHelpers [22].

Developing a library of digital therapy materials can be more effective than materials typically used in "tabletop" speech therapy. Digital materials allow for a wide array of speech and language stimulation that is authentic and motivating for patients.

Experienced therapists know that a few core materials chosen carefully can serve to provide a range of treatment options as the therapist differentiates application of materials based on patient need.

Therapists can quickly develop an extensive selection of readily available therapy materials that can be accessed during the speech telepractice session with a "click."

1. Web-based materials: The best starting point for web-based materials, to be accessed and used in telepractice sessions, is found on the website of Judith Maginnis Kuster [25].

   Examples of materials that can be adapted for therapy is a collection by Kuster [25] that has dozens of links to treatment materials for all disorders. This site is regularly updated and is a valuable starting place.

   Tip: Most of these materials can be used if the selected telepractice system allows sharing of web content on the therapist's desktop.

   Hint: When selecting online web-based material, interactive features, including animation and audio, are often part of the program. This is desirable because it creates multimedia material for use. However, in a therapy session, the therapist will need to control these features. Look for program that allows the therapist to pause the program or that automatically pauses as the patient makes a response (either verbally or using the digital cursor).

   Material that can be printed, e-mailed, or recorded for later use by the patient is very helpful.
2. Using Microsoft PowerPoint (PPT) to create authentic digital materials: This program is the backbone for developing speech telepractice material at WCGH.

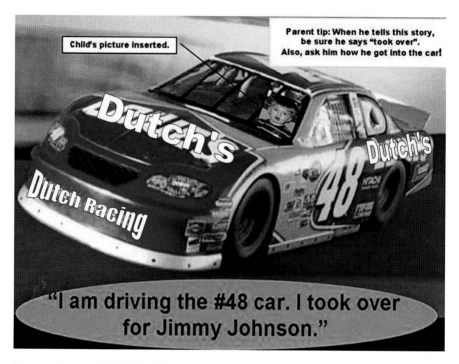

Fig. 8.4 Custom digital PPT teletherapy materials recorded for practice in multiple settings

Therapists at WCGH make extensive use of powerful PPT features to add custom photos and insert open-source images found on the Internet to create high-interest stimulation materials.

Tip: PPT easily allows adding of text for practice in therapy sessions as well as patient repetition later on. Especially helpful is the use of text boxes to let caregivers know exactly what to target.

In Fig. 8.4, the PPT slide has been customized with a caregiver reminder. The child's photo has been placed in the race car and his utterance is inserted on the slide, with the child's recorded narration. Correct language models and a complete therapy session were created using successive custom slides. The session was recorded and the child's family could access the entire session online, for repeated practice. This creates opportunities for the therapy to be continued, even when the therapist is not there!

Hint: Produce custom patient and therapist recorded narration. On the PPT toolbar find/Slide Show-Record Narration/. Produce custom narration on as many slides as desired and match the narration with the text. Produce the custom narration and text to target specific speech therapy objectives. Then the material is saved. The entire PPT can be e-mailed or uploaded to the patient to work on before the next treatment session (including narrated speech models).

Hint: Upload the PPT to an online site such as YouTube, send to smart phones or tablets, or use in subsequent speech telepractice sessions. Using the narration feature allows both the therapist and the patient to record therapy targets for multiple practice opportunities.

Hint: When recording/saving to make a home DVD, use the PPT feature File/Package for CD. This allows the material to play on any computer, even if PowerPoint is not installed.

3. Authentic materials - pictures: Utilize the easy accessibility of capturing pictures on smart phones, tablets, and digital cameras. Both therapists and family members can take pictures of authentic objects, people, locations, and events. Most cameras allow easy uploading of images. These images can also be e-mailed to the therapist before the speech telepractice session. It is easy and fast to copy and paste the photos into PowerPoint, add text, and have highly stimulating materials readily available for speech telepractice sessions.

4. Authentic materials - video: Patients/caregivers can make videos of their interactions with patients. Smart phones and tablets have very good video capabilities. Short videos can be quickly e-mailed or uploaded to an online site. Upload the video to a private YouTube channel or online service like yousendit.com. These videos can be especially helpful monitoring home activities including swallowing/feeding, giving feedback to caregivers for coaching purposes, and developing follow-up activities.

Tip: An easy-to-operate document scanner is important in building a good library of therapy materials. A document scanner can convert paper materials to digital very easily. Choose a mid-quality scanner, like the Epson WorkForce GT-1500, costing around $250. A scanner like this is a workhorse, converting paper materials, pictures and drawings to color or b/w digital formats. It has easy desktop settings for converting and storing materials.

Hint: Uploading to YouTube can be safe and private. Register for a YouTube channel. It is free. The settings allow the therapist to restrict access to video to only those identified by the therapist. Other online sites like yousendnit.com have similar services for free and may charge a fee for large file uploads. The advantage of these sites is that the video is easier to download and store than YouTube video.

8.5 eHelpers

An eHelper is anyone who assists the patient during the speech therapy telepractice session. eHelpers might be a caregiver, family member, nurse, or teacher.

A speech therapy teletherapy model can focus on coaching the eHelper to follow through with treatment in a variety of contexts. For example, the eHelper can help display assessment materials or can communicate to others how to access online recorded treatment materials.

eHelpers are not passive observers, but are actively involved in helping mediate the session, learning treatment techniques, and developing a sense of independence of their abilities to continue with therapy carryover activities embedded in authentic activities throughout the day.

8.6   Speech Therapy Telepractice Competencies

At WCGH, training and assessment of clinical competencies for both speech-language pathologists and eHelpers are at the core of treatment success.

The effectiveness of speech therapy telepractice is not the technology. The single most important predicative factor of therapy success is the skill of the therapist [28].

Therapists who fail to acquire training in the minimum competencies required for speech therapy telepractice risk tainting the credibility of this emerging service delivery model and make it indistinguishable from an online video chat.

The effectiveness of therapy outcomes depends on the skill of the therapist in the clinical application of effective digital therapy material and in motivating the patient for change.

The minimal competencies for quality speech therapy telepractice [14] are listed in Tables 8.1, 8.2, 8.3, 8.4, 8.5, 8.6, and 8.7.

Table 8.1 Competencies for eHelpers: eHelper technical skills

Set up a schedule that provides an optimal and consistent time for the patient to offer best responses	Troubleshoot basic audio and video difficulties
Can access e-mail and Internet to locate the links and online connections for the telepractice session	Help patient access web-based therapy tools (highlighter, pointer, text tools, color palette, and documents)
Can establish the video and audio connection for the teletherapy session on the local computer	Provide feedback about quality of video, audio, materials being displayed, adjusting camera angles, and redirecting the patient when required

Table 8.2 eHelper instructional skills

Establish an adequate therapy environment for the patient, including positioning for privacy	Utilize e-mail, texting, and direct communication with other involved personnel, families, and caregivers about any pertinent updates before or after treatment sessions
Establish proper seating for the patient, allowing access to the computer, and establish appropriate lighting for video transmission of patient image	Understand therapeutic strategies, and provide timely cueing and strategies to help the patient become independent in responding to the teletherapy therapist
Attend solely to the patient's needs during teletherapy sessions, with no other job requirements (supervising or monitoring others)	Provide accurate feedback about patient response to materials, restate the patient's utterance if needed for clarification, and provide statements that will aid in completing tasks
Help patients transition from an existing activity to the area for telepractice, allowing them time to become comfortable and be ready for telepractice session	Provide feedback and restate expectations for behavior to patient at appropriate times during the session
Become aware of the patient's strengths and needs, acquire a basic understanding of the patient's communication needs, and have knowledge of the treatment goals	Assure privacy and confidentiality of the patient

Table 8.3 Competencies for speech-language pathologists therapy: technical skills

Can e-schedule appointments and send e-mail confirmation to eHelper	Demonstrate skills using text tools within a lesson
Can e-schedule recurring appointments and adjust e-mail confirmations to match the need of the eHelper	Demonstrate skills using pointer and electronic pen/crayon tool
Can create digital materials for use in a teletherapy session	Demonstrate skills using eraser tools within a lesson
Can locate, open, and load materials for use prior to a teletherapy session	Demonstrate skills passing the presenter role to the patient
Demonstrate the ability to record sessions or parts of a session	Demonstrate skills retrieving presenter role from the patient
Demonstrate the ability to store recorded sessions and provide patients or caregivers with links to the recording	Demonstrate skills adjusting video quality of image
Demonstrate skills in sharing whiteboard with patient	Demonstrate ability to password protect the meetings
Demonstrate skills in sharing desktop with patient	Demonstrate ability to manage accounts, personal settings, and privacy controls in online telepractice application
Demonstrate skills in sharing documents with patient	Demonstrate skills managing the desktop to provide optimum video for the patient
Demonstrate skills in sharing web content with patient	Demonstrate skills ending a session by saving documents and recordings
Demonstrate skills in sharing applications with patient	Demonstrate skills selectively using chat instant messages to the eHelper
Demonstrate skills in using highlighter tools within a lesson	Can demonstrate cross-platform skill in providing teletherapy using Mac and PC operating systems

Table 8.4 Connecting and digital management

Solve problems on local computer and with video at distant sites	Assure privacy and confidentiality of services through careful location and screening of computer
Solve problems on local computer and with audio at distant sites	Provide eHelper with guidelines to assure privacy and confidentiality of services of each patient
Solve problems related to the location of local computer and maximize optimal image lighting at distant sites	Establish a schedule mutually helpful to and agreed upon by the eHelper and the patient
Solve problems related to the location of local computer and reduce distractibility and background noise at distant sites	

Table 8.5 Interpersonal skills

Develop rapport quickly within a teletherapy session to engage each patient	State expectations of role of a therapist in the therapy process
Establish a relationship to coach the eHelper in providing support in the therapy process	State expectations of an eHelper within the therapy process

Table 8.6 Therapeutic skills

Support repetition and deliberate practice of vital target behaviors within teletherapy sessions	Demonstrate coaching skills in working with caregivers and eHelpers, including developmental feedback, removing obstacles, creating sense of success to build change, and creating coalitions to support patient goals
Demonstrate flexibility in adjusting preplanned lesson to meet a current need within a teletherapy session	Clinicians demonstrate adequate documentation of services, written daily notes, and progress reports
Can identify which patients could benefit from teletherapy services	Clinicians use strategies to aid e-learner with transitions
Document the need and rationale for providing teletherapy services to each patient	Clinicians use appropriate vocal loudness and animation to match the need of the client within each session
Provide opportunities for caregivers and others staff to observe and join teletherapy sessions though shared online connection	Demonstrate skill in Internet search and custom use of video/photo capture (digital cameras, smart phones), uploading, file conversion, editing, presentation applications, screen capture software, and electric scanning materials in developing and making theory materials and programs of store-forward therapy

Table 8.7 Regulatory knowledge

Clinicians understand scope of practice and comply with all requirements of ASHA within the delivery of services	Demonstrate knowledge of specialized billing codes and practices for teletherapy services with state and federal regulatory agencies and commercial insurance companies
Understand copyright and intellectual property laws when creating and using digital therapy materials	Demonstrate understanding of licensing laws affecting speech therapy telepractice, across state and international boundaries

8.6.1 Telepractice Outcomes and Attitudes: Better Than Expected

Speech telepractice at WCGH has produced encouraging and surprising results in a small cohort (N10) of preschool language-disordered children (ages 3–5 years) receiving telepractice in a rural area in Maine. All the children were diagnosed with moderate-to-severe disorders, two are diagnosed with autism, and all had been without services from 6 months to more than a year.

Results reported in Fig. 8.5 identify children receiving speech telepractice to be progressing faster and achieving greater gains than children seen in a more traditional model.

These data report outcomes for children with similar disorders and demographic backgrounds, with service delivery by the same therapists delivering both the speech telepractice and more traditional onsite treatment to different groups of children [14].

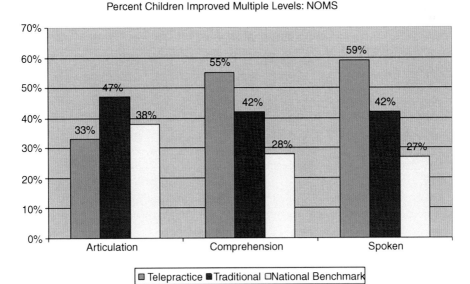

Fig. 8.5 Children receiving speech therapy telepractice compared to traditional model

These outcomes are compared to results reported by other similar faculties nationwide on the National Outcomes Measurement Survey (NOMS) [5, 6].

These data were collected using the NOMS Functional Communication Measures (FCMs) and report multiple levels of improvement for children when compared to local and national benchmarks. The reported children are diagnosed with language and articulation disorders. Speech therapy treatment is targeted primarily at language and literacy skills, with secondary focus on speech articulation.

Data related to changes in functional communication levels from time of therapy admission to date of therapy discharge for the speech telepractice children (average time in treatment 6.7 months) were compared with that of all children (N53) with similar disorders undergoing traditional therapy at Waldo County General Hospital for a year, and also compared with other similar reporting facilities nationwide.

The FCMs are a series of seven-point rating scales, ranging from (1) least functional to (7) most functional levels, developed to describe different levels of speech and language function.

Therapists have provided speech telepractice service to children located in a rural area of Maine for an average of 6.7 months. Services are provided for 30 min, two times a week, utilizing an eHelper in the child's preschool setting. Progress is measured using the FCMs.

These results demonstrate that this cohort of children is progressing better than would be expected, even if seen by the same therapists at WCGH or at their preschools. Child progress in this period exceeds national benchmarks measured by NOMS.

8.6.1.1   eHelpers: Attitudes of Supportive Personnel

The eHelpers in three remote locations were surveyed to identify any changes in their approach or attitude since starting to provide assistance with speech telemedicine.

At the start, 100 % were "not sure or were very apprehensive" about "telepractice being successful." Most (83.4 %) reported being "uncomfortable or very uncomfortable" in setting up a teletherapy session.

When recently resurveyed, 100 % report being comfortable in setting up a teletherapy session.

All the respondents report speech teletherapy being effective, with 50 % rating it "highly effective."

In rating the effectiveness of teletherapy in helping classroom follow-up, 100 % of the eHelpers were using the treatment strategies regularly and were continuing to learn new strategies each week.

Of all, 66.7 % rated the quality of the video/audio telepractice connection as very good and 33.3 % as excellent.

In total, 83.3 % of the eHelpers would "highly encourage" other students receive teletherapy services.

Several factors may have influenced this promising application of speech therapy telepractice with preschool children.

The influencers appear to be:

- the application of a strongly emerged teacher–parent coaching model;
- improved therapy engagement and learning of digital natives with computer technology;
- more authentic digital materials than typical speech therapy pictures on a table;
- therapist's ability to digitally customize treatment materials for authentic therapy;
- the active and required involvement of eHelpers in assisting the children in the speech therapy sessions;
- the ability of parents and other caregivers to participate by joining online sessions from other locations;
- parent/teacher/child access to store-forward therapy treatment sessions and supportive digitized treatment materials.

Summary

- Speech therapy telepractice requires very little cost and no investment in specialized hardware or software programs, and can be delivered virtually anywhere patients live, work, and learn.
- Telepractice has emerged as a credible service delivery method, with many early adopters from around the world reporting good patient success and satisfaction.

- It is not difficult to envision that speech therapy telepractice will disrupt current service delivery methods and expand rapidly from the fringes of rural service delivery to a preferred method of speech therapy delivery [10, 11].
- Speech therapy telepractice costs less and is convenient, accessible, and emerging as a treatment model better than traditional speech therapy.

Abbreviations/Acronyms

ARF	WebEx Advanced Recording Format
ASHA	American Speech-Language-Hearing Association
AVI	Audio Video Interleaved
FCM	Functional Communication Measure
FERPA	Family educational Rights and Privacy Act
FLV	Flash Video File
GIAC	Global Information Assurance Certification
HIPAA	Health Insurance Portability and Accountability Act
NOMS	National Outcomes Measurement Survey
PPT	Microsoft PowerPoint
SSL	Secure Sockets Layer
VOiP	Voice-over Internet protocol
WCGH	Waldo County General Hospital
WMV	Windows Media Video

References

1. Adobe Connect. 2011. Available at: http://www.adobe.com/products/adobeconnect.html. Accessed 1 Jan 2011.
2. American Speech-Language-Hearing Association. Survey of telepractice use among audiologists and speech-language pathologists. Rockville: American Speech-Language-Hearing Association; 2002.
3. American Speech-Language-Hearing Association. Speech-language pathologists providing clinical services via telepractice: position statement. 2005. Available at: http://www.asha.org/docs/html/PS2005-00116.html. Accessed 29 Jan 2011.
4. American Speech-Language-Hearing Association. Schools survey report: workforce and work conditions trends 2000–2008. Rockville: American Speech-Language-Hearing Association; 2008.
5. American Speech-Language-Hearing Association. National outcomes measurement system (NOMS). 2011. Available at: http://www.asha.org/members/research/NOMS/. Accessed 29 Jan 2011
6. American Speech-Language-Hearing Association. Articles about telepractice for speech language pathology and audiology. 2011. Available at: http://www.asha.org/practice/telepractice/TelepracticeReferences.htm. Accessed 5 Feb 2011.
7. American Telemedicine Association. A blueprint for telerehabilitation guidelines. 2010. Available at: http://www.americantelemed.org/files/public/standards/ATA%20Telerehab%20Guidelines%20v1%20(2).pdf. Accessed 19 Dec 2010.

8. Anderson J, Rainie L. The future of social relations. Pew Internet and Family Life Project. 2010. Available at: http://pewinternet.org/Reports/2010/The-future-of-social-relations/Overview/Overview-of-responses.aspx. Accessed 1 Jan 2011.

9. Baron C, Hatfield B, Georgeadis A. Management of communication disorders using family member input, group treatment, and telerehabilitation. Top Stroke Rehabil. 2005;12(2):49–56.

10. Christensen C. The innovator's dilemma: the revolutionary book that will change the way you do business. New York: Harper; 2003.

11. Christensen C, Johnson C, Horn M. Disrupting class: how disruptive innovation will change the way the world learns. New York: McGraw Hill; 2008.

12. Cisco. WEBEX conferencing. 2011. Available at: http://www.webex.com/lpintl/us/sem/sem-together.html?CPM=KNC-sem&TrackID=1021381&semid=sWYmpndQV_4560000266. Accessed 6 Feb 2011.

13. Crutchley S, Campbell M. Telespeech therapy pilot project: stakeholder satisfaction. Int J Telerehabil. 2010;2:23–30. doi:10.5195/ijt.%Y.6049.

14. Curtis N, Whitcomb J, Wilbur J. Speech telepractice outcomes in northern Maine, Waldo County General Hospital (unpublished). 2011.

15. Denham C. The no outcome-no income tsunami is here: are you a surfer, swimmer or sinker. J Patient Saf. 2009;5(1):42–52. doi:10.1097/PTS.0b013e31819b0fbb.

16. Denton D. Ethical and legal issues related to telepractice. Semin Speech Lang. 2003;24(4):313–22.

17. Duchan J. Getting here: a short history of speech pathology in America. 2010. Available at: http://www.acsu.buffalo.edu/~duchan/history.html. Accessed 5 Feb 2011.

18. Duffy JR, Werven GW, Aronson AE. Telemedicine and the diagnosis of speech and language disorders. Mayo Clin Proc. 1997;72:1116–22.

19. Forducey PG. Speech telepractice program expands options for rural Oklahoma schools. The ASHA Leader. 2006. Available at: http://www.asha.org/Publications/leader/2006/060815/060815f.htm. Accessed 29 Jan 2011.

20. Givens GD, Elangovan S. Internet application to Tele-audiology – "Nothin' but Net". Am J Audiol. 2003;12:59–65.

21. Glanz W. Telehealth touted as untapped resource. The Washington Times, 2004.

22. Heath C, Heath D. Made to stick: why some ideas survive and others die. New York: Random House; 2007.

23. iHAS. iHAS MD integrated healthcare access. 2011. Available at: http://www.ihasmd.com/index.jsp. Accessed 6 Feb 2011.

24. Krumm M, Ribera J, Schmiedge J. Using a telehealth medium for objective hearing testing: implications for supporting rural universal newborn hearing screening programs. Semin Hear. 2005;26:3–12.

25. Kuster JM. Net connections for communication disorders and sciences. An internet guide. 2010. Available at: http://www.mnsu.edu/comdis/kuster2/sptherapy.html. Accessed 28 Jan 2011.

26. Madden M. Eating, thinking and staying active with new media. Pew Internet and Family Life Project. 2009. Available at: http://www.pewinternet.org/Presentations/2009/15--Eating-Thinking-and-Staying-Active-with-New-Media.aspx. Accessed 6 Feb 2011.

27. Madden M. Older adults and social media. Pew Internet and Family Life Project. 2010. Available at: http://www.pewinternet.org/Reports/2010/Older-Adults-and-Social-Media.aspx. Accessed 6 Feb 2011.

28. Miller W, Rollnick S. Motivational interviewing. Preparing people for change. New York: Guilford Press; 2002.

29. OMNIE Ohio Master's Network Initiatives in Education. Information for school district administrators. 2009. Available at: http://www.omnie.org/For%20Ohio%20School%20Admin/Staffilino%20letter.html. Accessed 19 Dec 2010.

30. Pogue D. Are you taking advantage of web 20. New York Times. 2008. Available at: http://www.nytimes.com/2008/03/27/technology/personaltech/27pogue-email.html. Accessed 6 Feb 2011.

31. Prensky M. Digital natives, digital immigrants part 2: do they really think differently? On the Horizon. 2001;9(6). doi:10.1108/10748120110424843.

32. Prensky M. Turning on the lights. Educational leadership. 2008. Available at: http://www.ascd.org/publications/educational-leadership/mar08/vol65/num06/Turning-On-the-Lights.aspx. Accessed 5 Dec 2010.
33. Prensky M. Teaching digital natives. Thousand Oaks: Corwin; 2010.
34. Saptono A, Schein R, Parmanto B, et al. Methodology for analyzing and developing information management infrastructure to support telerehabilitation. Int J Telerehabil. 2009;1(1):39–46. doi:10.5195/ijt.2009.6012.
35. Sicotte C, Lehoux P, Fortier-Blanc J, et al. Feasibility and outcome evaluation of a telemedicine application in speech-language pathology. J Telemed Telecare. 2003;9(5):253–8.
36. Smith A. Home broadband 2010. Pew Internet Family Life Project. 2010. Available at: http://www.pewinternet.org/Reports/2010/Home-Broadband-2010.aspx. Accessed 9 Jan 2011.
37. Tindall LR, Huebner RA, Stemple JC, et al. Videophone-delivered voice therapy: a comparative analysis of outcomes to traditional delivery for adults with Parkinson's disease. Telemed J E Health. 2008;14(10):1070–7.
38. Towey M. Maine advocacy wins telepractice coverage. The ASHA Leader. 2009. Available at: http://www.asha.org/Publications/leader/2009/090901/090101a1.htm. Accessed 19 Dec 2010.
39. Vaughn GR. Tele-communicology: health care delivery system for persons with communicative disorders. ASHA. 1976;18:13–7.
40. Vygotsky LS. Mind and society: the development of higher psychological processes. Cambridge: Harvard University Press; 1978.
41. Waite M, Cahill L, Theodoros D, et al. A pilot study of online assessment of childhood speech disorders. J Telemed Telecare. 2006;12 Suppl 3:92–4.
42. Waite MC, Theodoros DG, Russell TG, et al. Internet-based telehealth assessment of language using the CELF. Lang Speech Hear Serv Sch. 2010;41:445–58.
43. Zickuhr K. Generations 2010 Pew internet and family life project. 2010. Available at: http://www.pewinternet.org/Experts/~/link.aspx?_id=B821B38A148E4EFC81BE8EC5A9BB59A4&_z=z. Accessed 9 Jan 2011.
44. Zickuhr K. Generations and their gadgets. Pew Internet and Family Life Project. 2011. Available at: http://pewinternet.org/Reports/2011/Generations-and-gadgets.aspx. Accessed 6 Feb 2011.

Chapter 9
Applications in Teleaudiology

Mark Krumm and Barbara A. Vento

Abstract Teleaudiology, the delivery of audiology services at a distance using telecommunications technologies, represents a growing area of opportunity for clinical practice. While audiology is a mature discipline whose development was fueled by World Wars I and II, advances in teleaudiology are relatively recent, having occurred over the past decade. Teleaudiology service delivery models include synchronous, asynchronous (i.e., store-and-forward) and hybrid approaches. As examples, computer-based teleaudiology technologies have been demonstrated to: perform puretone audiometry; measure otoacoustic emissions; program cochlear implants via neural response/telemetry assessment; and perform video-otoscopy. With further development of computer-based tympanometry, synchronous impedance testing via teleaudiology is soon to become a reality. Low technology teleaudiology applications are also developing. Teleaudiology appears very promising, as most of the teleaudiology applications reported upon thus far have demonstrated outcomes comparable to in-person interactions.

9.1 Introduction

Teleaudiology is the delivery of hearing services using a telecommunication medium to assess or provide treatment to consumers situated at a distant location [2, 27]. Most audiologists believe that teleaudiology is useful for those individuals who live

M. Krumm, Ph.D.(✉)
Department of Speech Pathology and Audiology, School of Health Sciences,
Northeast Ohio Au.D. Consortium, Kent, OH 44242-001, USA
e-mail: mkrumm@kent.edu

B.A. Vento, Ph.D.
Department of Communication Science and Disorders,
School of Health and Rehabilitation Sciences, University of Pittsburgh,
5061 Forbes Tower, 3600 Forbes Avenue, Pittsburgh, PA 15260, USA
e-mail: barbv@pitt.edu

S. Kumar, E.R. Cohn (eds.), *Telerehabilitation*, Health Informatics,
DOI 10.1007/978-1-4471-4198-3_9, © Springer-Verlag London 2013

in rural communities where hearing health-care services are lacking or absent. However, in a recent paper, Ciccia et al. [5] reported that teleaudiology was used to provide services to individuals in inner-city clinics. Therefore, we need to expand our current notion and definition of teleaudiology. Audiologists need to see the benefit of audiology telehealth as a literal extension of a clinician's hands to patients who cannot access the traditional clinic for services easily for a variety of reasons.

The concept of telehealth is relatively new to audiology; however, a number of medical professions have been using telehealth technology over a long period of time. These professions include otology, pediatrics, radiology, psychology, and psychiatry [2, 3, 23]. Telehealth services are becoming increasingly cost effective and feasible. Today's high-speed Internet connectivity allows clinicians to realistically consider using affordable real-time video either from dedicated video systems or from a web cam [5]. In addition, hearing health-care professionals have the capability to control audiology equipment with "real-time" remote computing applications across considerable distances [16, 24]. Unfortunately, reimbursement for teleaudiology services is limited or non-existent at this time, which has created a substantial barrier for adoption of teleaudiology as a standard clinical practice. More evidence is needed to show third-party payers that these methods of service are reasonable and reliable, and can be cost-effective options for audiologic services, particularly when the patient is unable to come physically to the audiology office for care.

9.2 History of Teleaudiology

Telemedicine is the historic term describing the provision of health-care services using a telecommunication system. The term telemedicine suggested sole service provision by physicians. However, this definition was expanded through the Comprehensive Telehealth Act of 1997 to include the term *telehealth*. As a consequence, all health-care professionals including audiologists were encouraged to employ telehealth technology for health-care delivery. Subsequently, both the American Academy of Audiology (AAA) [1] and the American Speech-Language Hearing Association (ASHA) [2] developed position statements on telepractice in audiology. However, it should be noted that these organizations are supportive of teleaudiology services only if the results are equal to those provided in person under typical clinic conditions. Research to support the feasibility and reliability of teleaudiology has been completed, but more data are necessary. Specifically, teleaudiology literature lacks research with large sample sizes, field-based research, and a comprehensive hearing health-care model.

Researchers began to conduct teleaudiology studies in the mid-1990s, successfully demonstrating that this technology could be used to fit hearing aids, conduct otoacoustic measurements, and provide pure-tone threshold testing. All of these procedures were achieved using remote computing technology with "off-the-shelf" computerized equipment and remote computing software [14, 16]. At the turn of the millennium the first dedicated teleaudiology system was described, with several others appearing later in the decade [12, 13]. Consequently, within the past 5 years, there have been significant gains in teleaudiology applications. Research projects incorporating telehealth technology have validated a number of teleaudiology applications with auditory brainstem response (ABR), otoacoustic emissions (OAE), pediatric hearing screening, real ear measurements, and the development of several audiometric systems for exclusive hearing testing over the Internet [4, 5, 10, 24, 25].

9.3 Technology Framework in Teleaudiology

A review of teleaudiology literature shows an emphasis on live services. Specifically, researchers have attempted to provide services to patients as if they were face to face in a typical clinical setting. Consequently, most teleaudiology services and research have incorporated interactive video, remote computing technology, modified audiology systems interfaced to personal computers, and the use of high-speed networks. Naturally, an Internet or a wide area network (WAN) must be available on both the clinician and the patient sites for remote computing applications. Dedicated teleaudiology systems have been developed to use relatively modest bandwidth and, more recently, have been used with Wi-Fi. An excellent example of such a system was described and validated by Swanepoel et al. [24]. Web cams are now commonly used in dedicated audiology telehealth systems. These outcomes are very interesting, as a decade ago interactive video resolution was usually poor unless a standalone video system was used. Such standalone systems cost tens of thousands of dollars. Contemporary web cam systems cost approximately $100 and can deliver clear interactive video images appropriate for teleaudiology applications.

9.3.1 Asynchronous Services

Asynchronous technology is used when client data are collected and sent to an expert at a separate location for diagnosis or interpretation. This method of service delivery is also known as "store-and-forward." Store-and-forward technology is commonly used in telehealth but has been used sparingly in teleaudiology paradigms. Store-and-forward technology may be used for a variety of reasons. If analog audiology equipment is used, such as a tympanometer that cannot be interfaced to a computer, a tympanogram can still be printed out, scanned into a computer, and sent via e-mail to an expert for interpretation. Similarly, a digital video-otoscopy image or even a video clip of video-otoscopy may be sent through a store-and-forward service for evaluation.

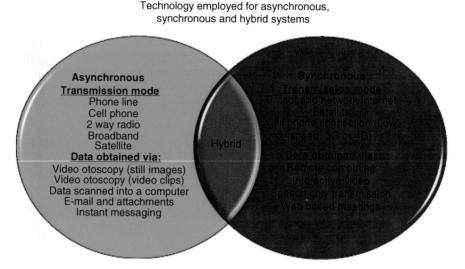

Technology employed for asynchronous,
synchronous and hybrid systems

Fig. 9.1 Services delivery modes that can be delivered in a synchronous, asynchronous, or hybrid environment. The hybrid environment occurs when both synchronous and asynchronous modes are used together or overlap

9.3.2 Synchronous Services

Synchronous services are characterized by the clinician delivering services to clients in real time using interactive video, and are intended to simulate in-person services. In addition, interactive video provides a means to ensure that audiometric equipment is properly configured and fit to the client for diagnostic or treatment services. The appeal of synchronous services is the look and feel of onsite services to clients that cannot be otherwise accomplished unless enormous resources are employed.

9.3.3 Hybrid Technology

The hybrid model incorporates the use of both synchronous and store-and-forward technologies often in an efficient service model. It is likely that audiology services will be administered best with a hybrid model to provide an array of audiology services. A flaw of the teleaudiology research at this time is the lack of models that permit comprehensive hearing assessment and service delivery as typically seen in audiology clinics. Likely, this issue will be solved as researchers grapple with comprehensive teleaudiology services in the future. Figure 9.1 indicates how synchronous, asynchronous, and hybrid technologies are differentiated.

an off-the-shelf PC-based OAE system, a web cam, and remote computing software to test newborns that required rescreening after not passing the screening at birth. All testing in this circumstance mirrored the results obtained at the infant testing site in a second set of test results conducted by an onsite audiologist. The most notable problem with the study was a consistent lack of bandwidth at the hospital location at which infants were rescreened. It is likely that this issue could have been solved with quality-of-service (QOS) enhancements of the hospital network, including larger bandwidth allocations.

9.3.7 Tympanometry

Tympanometry will frequently present problems for the clinician interested in providing telehealth services to clients. Typically, tympanometers are not easily connected to a computer for remote computing purposes. Most likely, the only method available will be the use of store-and-forward technology. Specifically, the tympanometry results will have to be obtained by a technician at the client site, scanned into a computer, and sent via e-mail to the evaluator for interpretation. Such a procedure was carried out by Lancaster et al. [17] for a hearing screening of third-grade children and was effective. As it is unlikely that tympanometry will be used in isolation, effective use of this procedure is probably relegated to a hybrid model that incorporates both synchronous and asynchronous technologies, similar to the method used by Lancaster et al. [17] in their study.

9.3.8 ABR Testing

One area of audiology assessment in which little research has been conducted is electrophysiology. With an emphasis on early hearing detection and intervention (EDHI) programs in the United States and abroad, the ABR might be used in conjunction with telehealth technology for screening, diagnostics, and training personnel. Two publications exist today that successfully incorporate teleaudiology and the ABR.

The first study was conducted by Towers et al. [25], in which ABR tests were recorded on subjects situated approximately 1,000 miles from the evaluator. In this study, normal-hearing subjects were evaluated locally by an audiologist whose results were compared with those of an evaluator obtaining data remotely. Both click and tone burst stimuli were used to elicit ABR results. The data obtained at the remote site mirrored the results obtained onsite. While this was an excellent study in many respects, further investigation is needed in the populations most likely to benefit from ABR testing. Specifically, research is needed in individuals with hearing loss, infants, and young children and, possibly, in interoperative monitoring.

The second study by Krumm and colleagues [15] that assessed remote OAEs also conducted automated ABR (AABR) in the infants as a proof of concept study. Using an off-the-shelf AABR system, a web cam, and remote computing software, these researchers found no differences between onsite and remote computing results for infants less than 1 month of age. While the use of AABR technology in this study does not approximate typical diagnostic ABR conditions, the results did suggest that remote computing with ABR was technically feasible with newborns. However, more data are needed for this type of application. Specifically, with AABR the results obtained are objective in nature in that the decision for pass or fail is determined by the built-in template of the equipment. With diagnostic ABR, test results are subjective requiring the audiologist to interpret results. Consequently, more data are needed for this type of application, particularly with hearing-impaired populations.

9.3.9   Hearing Aids and Verification

It is likely that remote computing was first used clinically to program analog digital hearing aids in the mid-1990s [8, 9]. Specifically, Fabry described a project in which he programmed analog digital hearing aids from his primary clinic location to various satellite clinics in Minnesota. Using off-the-shelf remote computing software and hearing aid programming software, he demonstrated the ability to program the analog digital hearing aids of veterans in Veteran Affairs (VA) facilities using a WAN. The success of this project in the mid-1990s with what was, at the time, a new form of technology is amazing. It assured everyone that remote computing technology was going to work and would continue into other applications. Fabry's work was later followed up by Wesendahl [26]. More recently, Ferrari and Hernardez-Braga [10] published an article describing how verification of hearing aid technology could be accomplished using real ear technology in a telehealth environment.

9.3.10   Speech Testing

One of the most elemental aspects of a basic hearing evaluation is speech testing. While some research has been completed with speech audiometry and teleaudiology technology, this remains a critical area of investigation. A study by Ribera [19] described administration of the Hearing in Noise Test (HINT) to subjects situated over 1,000 miles away from his location. Once again, by using a web cam and remote computing software, he was able to administer the HINT test to his subjects and obtain results similar to those obtained when the subjects were onsite. Obviously, the HINT is not considered a part of the speech battery commonly used by audiologists for basic assessment. However, Ribera's results supported the hypothesis in this proof of concept study that recorded speech tests could be used effectively with telehealth technology to assess speech perception capabilities of clients at a distant location.

9.3.11   Cochlear Implants

Use of cochlear implant technology and telehealth technology is rapidly developing. Several studies have been published concerning the programming of cochlear implants remotely and also the use of remote technology to determine implant functionality during surgery. Franck et al. [11] were the first to describe programming cochlear implants. Using a broadband connection to a distant clinic site with off-the-shelf remote computing software and a cochlear implant programming module (placed at the site of the client) they reported satisfactory results. Another study by Ramos et al. [18] that appears to have replicated the work of Franck et al. [11] was conducted with similar positive outcomes.

That remote computing technology can be used to program cochlear implants is probably intuitive. However, assessing the function of the cochlear implant after surgery is important as well. Typically, cochlear implant functioning is determined objectively with either neural response telemetry (NRT) or neural response imaging (NRI). Given that NRT and NRI are desirable measurements and that the length of cochlear implant surgery is not easily predicted, audiologists could administer these measures remotely from their offices on an as-needed basis. Such a hypothesis was tested by Shapiro et al. [21], who used off-the-shelf remote computing software, along with a typical cochlear implant programming module to accomplish NRT recordings. They found that the remote computing technology was suitable for initial cochlear implant function assessment.

9.3.12   Self-Assessment

There is yet another consideration for teleaudiology: the use of self-assessment and screening tools online. Websites are available that provide common self-assessment tools, including questionnaires, and speech in noise tests with automatic scoring. While the use of self-assessment tools seems reasonable, comprehensive evaluation of these tools has not been described. Therefore, these forms of self-assessment tools require further investigation to determine their efficacy. At the very least, clients should be encouraged to use screening tools only under the care of a qualified audiologist.

Phone-based systems are an option for audiology self-screening. Phone-based hearing screening systems have been described by researchers, particularly in the Netherlands [22]. These researchers used speech and noise procedures to determine the levels of handicap of incoming callers. Results of this study suggested that the use of such hearing screening procedures over phone was valid. Similar hearing screening programs have been implemented to various degrees in other countries in Europe, including Britain, as well as in Australia. In Australia, the phone-based hearing screening system directed incoming callers with hearing loss to the appropriate local hearing health-care unit as a means for service continuity [6].

9.4   Teleaudiology Services Along a Continuum of Care

There is yet another way to view hearing health-care services. Instead of categorizing teleaudiology services in terms of synchronous, asynchronous, and hybrid services, perhaps researchers should consider this technology as it is used across a continuum of increasingly complex hearing health-care services. In actual practice, it is likely that screening and self-screening service can be provided primarily with store-and-forward technology. Diagnostic services would likely be primarily synchronous with a mixture of store-and-forward applications. And for the complex cases, a regional expert would need to see clients face to face and perhaps supplement services with a synchronous, asynchronous, or hybrid system (see Fig. 9.3).

9.5   Evidence to Support Teleaudiology

The incidence of hearing loss worldwide has been estimated to be as high as 10 % of the population [24]. However, accessibility to hearing care from identification to intervention is varied. The underserved in the inner cities and the residents of rural areas across the globe will benefit from an efficient and reasonable use of teleaudiology. Third-party payers have asked for evidence to show that remote audiologic services is as reliable as the assessment and intervention conducted in a typical audiology clinic.

Fortunately, much is known about teleaudiology at this time. The tests that we use routinely to evaluate auditory function—pure-tone audiometry, tympanometry, OAE, and electrophysiologic testing—have been well established as reliable means of assessing hearing and auditory function [15] Many of these tests have already been tested successfully with remote test methods as mentioned earlier in this chapter. If the tests can be validated, and the remote systems can be set up and it actually works, the barriers to teleaudiology can be overcome. Let us consider the following:

1. Patient-examiner interaction

    The truth is that audiologists are routinely separated from their patients by a soundproof wall. In fact, in some clinics, the patients are actually turned away from the window, so they cannot get "clues" from the examiner. "Hands-on" interaction is when we place the head phones, insert test probes, and attach

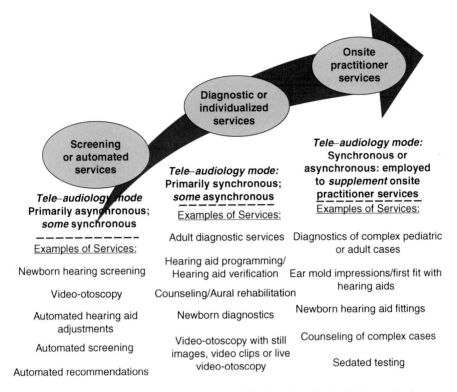

Onsite practitioner services

Diagnostic or individualized services

Screening or automated services

Tele–audiology mode:
Primarily asynchronous;
some synchronous
– – – – – – – – – – –
Examples of Services:

Newborn hearing screening

Video-otoscopy

Automated hearing aid adjustments

Automated screening

Automated recommendations

Tele–audiology mode:
Primarily synchronous;
some asynchronous
– – – – – – – – – –
Examples of Services:

Adult diagnostic services

Hearing aid programming/
Hearing aid verification

Counseling/Aural rehabilitation

Newborn diagnostics

Video-otoscopy with still images, video clips or live video-otoscopy

Tele–audiology mode:
Synchronous or asynchronous: employed to *supplement* onsite practitioner services
– – – – – – – – – – – –
Examples of Services:

Diagnostics of complex pediatric or adult cases

Ear mold impressions/first fit with hearing aids

Newborn hearing aid fittings

Counseling of complex cases

Sedated testing

Fig. 9.3 A continuum of teleaudiology services and likely modes of teleaudiology technology

electrodes, or deliver hearing aids. All of which can be reliably done by a first-year student or an assistant in a remote location with minimal training time.

The greater problems with remote audiology appear to be with the behavioral assessment of infants and children and in counseling situations. Behavioral testing of the pediatric patient often requires "hands-on" and close interaction of the examiner. Certainly, further research on the feasibility of this level of remote assessment is necessary.

Counseling would also be different and possibly not as effective as in a remote situation. Telling a parent that the infant is hearing impaired over a video connection would not be an ideal situation. However, for those situations where audiologists are limited and distance is an issue this would be preferable to not identifying the infant's hearing loss.

Delivery of hearing aids and teaching of how to use the aid would most likely be delegated to the assistant at the remote facility. Although visual oversight of the training would certainly need to be established for quality control purposes, it would also be possible to set up computer communications to programming software of both hearing aids and cochlear implants to reduce the need for patients to travel.

2. Cost of the equipment

   The cost of the equipment is a potential stumbling block in this service delivery model. Although there are a few commercially available options for remote testing, there is the added cost of the equipment at the testing location and that at the remote location. This may not be cost prohibitive, but would be more expensive than establishing an onset test environment without the added expense of the remote connection. In addition, there would be a need to establish a place for testing or consider mobile equipment options.

3. Recruitment and training of the technical assistants

   This need is obviously a big concern and can make or break the success of the teleaudiology clinic. An "ideal" option would be to use well-trained individuals with hearing aid licenses or audiometric technician certification. More likely, it will be local technicians or perhaps nurses who will facilitate teleaudiology services at the client site. Unfortunately, there is virtually no literature in teleaudiology that addresses this issue in a systematic way.

4. Internet connectivity

   Reliable Internet connectivity is the one requirement that must be met. In addition, sufficient bandwidth to allow video streaming must be provided. Obviously in some remote sites or even in the inner city this is a potential problem as the bandwidth may be limited. Bandwidth can be allocated for teleaudiology services, but this issue must be solved before teleaudiology services are planned.

9.6 Conclusion

There is no doubt that teleaudiology research has expanded considerably over the past decade. It is likely that dedicated teleaudiology systems will be used to provide consumer services in distant communities. And the research to this point has supported teleaudiology well as a potential practice. But there will always be areas of audiology that require face-to-face interaction. That would include behavioral testing of infants and young children, and initial delivery sessions with hearing aids. Researchers have not offered an opinion regarding when traditional services should be used instead of teleaudiology. In addition, much of the teleaudiology research has been proof of concept in nature; therefore, virtually no field-based research exists in teleaudiology. Further hampering teleaudiology are the lack of research on individuals with hearing loss and studies with small subject sizes. While these issues are not unusual in telehealth research, teleaudiology still requires vigorous research with appropriate subject sizes and populations. Furthermore, the model of teleaudiology must include all typical audiology services instead of a single audiometric test or service. Audiology has always been a profession in which a battery of tests is used and considered desirable. Finally, teleaudiology must consider models along a continuum of services including self-testing, comprehensive assessment, and a full array of treatment services.

Summary

- Teleaudiology is the delivery of audiology services using a telecommunication medium to assess or provide treatment to consumers placed at a distant location.
- Telehealth services can be delivered by synchronous or asynchronous methods. Asynchronous technology is used when client data are collected and sent to an expert at a remote location for diagnosis or interpretation. In synchronous services, clinician delivers services to clients in real time and simulates face-to-face services using interactive video.
- Audiology services may be administered best with a hybrid model that incorporates both synchronous and store-and-forward technologies.
- At present, reimbursement for teleaudiology services is limited or non-existent, which restricts its adoption as a standard clinical practice. More evidence is needed to prove its reliability and efficiency to third-party payers.
- Teleaudiology research has expanded considerably over the past decade. It is likely that the underserved in the inner cities and the residents of rural areas across the globe will benefit from its use. However, certain areas of audiology will always require face-to-face interaction.

Abbreviations/Acronyms

AAA	American Academy of Audiology
AABR	Automated auditory brainstem response
ABR	Auditory brainstem response
ASHA	American Speech-Language Hearing Association
EDHI	Early hearing detection and intervention
HINT	Hearing in Noise Test
NRI	Neural response imaging
NRT	Neural response telemetry
OAE	Otoacoustic emissions
QOS	Quality of service
VA	Veteran Affairs
WAN	Wide area network

References

1. American Academy of Audiology Resolution 2008–06. The use of telehealth/telemedicine to provide audiology services. (2008) Available at: http://www.audiology.org/advocacy/publicpolicyresolutions/Documents/TelehealthResolution200806.pdf. Accessed Mar 2012.
2. American Speech-Language-Hearing Association. Audiologists providing clinical services via telepractice: technical report. 2005. Available at: www.asha.org/policy.

3. Blackham R, Eikelboom RH, Atlas MD. Assessment of utilization of ear, nose and throat services by patients in rural and remote areas. Aust J Rural Health. 2004;12:150–1.
4. Choi J, Lee H, Park C, Oh S, et al. PC-based tele-audiometry. Telemed J E Health. 2007; 13(5):501–8.
5. Ciccia A, Whitford B, Krumm M, et al. Improving the access of young urban children to speech, language and hearing screening via telehealth. J Telemed Telecare. 2011;17:240–4.
6. Dillon H. Self fitting hearing aid (and publicly available automated hearing tests). Presented at the NIDCD Research Working Group on accessible and affordable hearing health care for adults with mild to moderate hearing loss, Bethesda, 25–27 Aug 2009.
7. Elangovan S. Telehearing and the Internet. Semin Hear. 2005;26:19–25.
8. Fabry D. Remote hearing aid fitting applications. Presented at the 8th annual Mayo Clinic audiology videoconference, Rochester, Nov 1996.
9. Fabry D. Applications of telehealth for hearing care. Audiol Today. 2010;6:18–24.
10. Ferrari DV, Bernardez-Braga GR. Remote probe microphone measurement to verify hearing aid performance. J Telemed Telecare. 2009;15:122–4.
11. Franck K, Pengelly M, Zerfoss S. Telemedicine offers remote cochlear implant programming. Volta Voices. 2006;13(1):16–9.
12. Givens GD, Blanarovich A, Murphy T, et al. Internet-based tele-audiometry system for the assessment of hearing: a pilot study. Telemed J E Health. 2004;9:375–8.
13. Givens G, Elangovan S. Internet application to Tele-audiology: "nothing but net". Am J Audiol. 2003;12:50–65.
14. Krumm M. Audiology telemedicine. J Telemed Telecare. 2007;13:224–9.
15. Krumm M, Huffman T, Dick K, Klich R. Providing infant hearing screening using OAEs and AABR using telehealth technology. J Telemed Telecare. 2008;14(2):102–4.
16. Krumm M, Ribera J, Klich R. Providing basic hearing tests using remote computing technology. J Telemed Telecare. 2007;13(8):406–10.
17. Lancaster P, Krumm M, Ribera J. Remote hearing screenings via telehealth in a rural elementary school. Am J Audiol. 2008;17(2):114–22.
18. Ramos A, Rodriguez C, Martinez-Beneyto P, et al. Use of telemedicine in the remote programming of cochlear implants. Acta Otolaryngol. 2009;129:533–40.
19. Ribera J. Interjudge reliability and validation of telehealth applications of the hearing in noise test. Semin Hear. 2005;26:13–8.
20. Schmiedge J. Distortion product otoacoustic emissions testing using telemedicine technology. Thesis, Minot State University; 1997. p. 97.
21. Shapiro W, Huang T, Shaw T, et al. Remote intraoperative monitoring during cochlear implant surgery is feasible and efficient. Otol Neurotol. 2008;29:495–8.
22. Smits C, Kapteyn T, Houtgast T. Development and validation of an automatic speech-in-noise screening test by telephone. Int J Audiol. 2004;43(1):15–28.
23. Spooner AS, Gotlieb E, Steering Committee on Clinical Information Technology and Committee on Medical Liability. Telemedicine: pediatric applications. Pediatrics. 2004;113: e639–43.
24. Swanepoel D, Koekemoer D, Clark J. Intercontinental hearing assessment – a study in Tele-audiology. J Telemed Telecare. 2010;16:248–52.
25. Towers AD, Pisa J, Froelich TM, et al. The reliability of click-evoked and frequency-specific auditory brainstem response testing using telehealth technology. Semin Hear. 2005;26:19–25.
26. Wesendahl T. Hearing aid fitting: application of telemedicine in audiology. Int Tinnitus J. 2003;9(1):56–8.
27. Wootton R. Recent advances: telemedicine. Br J Med. 2001;60:557–60.

Chapter 10
Telehealth Opportunities in Occupational Therapy

Jana Cason and Tammy Richmond

Abstract Presently, utilization of telehealth is in its infancy within the profession of occupational therapy. However, the occupational therapy profession is poised to benefit from integrating this service delivery model across multiple practice settings and practice areas. Potential benefits of using a telehealth service delivery model within occupational therapy include increased accessibility of services to clients who live in remote or underserved areas, improved access to providers and specialists otherwise unavailable to clients, prevention of unnecessary delays in receiving care, and decreased isolation for practitioners through distance learning, consultation, and research. This chapter examines telehealth terminology and technologies, potential applications of telehealth across six practice areas of occupational therapy, reimbursement considerations, and standards and guidelines to support implementation of a telehealth service delivery model within occupational therapy. Adoption of telehealth as a service delivery model within occupational therapy will depend on continued efforts to fund and research the implementation of telehealth technologies across all occupational therapy practice areas, which, in turn, will promote policy change that results in expanded reimbursement and sustainability.

J. Cason (✉)
Auerbach School of Occupational Therapy, Spalding University,
845 S. 3rd Street, Louisville, KY 40203, USA
e-mail: jcason@spalding.edu

T. Richmond
Go 2 Care, Inc.,
Los Angeles, CA, USA
e-mail: tammyric@sbcglobal.net

S. Kumar, E.R. Cohn (eds.), *Telerehabilitation*, Health Informatics,
DOI 10.1007/978-1-4471-4198-3_10, © Springer-Verlag London 2013

10.1 Introduction

Technology is transforming health-care delivery from the use of electronic health records (EHRs) and videoconferencing to clinical health applications on smart phones and electronic tablets. Health informatics, the utilization of technology in the delivery of health-care services, emerged as a result of multiple contributing factors: the shortage of health-care professionals due to population growth, baby boomers aging and aging in place, the need to manage the staggering costs of chronic diseases, the disparity of quality of care by location, the fragmented continuum of care within our present medical delivery systems, and the ever-growing need to harness the power of information technologies to reach the consumer of health-care services in real time, at any location. Studies confirm that consumers already seek out health information through technology platforms. Pew Internet and American Life Project [61] reports that eight million people a day go online to research health-care topics and products, and 64 % of those online seek out information regarding specific diseases and conditions. According to the Global Mobile Health Market Report 2010–2015, 500 million people will be using mobile health applications by 2015 [57]. Research has demonstrated the capacity of technology to improve access to health-care services and facilitate care within local communities, enhance efficiency, increase effectiveness of chronic disease management, and promote individual adoption of healthy lifestyles [11]. The convergence of wireless technology, health-care services, and mobile devices may lead to a more effective medical and rehabilitative delivery system with a better continuum of care and wellness.

Occupational therapy (OT) practitioners and their clients are well poised to benefit from the use of emerging technologies to deliver health and wellness, habilitation, and rehabilitation services across multiple practice settings and within multiple practice areas. As defined by the American Occupational Therapy Association (AOTA), OT is a science-driven, evidence-based profession that enables people of all ages to live life to its fullest by helping them to promote health and prevent—or live better with—illness, injury, or disability. OT practitioners use meaningful therapeutic activities (occupations) to help people of all ages learn or regain skills needed to participate fully in daily life activities.

Potential benefits of a telehealth service delivery model within OT include increased accessibility of services to clients who live in remote or underserved areas, improved access to providers and specialists otherwise unavailable to clients, prevention of unnecessary delays in receiving care, and decreased isolation for occupational therapy practitioners through distance learning, consultation, and research.

10.2 Definition of Terms Related to Telehealth

Definitions associated with health informatics, including telehealth, are dynamic as the convergence of technology and health care changes rapidly to embrace the integration of administrative, clinical, and technical systems. The American Telemedicine

Association [9] defines telemedicine as the "use of medical information exchanged from one site to another via electronic communications to improve patients' health status" (para. 1). Telehealth is often used interchangeably with telemedicine, but is considered to be a broader term that encompasses both clinical and nonclinical health-related services. Schmeler et al. [69] defined telehealth as "the use of electronic information and telecommunications technologies to support long-distance clinical health care, patient and professional health-related education, public health, and health administration" (p. 12). Ultimately, telemedicine, telehealth, and telerehabilitation platforms will be integrated with electronic medical records (EMRs), electronic health records (EHRs), and personal health records (PHRs) to facilitate seamless delivery of health-related services.

Telerehabilitation falls under the broader term telehealth. The AOTA [7] defines telerehabilitation as "the application of evaluation, preventative, diagnostic, and therapeutic services via two-way or multipoint interactive telecommunication technology" (p. 1). Telerehabilitation is a service provided by rehabilitation professionals (e.g., occupational therapy practitioners, physical therapy practitioners, speech-language pathologists, etc.) delivered through telehealth technologies to clients at distant locations. Present telehealth models of care often describe services by what is being provided such as "tele-evaluation," "tele-consultation," "tele-intervention," "tele-therapy," "tele-monitoring," "tele-mentoring," "tele-supervising" and "tele-education" [21]. The national associations for rehabilitation professions have adopted different terms to describe services provided through telehealth technologies. The AOTA [7] uses the term telerehabilitation at the time of this writing, however, it is anticipated that the association will adopt the term telehealth to describe services provided remotely by occupational therapy practitioners using telehealth technologies. Therefore, the term telehealth will be promoted in this chapter. The Canadian Association of Occupational Therapists (CAOT) uses the term "tele-occupational therapy;" the American Speech-Hearing-Language Association (ASHA) uses the term "telepractice;" and the American Physical Therapy Association (APTA) uses the term "telehealth" to describe services delivered through telehealth technologies (Fig. 10.1).

10.3 Telehealth Applications and Technologies

Two main health-care application models are associated with telehealth: clinical and nonclinical. Clinical applications include consultation, evaluation, assessment, intervention, case management, and supervision. Nonclinical applications include distance learning and research. Telehealth applications are supported by various technologies including the Internet, videoconferencing, videophone, device monitoring, enhanced interactive systems (e.g. virtual reality; health monitoring devices), mobile devices, and wireless communications (see Table 10.1).

There are many technology options that can be incorporated into a telehealth service delivery model, and it is important for practitioners to understand the

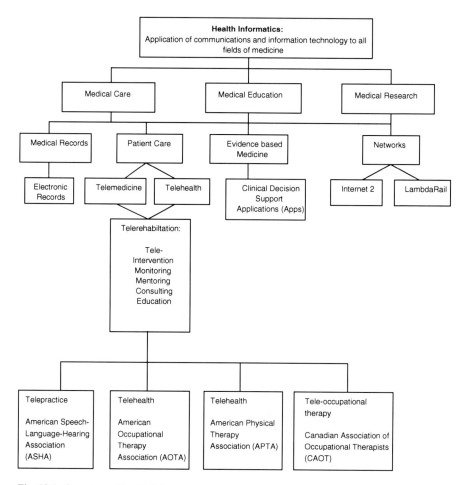

Fig. 10.1 Overview of health informatics

advantages and limitations of each before considering their use. Telehealth technologies may be classified as synchronous or asynchronous. Synchronous technologies permit real-time, live interaction between the health care provider and the patient/client located at a distant site. In contrast, asynchronous technologies capture patient/client data through recorded video, digital photographs, asynchronous monitoring and virtual technology devices, or electronic communication. Based on the recorded data, a health care provider may provide remote consultation, monitoring, evaluation, or intervention as part of a telehealth service delivery model.

Currently, occupational therapy services delivered through telehealth technologies predominantly involves the use of interactive videoconferencing. Videoconferencing is possible through voice-over Internet protocol (VoIP) software, mobile videoconferencing devices (e.g. smart phones, electronic tablets), Plain Old Telephone Service

Table 10.1 Telehealth Technologies

Technology	Example(s)	Considerations
Patient portal (web based, secure messaging)	MilitaryOneSource, Healthanywhere, MyCareTeam	Confidentiality (security, privacy)
VoIP technologies	Skype, Oovoo, iChat Google Voice and Video Chat, Tandberg Movi	Integrity (information protected from changes by unauthorized users)
Mobile videoconferencing	Apple IPhone	Availability (information, services)
Consumer HDTV videoconferencing	Cisco Umi; Galaxy Tabs (Samsung/Polycom)	Cost–benefit ratio
Home telemonitoring systems	Self-monitoring analysis and reporting technologies (SMART), Intel "Health Guide", Bosch "Health Buddy"	Socioeconomical considerations
POTS	Videophones, Honey Well HomMed, NextLINK	Leveraging existing infrastructure (equipment/ personnel)
Enhanced interactive gaming/virtual reality	Xbox Kinect; specialized VR therapeutic devices	Technology connection requirements (e.g., broadband, T1 line)
Mobile health vehicle	Mobile clinics/health units (health screenings, preventative education)	Sound and image quality
Telehealth network with commercial videoconferencing system	Polycom, Tandberg	Equipment accessibility
Wireless sensors	Patient monitoring; "Smart Cane", "CodeBlue"	Provider/end-user comfort, experience, and expertise with technology

Adapted from Ref. [19]

(POTS) videoconferencing devices (e.g. videophone), and high-definition television (HDTV) technologies. Videoconferencing through VoIP requires a computer and web-camera or a VoIP telephone (e.g. smart phone with VoIP capabilities, videophone, or a traditional telephone with adapter to convert voice into a digital signal that travels over the Internet) [29]. In addition to home-based and mobile technologies, many states have designated telehealth networks that utilize high-end videoconferencing technologies (e.g., Polycom, Tandberg) and fiber-optic telephone lines (e.g., T1 lines) or high-speed Internet to connect sites throughout the state. There is potential to leverage these existing networks to provide occupational therapy services using a telehealth service delivery model.

There are advantages and disadvantages associated with the different types of telehealth technologies. Synchronous technologies support live interaction between the patient/client and healthcare provider and facilitate the on-going gathering of information in real-time. Also, services can be provided in the client's natural environments. Disadvantages may include privacy, security, and confidentiality risks (unless utilizing a secure server/telehealth platform), limited interoperability between technology devices, lack of infrastructure for connectivity, diminished sound/image quality, and technological challenges associated with end-user experience and expertise with the telehealth technology. State telehealth networks with commercial videoconferencing systems are an exception to the disadvantages presented as the high-end technology affords videoconferencing sessions that meet security and privacy provisions outlined in the Health Insurance Portability and Accountability Act (HIPAA) and circumvents challenges associated with infrastructure, interoperability, socioeconomic barriers, and limited end-user experience and expertise with telehealth technology. Advantages of asynchronous technologies include having archived data that informs patient/client needs and progress; and flexibility in service provision as the patient/client and provider do not need to be connected at the same time.

10.4   Leveraging Telehealth in OT Across Practice Settings

The task at hand in adoption of a telehealth service delivery model across OT settings starts with educating various stakeholders (practitioners, payers, referral sources, funding sources, public agencies, government, consumers, and vendors) on what, where, how, and when services provided through telehealth technologies can be employed and studied. Traditional OT practice settings include hospitals, rehabilitation facilities, nursing homes, community mental health settings, school systems, home health, and early intervention (EI) programs. Some of these practice settings were early adopters of programs designed to provide health-care services through telehealth technologies; however, others are just beginning to explore its potential benefits. Locations of current telemedicine/telehealth programs include hospitals, remote clinics, Indian reservations, state prison systems, disaster sites, Veterans Affairs hospitals and community clinics, the National Aeronautics and Space Administration (NASA), and global health-care or public health foundations. Some of these settings offer traditional OT services; however, existing barriers associated with reimbursement, licensure portability, and limited research and educational support for the utilization of telehealth has impacted its use as a service delivery model by occupational therapy practitioners.

In addition to the traditional OT practice settings, the AOTA has identified six emerging practice areas: children and youth; health and wellness; productive aging; mental health; rehabilitation, disability, and participation; and work and industry. Current research supports opportunities for using a telehealth service delivery model in each of these areas (see Table 10.2). Kairy et al. [49], in their systematic review of telerehabilitation, concluded that telerehabilitation had comparable or better outcomes when compared to traditional interventions and a high level of satisfaction among clinicians and service recipients, regardless of population, setting, or study design. Similarly, the World Health Organization (WHO) and the World Bank [81] affirmed the efficacy of telerehabilitation in the *World Health Organization and World Bank's World Report on Disability*.

Table 10.2 Leveraging telehealth across OT practice areas

Practice areas	Potential OT services	Supportive telehealth/ telerehabilitation studies
Children and youth	Activity promotion in youth	Ref. [71]
	EI	Refs. [18, 39, 50, 79]
	Specialized intervention; cerebral palsy; school-based asthma; autism	Refs. [10, 33, 36, 80]
Health and wellness	Health promotion/life coaching	Ref. [73]
	Chronic disease management	Refs. [13, 15, 53]
	Disease prevention/education	Refs. [23, 63]
	Lifestyle redesign/obesity	Ref. [58]
	Home design, accessibility, and modifications	Ref. [38]
	Exercise/home exercise programs	Refs. [16, 37, 52, 78]
	Home mobility/safety	Refs. [41, 66]
Productive aging	Driver evaluation and rehabilitation services	Ref. [31]
	Low vision services	Ref. [22]
	Technology to promote aging in place	Ref. [13]
	Remote monitoring	Ref. [12]
	"Medical home"	Ref. [47]
	Cognitive strategies for dementia and Alzheimer's	Ref. [24]
	Caregiver support	Ref. [37]
	Home exercise programs	
Mental health	PTSDs	Refs. [64, 77]
	Life coaching	Ref. [73]
	Stress management	Ref. [76]
	Behavior management	Ref. [24]
	Social support	
Rehabilitation, disability, and participation	Stroke, multiple sclerosis, Parkinson's	Refs. [20, 21, 40, 44, 45, 75]
	Traumatic brain injury	Refs. [14, 74]
	Orthopedics	Refs. [28, 43, 65]
	Spinal cord injury	Refs. [62, 72]
	Wheel chair assessments	Refs. [51, 68]
	Disasters	Ref. [70]
Work and industry	Ergonomics	Ref. [48]
	Work-related injury prevention and rehabilitation	Ref. [26]
	Wound care	Ref. [69]
	Vocational rehabilitation, job modification	

10.4.1 Types of OT Opportunities: Children and Youth

EI services are designed to promote development of skills and enhance the quality of life of infants and toddlers who have been identified as having a disability or developmental delay. EI services are mandated by Part C of the Individuals with Disabilities Education Act (IDEA); however, personnel shortages, particularly in rural areas, limit access for children who qualify. This shortage of providers coupled with an increased need for services due to survival of preterm infants, many with chronic health conditions and disability, creates a unique challenge for EI program administrators. Telehealth is a service delivery model that demonstrates the potential to deliver EI services effectively and efficiently, thereby ameliorating the impact of provider shortages in underserved areas.

Several studies have investigated the use of telehealth as a service delivery model for EI services [18, 39, 50, 79]. Cason [18] investigated the use of telehealth technologies to provide EI OT to two families living in a rural community with limited access to services. The study demonstrated that telehealth is a feasible service delivery model that has the potential to improve access and reduce the cost associated with delivery of EI services in rural communities. Heimerl and Rasch [39] conducted 224 telehealth encounters between 2004 and 2006 and concluded that "telehealth services are not meant to replace face-to-face [in-person] services, but when in-person services are not feasible, they provide a viable alternative" (p. 3). Kelso et al. [50] used two-way interactive telecommunications technology over the Internet to supplement in-person EI services for four families living in a remote area. A high level of satisfaction among the interventionists and families and a cost–benefit analysis resulted in the authors concluding that telehealth "appears both feasible and beneficial" and that "early intervention programs could use this delivery method to more adequately serve young children with disabilities either instead of or in addition to making traditional home visits" (p. 339). Lastly, Vismara et al. [79] investigated the efficacy of telehealth technology as a training medium for EI providers. This study demonstrated that telehealth technology was as effective as in-person instruction. These studies provide evidence for the feasibility of telehealth as a delivery model in EI, particularly in areas where provider shortages limit access to services.

Similarly, a telehealth service delivery model has been used to provide therapy services to children in rural schools where access to onsite therapy services is limited. Telehealth provides an alternative service delivery model for school-based assistive technology consultation and follow-up for children with disabilities. The use of telehealth technologies reduces isolation and builds capacity among the local therapists, teachers, and administrators.

In the emerging OT practice area of prevention of violence among children and youth, OT practitioners can provide services using telehealth technologies as part of an interdisciplinary model to promote pro-social behaviors. Telehealth technologies also afford the opportunity to connect experts with school districts and students for educational workshops and one-on-one interventions.

10.4.2 Types of OT Opportunities: Health and Wellness

Health and wellness are defined as promoting healthy lifestyles through education, public policy, and healthy strategies in disease prevention and whole-person interventions. Present health-care delivery is based on impairment models. In 2007, $1.7 trillion were spent to care for patients with chronic conditions [17]. The National Council of Aging [56] reported that 57 % of people with chronic illnesses were not asked by their health-care provider whether or not they have help at home to manage their condition. Research shows that many of the physiological and social impairments of chronic diseases can be self-managed at home through telehealth technologies and could potentially decrease the staggering medical costs associated with repeat hospitalizations and long-term services in chronic diseases. In a landmark study associated with the Veterans Health Administration [23], veterans with chronic diseases such as diabetes mellitus, congestive heart failure, hypertension, and other long-term illnesses received care and self-management education through video, tele-monitoring, biometric devices, messaging devices, and digital cameras. The Care Coordination/Home Telehealth (CCHT) program involved over 31,000 veterans and showed a 25 % reduction in numbers of bed days in care, 19 % reduction in number of hospital admissions, and a patient satisfaction score of 86 %. In another study affiliated with the Department of Veterans Affairs, Harada et al. [37] implemented remote monitoring devices for physically inactive older adults to determine the feasibility of measuring exercise adherence. The study showed better adherence with the remote monitoring device and demonstrated monitoring feasibility. Other studies showed similar results utilizing remote monitoring with motivational and educational support tools for chronic disease management, including obesity [58] and other practice areas such as personal coaching [73].

There is a belief that the key element to reducing overall medical costs is engaging patients with chronic diseases in self-management. Telehealth technologies provide the opportunity and the vehicle in which patient participation in health and wellness is not only promoted but also necessary. One technology showing cost effectiveness, patient engagement, motivation, and improvement in self-care management of chronic diseases is an early warning behavior-based technology platform that consists of a remote web-based patient-monitoring system with interactive voice response [53]. Several medical settings such as the Henry Ford Health System are successfully using this technology for patients with heart failure to reduce hospital admissions and to provide remote education and motivational tools to improve continuum of care. As part of a multidisciplinary team, occupational therapy practitioners facilitate engagement, motivation, and participation through a holistic, client-centered approach.

10.4.3 Types of OT Opportunities: Productive Aging

Persons aged 65 years or older numbered 39.6 million in 2009, 12.9 % of the U.S. population, which will grow to 19 % of the population by 2030 [1]. Many older adults desire to remain in their home and communities throughout their life span. OT practitioners support the goals of aging in place by implementing various interventions and support strategies that allow older individuals to establish, restore, or maintain the skills used in activities of daily living and other meaningful occupations. These include universal design and environmental modifications in the home and communities, participation in healthy lifestyle changes, continued participation in meaningful activities at both work and social levels, and skilled services to prevent, rehabilitate, and educate individuals during changing physiological, cognitive, and emotional aging processes, and provide resources and support for their family and caregivers. A telehealth service delivery model allows continued access to care and support to take place wherever the older adult may live, play, or work. Harada et al. [37] demonstrated the feasibility of using text messaging through home-monitoring devices for physically inactive adults in their home. Videophone communication using Voice over the Internet Protocol (VoIP) software and a webcam was useful for providing cognitive rehabilitation for older adults with dementia, and good satisfaction by the family and caregivers was reported [47]. A survey by the National Alliance for Caregiving [55] examined family caregivers' receptivity to technology and assessed various types of technologies to support caregivers or to help them provide care. All the caregivers in the survey reported use of the Internet or some other technology for providing care. The researchers identified three areas of greatest potential for technology utilization: tracking PHRs, coordinating client care such as scheduling of medical appointments, and use of a medication reminder device.

Another area of productive aging that is receiving increasing attention is the promotion of the "patient-centered medical home" (PCMH). PCMHs are highly integrated, team-based practice models that promote care coordination through shared decision making with patients. Health information technologies are key components of the model and present several opportunities for OT practitioners to be involved in care management of chronic diseases and aging through homecare monitoring and interventions [12].

10.4.4   Types of Opportunities: Mental Health

OT is well founded on engaging individuals with mental health impairments in therapeutic strategies and interventions to promote recovery and well-being; psychological and social functioning within the home, work, and community; and participation in meaningful activities. The involvement of the U.S. military in Operation New Dawn, Operation Enduring Freedom, and Operation Iraqi Freedom combat operations has highlighted the need for mental health services for large numbers of individuals exposed to combat-related physical and emotional trauma. Psychological stressors are contributing to increased mental health issues among the civilian population as well. Existing barriers to accessing care and perceptions of stigma attached to mental health conditions have facilitated research, examining the use of telehealth technologies to provide therapeutic services for impairments such as major depression, post-traumatic stress disorder (PTSD), substance abuse, impairments in social functioning, and the inability to work and integrate into the community [46]. Germain et al. [34] and Tuerk et al. [77] demonstrated the effectiveness of a telehealth service delivery model via videoconferencing for improved functioning in individuals with PTSD. Studies implementing virtual reality [64] and telephone technologies [54] showed similar capabilities and high satisfaction with the use of a telehealth service delivery model to provide therapeutic services for individuals with PTSD and other mental health impairments.

Empowerment is vital for enhancing quality of life and health among individuals with mental, physical, and social disabilities, and is a core element of "client-centered" health-care delivery systems. Through the use of telehealth technologies, occupational therapy practitioners promote client empowerment and wellness. A telehealth service delivery model can also be used to support family and caregivers as part of the therapy process. DeVany et al. [24] examined the ability of telehealth technologies to assist the client, their family, and extended support system. Similarly, Suter et al. [73] described the benefits of a telehealth service delivery model, specifically tele-monitoring, to promote patient self-efficacy with disease management. Increased self-efficacy, empowerment, and caregiver and family support using telehealth technologies may lead to improved health, participation in meaningful activities, and quality of life for clients dealing with chronic disability and mental health issues.

10.4.5   Types of OT Opportunities: Rehabilitation, Disability, and Participation

Telehealth has proven to be a beneficial service delivery model to provide therapeutic services for individuals with spinal cord injuries (SCIs), traumatic brain injuries (TBIs), Parkinson's disease, and cerebrovascular accident (CVA)/stroke among other health conditions. (see Table 10.2).

10.4.5.1   Spinal Cord Injury

According to the Foundation for Spinal Cord Injury Prevention, Care & Cure [32], approximately 259,000 individuals live with SCI and 12,000 new SCIs occur every year. Shortened hospital stays due to reimbursement restrictions has resulted in many patients being discharged with continued need for therapeutic services, in either an outpatient or a home health setting. Unfortunately, many patients, particularly those with complex SCIs, may have difficulty accessing follow-up care from specialized rehabilitation facilities due to distance and travel limitations associated with the injury. Although home health services may be available within the individual's community, local practitioners may lack expertise working with individuals with SCIs. Telehealth provides a means for expert consultation (tele-consultation) with local providers, in-home consultation for home modifications, monitoring of functional status, evaluation for assistive technology and wheel chair seating, and prevention of pressure ulcers [69].

10.4.5.2   Traumatic Brain Injury

Occupational therapy practitioners commonly work with individuals with TBI. Approximately 1.4 million individuals sustain a TBI each year. According to Fischer [30], in the report *U.S. Military Casualty Statistics: Operation New Dawn, Operation Iraqi Freedom, and Operation Enduring Freedom*, a Congressional Research Service report to Congress, a total of 178,876 TBI cases were reported among U.S. military members between 2000 and 2010. Bergquist et al. [14] investigated patient satisfaction with Internet-based cognitive rehabilitation in persons with memory impairments, and found that the study participants were willing to use the Internet and that some compensatory strategies were well suited to a telehealth service delivery model. Diamond et al. [25] built an Internet-based "virtual rehabilitation center" (VRC) for individuals with TBI to provide rehabilitation, education, and support services. All eight participants successfully learned to use the VRC, and generalization of skills into the community for one study participant was demonstrated. Owing to a growing need for TBI management, shortage of specialists, and increased risk for secondary injury among individuals with TBI, Girard [35] concluded that the use of telehealth technologies to provide interventions will continue to be an important component in patient care.

10.4.5.3   Parkinson's Disease

An estimated one million Americans live with Parkinson's disease and an additional 60,000 Americans are diagnosed with Parkinson's disease each year [60]. Occupational therapists have traditionally worked with individuals with Parkinson's disease to facilitate movement, improve coordination and fine motor skills, practice safe transfer techniques, incorporate adaptive techniques and adaptive equipment, explore new ways to engage in meaningful activities, and modify the home to improve safety and performance in activities of daily living [3, 4]. Many of these interventions are consultative in nature and may be effectively delivered through telehealth technologies. Some assessments also lend themselves to effective administration through telehealth technologies. Hoffman et al. [45] concluded that ADL status and fine motor skills using the motor component of the Functional Independence Measure, the Unified Parkinson's Disease Rating Scale (UPDRS), Nine Hole Peg Test, Preston Pinch Gauge, and Jamar dynamometer could be assessed with good validity and reliability using a low-bandwidth Internet-based telerehabilitation system.

10.4.5.4   Cerebrovascular Accident (CVA)/Stroke

Stroke is the leading cause of serious, long-term disability in the United States and the third leading cause of death [2]. Hermann et al. [40] examined the efficacy of using a telehealth service delivery model, Internet-based videoconferencing, to supervise a home program using functional electrical stimulation (FES) with a client who had experienced a stroke resulting in residual upper-extremity impairment and functional limitations. The researchers concluded that telehealth is a promising service delivery model for individuals who live in remote areas or who experience transportation challenges. Similarly, Chumbler et al. [20] concluded that the use of telehealth technologies is an innovative way to meet the therapeutic needs of individuals who have had a stroke and would otherwise encounter barriers to timely healthcare services.

Telehealth technologies provide a means for care coordination among remote experts and local practitioners and reduce the burden of travel to specialized facilities for individuals living in rural and underserved communities. Despite positive outcomes associated with the research presented, practitioners must be aware of the complexity of using telehealth technologies to provide interventions including barriers and considerations associated with rapidly changing technologies, equipment reliability, interdepartmental coordination, and procedural safeguards designed to protect recipients of services [20]. Consideration of service recipients' needs and post-discharge environment is also critical.

10.4.6   Types of OT Opportunities: Work and Industry

OT practitioners have expertise in providing services in ergonomics, work performance, and vocational rehabilitation due to a holistic approach that encompasses occupational performance and how the environment, technology, and tools support or hinder occupational performance. Individuals with disabilities are confronted with barriers, such as accessibility and decreased resources, to participate in education, employment, and independent living. Telehealth technologies would provide obvious access to services presently limited by geography and resources, including access to specialists. However, very few telehealth applications have been reported in this occupational therapy practice area. Schmeler et al. [69] identified two studies using technologies for vocational rehabilitation. The first study looked at the potential of employing video technology as a medium for vocational training, and the results supported the feasibility of the application in areas of job development, client monitoring, and support. Another study used remote technologies such as teleconferencing, web-based applications, and phone calls to assess the feasibility of the participants to reach their vocational goals. Both studies demonstrate the potential of using a telehealth service delivery model to facilitate attainment of vocational outcomes.

10.4.7   Service Delivery Model Considerations

The goal of a telehealth service delivery model is to provide client-centered, quality OT services that assimilate in-person interactions. Regardless of the practice area, an OT practitioner must use clinical reasoning skills to determine the appropriateness of using a telehealth service delivery model and the best technology to maximize therapeutic outcomes for clients receiving OT. As a general guideline, factors in determining if a telehealth service delivery model is appropriate includes consideration of all stakeholders involved and the clinical, technical and administrative needs and requirements of both the originator (practitioner) and end user (client) of OT services. Stakeholders may include practitioners, payers, referral sources, funding sources, public agencies, government organizations, clients, client's caregivers or social support, and technology vendors.

Context considerations include the client's location, ability to access OT services, diagnosis and therapeutic needs, the client's capability to use and engage in specific technologies, the client's support system, access to and availability of technology, and the ability to measure outcomes. Studies support several OT assessments as appropriate and reliable for use in a telehealth service delivery model including the Functional Reach Test and European Stroke Scale [59]; the Kohlman Evaluation of Living Skills and the Canadian Occupational Performance Measure [27]; the FIM, the Jamar Dynamometer, the Preston Pinch Gauge, the Nine Hole Peg Test, and the Unified Parkinson's Disease Rating Scale [45].

Appropriate technical selection includes technological, human, and logistical components. Items to consider are appropriateness and maintenance of the technology, and the sustainability of participation by the client [67]. This includes knowledge of Internet requirements such as bandwidth and video resolution, application requirements such as enhanced multimedia and interactive format integration (i.e. Flash, Silverlight), equipment safety and effectiveness to meet requirements of OT services implementation, the client's ability to interface with the technology selected, and privacy and security compliance.

Administration considerations include safety and effectiveness of interventions provided through telehealth technologies, policies and procedures, reimbursement structure, payer source, and return on investment along with legal and ethical requirements such as practitioner qualifications, informed consent, and adherence to standards of practice, scope of practice, licensure issues, and cultural competency [7].

10.5   Practitioner Qualifications and Ethical Considerations

OT practitioners considering the use of telehealth as a service delivery model for OT should become familiar with the AOTA's official position on the use of telehealth within occupational therapy (i.e., AOTA *Telerehabilitation Position Paper* [7] and subsequent updated position papers on the topic). Additionally, the American Telemedicine Association's Telerehabilitation Standard and Guideline document, *A Blueprint for Telerehabilitation Guidelines,* outlines important administrative, clinical, technical, and ethical principles associated with telerehabilitation [8]. OT services provided through telehealth technologies are held to the same professional, legal, and ethical standards as in-person services. OT practitioners must adhere to the AOTA's *Standards of Practice for Occupational Therapy* [6] and *Occupational Therapy Code of Ethics and Ethics Standards* [5], as well as pertinent licensure and reimbursement requirements. In general, an OT practitioner providing services across state lines using telehealth technologies is required to be licensed in both the state where the OT practitioner is located and the state where the client is located. Ultimately, a national licensure model, expedited license process, or license compact between states where a license from one state is accepted in another (e.g., Nurse Licensure Compact) would facilitate provision of services across state lines to better meet the therapeutic needs of underserved communities, enable access to highly specialized practitioners, and mobilize resources in times of disaster.

10.6   Reimbursement and Funding

Reimbursement is vital to the adoption and sustainability of the integration of telehealth delivery models within health care and is dependent on several key legislative measures. Senate Bill 1665 enacted the "Telemedicine Development Act of 1996," which imposed requirements for health-care services delivered through telemedicine platforms. It required insurance companies to reimburse providers for qualifying services and also stipulated that third-party payers, including Medicaid and HMOs, cannot require in-person contact as a condition for payment. Currently, Medicare and Medicaid continue to restrict services and location of qualifying services to remote sites that lack health-care professionals or are sites that are considered "rural." The Balanced Budget Act of 1997 included the first national policy for Medicare coverage of telehealth services and further revisions in 2000 specified providers, services, and locations applicable for telehealth such as rural areas with professional shortages. Thereafter, states began to pass their own legislative measures to define and specify further covered services such as tele-dermatology and tele-ophthalmology, and related technology transmission modes. Advancement in health-care delivery technology platforms received a large boost when the American Recovery and Reimbursement Act (ARRA) of 2009 was passed, giving about $150 billion to expand broadband and promote the adoption of health information technology and fund chronic disease management projects. Despite all the legislative support for telehealth, at the time of this writing OT practitioners are not listed as eligible providers under Medicare Medicaid reimbursement for occupation therapy is state driven and is subject to state policy requirements or restrictions. It has been up to the advocacy of OT practitioners and their state licensure boards to include telehealth within their practice acts.

Current reimbursement for OT services provided through a telehealth service delivery model is primarily through private pay and state-funded initiatives. Billing and coding for services use the same coding methodology except for the addition of a unique modifier to differentiate the encounter from a traditional, in-person encounter. These modifiers enable states to track frequency and types of services provided through a telehealth service delivery model and may be used to support research associated with telehealth outcomes.

Other funding is possible through grants provided by state health-care foundations and agencies such as Department of Health and Human Services, as a result of the American Recovery and Reinvestment Act of 2009 and federal health-care reform and economic stimulus initiatives. Funds support the implementation of innovative telehealth approaches and research to promote accessibility to care, cost effectiveness, and continuum of delivery of care. Furthermore, congressional monies awarded to the Department of Defense and the Department of Veterans Affairs to provide health care to our wounded warriors have resulted in numerous opportunities for applications, including some occupational therapy services delivered through telehealth technologies (https://fbo.gov/).

OT practitioners can participate in these and other funding opportunities to integrate and advance the use of telehealth technologies within traditional and emerging practice areas of OT.

10.7 Discussion

Despite the emerging research that supports the use of a telehealth service delivery model within occupational therapy (see Table 10.2), there are several barriers to the overall adoption of telehealth as a service delivery model within the present health-care delivery system. Those include, but are not limited to, the following:

- Limited broadband coverage to remote and rural areas
- Lack of reimbursement and sustained funding
- End-user acceptance of interactive technologies
- Lack of OT practitioners on payers' telehealth provider lists
- Lack of rigorous research supporting effectiveness and utility of services provided through telehealth technologies
- Privacy and security concerns with various technology platforms
- Lack of incentives to promote inclusion of telehealth technologies within existing rehabilitation mechanisms, especially in allied health-care professions
- Inter-state licensure concerns related to telehealth and lack of licensure portability

Presently, utilization of telehealth as a service delivery model is in its infancy in OT. There is a need to increase awareness, education, and advocacy for the application of telehealth technologies within the profession. Adoption of telehealth as a service delivery model within the profession will depend on continued efforts to fund and research the implementation of telehealth applications across all OT practice areas, which, in turn, will promote policy changes that result in expanded reimbursement and sustainability. Additionally, creation of standards and guidelines related to the use of a telehealth service delivery model within OT, development of provider competency standards, assimilation of telehealth within educational standards for entry-level practitioners, continuing education opportunities, model language for inclusion in state practice acts, and materials to educate stakeholders on the benefits of using telehealth technologies within OT are needed to facilitate the integration of telehealth as a service delivery model within OT and promote a climate conducive for its sustainability.

10.8 Case Examples

The following are hypothetical case examples designed to demonstrate potential applications of a telehealth service delivery model within EI, neurological rehabilitation, and mental health practice settings.

10.8.1 Pediatric OT

Katelyn,[1] a 2-year-old child, qualified for EI services to address delays in motor skills, adaptive (self-help) skills, and communication. Additionally, concerns related to Katelyn's ability to process sensory information were identified as having an impact on her ability to self-regulate and participate in daily routines. The EI service team consisted of a service coordinator, a physical therapist, and a speech-language pathologist. OT was recommended; however, an occupational therapist was not available within Katelyn's community. After obtaining appropriate informed consent, the service coordinator used an electronic tablet wtih videoconferencing software to virtually connect an occupational therapist with Katelyn's caregiver and EI service providers. During this meeting, the occupational therapist collaborated with the EI service team, discussed concerns, and identified therapeutic techniques and strategies that could be embedded by Katelyn's caregiver and service providers into Katelyn's naturally occurring routines (mealtime, play time, bath time, etc.). The occupational therapist offered recommendations to promote Katelyn's development within the motor, adaptive, and sensory areas and, through technology, provided a professional perspective that would otherwise have been unavailable. During subsequent virtual meetings, the occupational therapist was able to recommend and virtually demonstrate new strategies and techniques for Katelyn's caregiver and service providers to implement with Katelyn. As a result of mobile videoconferencing, Katelyn was able to benefit from the expertise of an occupational therapist with specialized knowledge and skills in the area of pediatric therapy and sensory processing. Additionally, Katelyn's local service providers benefitted from mobile videoconferencing with the occupational therapist as their knowledge and skills were enhanced through remote consultation.

---

[1] This case study was originally published in Cason, J. (2011). Telerehabilitation: An adjunct service delivery model for early intervention services. *International Journal of Telerehabilitation,* *3*(1), 19-30. doi: 10.5195/IJT.2011.6071

10.8.2   Neurological Rehabilitation

Mildred, a 68-year old patient with long-term diabetes, was discharged home after a mild stroke that resulted in right-sided weakness in her upper extremity, balance problems, minimal assistance needed to complete activities of daily living, and the inability to drive to follow up therapy appointments. Mildred lived alone but was set up to receive caregiving services for some period of time. The occupational therapist recommended continued OT services through a home telemonitoring system with interactive audio/video mechanisms, alert systems, and educational and motivational tools. Once a week the occupational therapist contacted Mildred via videoconferencing to guide her through her home exercise program, provide recommendations for home safety and environmental modifications, and provide caregiver training to assist Mildred with activities of daily living. She also received adjunct instructional materials through her telemonitoring device as needed. As a result of home telemonitoring and videoconferencing with the occupational therapist, Mildred made an excellent recovery and is now able to function independently at home and within her community.

10.8.3   Mental Health

Sam, a young soldier, returned home from his military deployment in Iraq with mild TBI and PTSD after his military vehicle was hit by an improvised explosive device (IED). He lives with his family, who is very supportive. The nearest Veterans Administration hospital is over 150 miles from the family home. Sam has been assessed and admitted into the Assisted Living Pilot Project through the Defense and Veterans Brain Injury Center [42], which incorporates therapeutic services provided through a web-based, secure portal with teleconferencing capabilities. The multidisciplinary approach includes OT among other support services. Sam and his therapist will have weekly telerehabilitation sessions to work on his executive functioning, vocational rehabilitation through teleconferencing, and follow up home-management programming through secure e-mail messaging and instructional attachments. Sam will be reassessed every 4 weeks for progress of short-term goals until he achieves successful re-entry into the community and can return to gainful employment and independent living.

10.9   Conclusion

Telehealth opportunities in occupation therapy reach across multiple practice settings and practice areas. Research is beginning to show increased access to services, improved functional outcomes, high levels of satisfaction with remote services, enhanced communication and continuity of care, increased management of chronic diseases, and adoption of healthy lifestyles when a telehealth service delivery model is incorporated. Telehealth technologies allow OT practitioners to assess, educate, provide interventions, monitor, and modify services regardless of where the client works or lives, thus promoting participation in daily life activities.

Summary

- The American Occupational Therapy Association (AOTA) defines occupational therapy (OT) as a science-driven, evidence-based profession that enables people of all ages to promote health and prevent illness, injury, or disability.
- The potential benefits of a telehealth service delivery model within OT include increased accessibility of services to clients who live in remote or underserved areas; improved access to providers and specialists otherwise unavailable to clients; prevention of unnecessary delays in receiving care; and decreased isolation for therapists through distance learning, consultation, and research.
- OT practitioners can use telehealth technologies to promote pro-social behaviors among children and youth, provide older adults with continued access to care and support irrespective of their location, and promote recovery and well-being in individuals with mental health impairments.
- Despite the emerging research that supports the use of a telehealth service delivery model; there are several barriers to the overall adoption of telehealth as a service delivery model within the present health-care delivery system.
- Presently, use of telehealth as a service delivery model is in its infancy in OT. Adoption of telehealth will depend on continued efforts to fund and research the implementation of telehealth technologies across all OT practice areas.

Abbreviations/Acronyms

ADL   Activities of Daily Living
AOTA   American Occupational Therapy Association
APTA   American Physical Therapy Association
ARRA   American Recovery and Reimbursement Act
ASHA   American Speech-Hearing-Language Association
CAOT   Canadian Association of Occupational Therapists
CCHT   Care Coordination/Home Telehealth
CVA   Cerebrovascular accident
EHR   Electronic health record
EI   Early intervention
EMR   Electronic medical record
FES   Functional electrical stimulation

HDTV	High-definition television
HIPAA	Health Insurance Portability and Accountability
IDEA	Individuals with Education Act
IED	Improvised explosive device
NASA	National Aeronautics and Space Administration
OT	Occupational therapy
PCMH	Patient-centered medical home
PHR	Personal health records
PTSD	Post-traumatic stress disorder
POTS	Plain Old Telephone Service
SCI	Spinal cord injury
TBI	Traumatic brain injury
UPDRS	Unified Parkinson's Disease Rating Scale
VoIP	Voice-over Internet protocol
VRC	Virtual rehabilitation center

References

1. Administration on Aging. Aging statistics. 2010. Available at: http://www.aoa.gov/aoaroot/aging_statistics/index.aspx. Accessed 11 Feb 2011.
2. American Heart Association. Stroke statistics. 2011. Available at: http://www.americanheart.org/presenter.jhtml?identifier=4725. Accessed 5 Feb 2011.
3. American Occupational Therapy Association. Living with Parkinson's disease. 2007. Available at: http://www.aota.org/featured/area6/links/link02am.asp. Accessed 5 Feb 2011.
4. American Occupational Therapy Association. Obesity and occupational therapy position paper. Am J Occup Ther. 2007;61:701–3. doi:10.5014/ajot.61.6.701.
5. American Occupational Therapy Association. Occupational therapy code of ethics and ethics standards. Am J Occup Ther. 2010;64:S17–26. doi:10.5014/ajot.2010.64S17.
6. American Occupational Therapy Association. Standards of practice for occupational therapy. Am J Occup Ther. 2010;64:S106–11. doi:10.5014/ajot.2010.64S106.
7. American Occupational Therapy Association. Telerehabilitation position paper. Am J Occup Ther. 2010;64:S92–102. doi:10.5014/ajot.2010.64S92.
8. American Telemedicine Association. A blueprint for telerehabilitation guidelines. 2010. Available at: http://www.americantelemed.org/files/public/standards/ATA%20Telerehab%20Guidelines%20v1%20(2).pdf. Accessed Feb 2011.
9. American Telemedicine Association. Telemedicine defined. 2011. Available at: http://www.americantelemed.org/i4a/pages/index.cfm?pageid=3333. Accessed 5 Feb 2011.
10. Baharav E, Reiser C. Using telepractice in parent training in early autism. Telemed J E Health. 2010;16:727–31.
11. Bashshur R, Shannon G. National telemedicine initiatives: essential to healthcare reform. Telemed J E Health. 2009;15:600–10. doi:10.1089/tmj.2009.9960.
12. Bates D, Bitton A. The future of health information technology in the patient-centered medical home. Health Aff. 2010;29(4):614–21. doi:10.1377/hithall.2010.0007.
13. Bendixen R, Horn K, Levy C. Using telerehabilitation to support elders with chronic illness in their homes. Top Geriatr Rehabil. 2007;23(1):47–51.
14. Bergquist TF, Thompson K, Gehl C, et al. Satisfaction ratings after receiving internet-based cognitive rehabilitation in persons with memory impairments after severe acquired brain injury. Telemed J E Health. 2010;16:417–23.

15. Biswas-Diener R. Personal coaching as a positive intervention. J Clin Psychol. 2009;65:544–54.
16. Burns RB, Crislip D, Daviou P, et al. Using telerehabilitation to support assistive technology. Assist Technol. 1998;10:126–33.
17. California Healthcare Foundation. Participatory health: online and mobile tools help chronically ill manage their care. 2009. Available at: http://www.chcf.org/publications/2009/09/participatory-health-online-and-mobile-tools-help-chronically-ill-manage-their-care. Accessed 16 Dec 2010.
18. Cason J. A pilot telerehabilitation program: delivering early intervention services to rural families. Int J Telerehabil. 2009;1:29–37.
19. Cason J. Telerehabilitation: an adjunct service delivery model for early intervention services. Int J Telerehabil. 2011;3(1):19–30. doi:10.5195/ijt.2011.6071telerehab.pitt.edu/ojs/index.php/Telerahab/article/view/6071/6315.
20. Chumbler N, Quigley P, Sanford J, et al. Implementing telerehabilitation research for stroke rehabilitation with community dwelling veterans: lessons learned. Int J Telerehabil. 2010;2:15–2. doi:10.5195/ijt.2010.6047.
21. Clark P, Dawson S, Scheiderman-Miller C, et al. TeleRehab: stroke teletherapy and management using two-way interactive video. Neuroreport. 2002;26:87–93.
22. Crossen-Sills J, Toomey I, Doherty ME. Technology and home care: implementing systems to enhance aging in place. Nurs Clin North Am. 2008;44:230–46.
23. Darkins A, Ryan P, Kobb R, et al. Care coordination/hometelehealth: the systematic implementation of health informatics, home telehealth, and disease management to support the care of veteran patients with chronic conditions. Telemed J E Health. 2008;14:1118–26.
24. DeVany M, Alverson D, D'Iorio J, et al. Employing telehealth to enhance overall quality of life and health for families. Telemed J E Health. 2008;14:1003–7. doi:10.1089/tmj.2008.0107.
25. Diamond B, Shreve G, Bonilla J, et al. Telerehabilitation, cognition and user-accessibility. NeuroRehabilitation. 2003;18:171–7.
26. Dobke M, Bhavsar D, Gosman A, et al. Pilot trial of telemedicine as a decision aid for patients with chronic wounds. Telemed J E Health. 2008;14:245–9. doi:10.1089/tmj.2007.0038.
27. Dreyer N, Dreyer K, Shaw D, et al. Efficacy of telemedicine in occupational therapy: a pilot study. J Allied Health. 2001;30(1):39–42.
28. Eriksson L, Lindstrom B, Ekenberg L. Patient's Experiences of telerehabilitation at home after shoulder joint replacement. J Telemed Telecare. 2011;17:25–30.
29. Federal Communications Commission. Voice-over-Internet protocol. 2010. Available at: http://www.fcc.gov/voip/. Accessed 5 Feb 2011.
30. Fischer H. U.S. military casualty statistics: operation new dawn, operation Iraqi freedom, and operation enduring freedom. 2010. Available at: http://www.fas.org/sgp/crs/natsec/RS22452.pdf. Accessed 5 Feb 2011.
31. Fonda SJ, Bursell SE, Lewis DG, et al. The relationship of a diabetes telehealth eye care program to standard eye care and change in diabetes health outcomes. Telemed J E Health. 2007;13:635–44.
32. Foundation for Spinal Cord Injury Prevention, Care & Cure. Spinal cord injury statistics. 2009. Available at: http://www.fscip.org/facts.htm. Accessed 5 Feb 2011.
33. Gallagher TE. Augmentation of special-needs services and information to students and teachers "ASSIST"—a telehealth innovation providing school-based medical interventions. Hawaii Med J. 2004;63:300–9.
34. Germain V, Marchand A, Bouchard S, et al. Effectiveness of cognitive behavioural therapy administered by videoconference for posttraumatic stress disorder. Cogn Behav Ther. 2009;38(1):42–53.
35. Girard P. Military and VA telemedicine systems for patients with traumatic brain injury. J Rehabil Res Dev. 2007;44:1017–26.
36. Golomb MR, McDonald BC, Warden SJ, et al. In-home virtual reality videogame telerehabilitation in adolescents with hemiplegic cerebral palsy. Arch Phys Med Rehabil. 2010;91(1):1–8.
37. Harada N, Dhanani S, Elrod M, et al. Feasibility study of home telerehabilitation for physically inactive veterans. J Rehabil Res Dev. 2010;47:465–76.

38. Haugen HA, Tran ZV, Wyatt HR, et al. Using telehealth to increase participation in weight maintenance programs. Obesity. 2007;15:3067–77.
39. Heimerl S, Rasch N. Delivering developmental occupational therapy consultation services through telehealth. Dev Disabil Spec Interest Sec Q. 2009;32(3):1–4.
40. Hermann V, Herzog M, Jordan R, et al. Telerehabilitation and electrical stimulation: an occupation-based, client-centered stroke intervention. Am J Occup Ther. 2010;64:73–81.
41. Hoenig H, Sanford JA, Butterfield T, et al. Development of a teletechnology protocol for in-home rehabilitation. J Res Dev. 2006;43:287–98.
42. Hoffman SW, Shesko K, Harrison CR. Enhanced neurohabilitation techniques in the DVBIC assisted living pilot project. NeuroRehabilitation. 2010;26:257–69.
43. Hoffman T, Russell T. Pre-admission orthopaedic occupational therapy home visits conducted using the internet. J Telemed Telecare. 2008;14:83–7.
44. Hoffman T, Russell T, Cooke H. Remote measurement via the internet of upper limb range of motion people who have had a stroke. J Telemed Telecare. 2007;13:401–5.
45. Hoffman T, Russell T, Thompson L, et al. Using the internet to assess activities of daily living and hand function in people with Parkinson's disease. NeuroRehabilitation. 2008;23:253–61.
46. Hoge C, Castro C, Messer S, et al. Combat duty in Iraq and Afghanistan, mental health problems, and barriers to care. N Engl J Med. 2004;351:13–22.
47. Hori M, Kubota M, Kihara T, et al. The effect of videophone communication (with Skype and webcam) for elderly patients with dementia and their caregivers. Gan To Kagaku Ryoho. 2009;36S:36–8.
48. Huis in't Veld R, Huijgen B, Schaake L, et al. Staged approach evaluation of remotely supervised myofeedback treatment (RSMT) in women with neck – shoulder pain due to computer work. Telemed E Health. 2008;14:545–51. doi:10.1089/tmj.2007.0090.
49. Kairy D, Lehoux P, Vincent C, et al. A systematic review of clinical outcomes, clinical process, healthcare utilization and costs associated with telerehabilitation. Disabil Rehabil. 2009;31:427–47.
50. Kelso G, Fiechtl B, Olsen S, et al. The feasibility of virtual home visits to provide early intervention: a pilot study. Infants Young Children. 2009;22:332–40.
51. Kim J, Brienza DM, Lynch RD, et al. Effectiveness evaluation of remote accessibility assessment system for wheelchair users using virtualized reality. Arch Phys Med Rehabil. 2008;89:470–9.
52. Lai JC, Woo J, Hui E, et al. Telerehabilitation – a new model for community-based stroke rehabilitation. J Telemed Telecare. 2004;10:199–205.
53. Monegain B. Henry Ford reduces hospital admissions with remote monitoring. 2009. Available at: http://www.healthcareitnews.com/news/henry-ford-reduces-hospital-admissions-remote-monitoring. Accessed 8 Feb2011.
54. Mozer E, Franklin B, Rose J. Psychotherapeutic intervention by telephone. Clin Interv Aging. 2008;3:391–6.
55. National Alliance for Caregiving. New study reveals family caregivers want web-based and mobile technologies to help them care for their loved ones. 2011. Available at: http://www.caregiving.org/. Accessed 11 Feb 2011.
56. National Council of Aging. Re-forming healthcare: Americans speak out about chronic conditions and the pursuit of health. 2009. Available at: http://www.ncoa.org/assets/files/pdf/FINAL_Survey_Fact_Sheet_DC.pdf. Accessed 16 Dec 2010.
57. Nerenberg J. 500 million people to use mobile health Apps by 2015: mHealth study. 2010. Available at: http://www.fastcompany.com/1701769/mhealth-summit-wraps-reveals-booming-industry. Accessed 20 Jan 2010.
58. Neubeck L, Redfern J, Fernandez R, et al. Telehealth interventions for the secondary prevention of coronary heart disease: a systematic review. Eur J Cardiovasc Prev Rehabil. 2009;16:281–9.
59. Palsbo SE, Dawson SJ, Savard L, et al. Televideo assessment using functional reach test and European stroke scale. J Rehabil Res Dev. 2007;44:659664.
60. Parkinson's Disease Foundation. Statistics on Parkinson's. 2011. Available at: http://www.pdf.org/en/parkinson_statistics. Accessed 5 Feb 2011.

61. Pew Internet and American Life Project. Online health search 2006. 2006. Available at: http://www.pewinternet.org/Reports/2006/Online-Health-Search-2006/03-113-Million-Internet-Users-Seek-Health-Information-Online/03-Fifteen-percent-of-internet-users-have-looked-online-for-information-about-dental-health.aspx. Accessed 5 Jan 2011

62. Philips VL, Temkin A, Vesmarovish S, et al. A feasibility study of video-based home telecare for clients with spinal cord injuries. J Telemed Telecare. 1998;4:219–23.

63. Polisena J, Tran K, Cimon K, et al. Home telehealth for chronic obstructive pulmonary disease: a systematic review and meta-analysis. J Telemed Telecare. 2010;16:120–7.

64. Reger GM, Holloway KM, Candy C, et al. Effectiveness of virtual reality exposure therapy for active duty soldiers in a military mental health clinic. J Trauma Stress. 2011;24(1):93–6. doi:10.1002/jts.20574.

65. Russell T, Buttrum P, Wooton R, et al. Internet-based outpatient telerehabilitation for patients following total knee arthroplasty: a randomized control trial. J Bone Joint Surg Am. 2011;93:113–20. doi:10.2106/JBJS.I.01375.

66. Sanford J, Hoenig H, Griffiths P, et al. A comparison of televideo and traditional in-home rehabilitation in mobility impaired older adults. Phys Occup Ther Geriatr. 2007;25(3):1–18.

67. Scheideman-Miller C. Rehabilitation. In: Stamm BH, Lauderdale D, Post M, et al., editors, Telemedicine technical assistance documents, p. 241–66. 2004. Available at: http://telehealth.muhealth.org/general%20information/getting.started.telemedicine.pdf. Accessed 11 Feb 2011.

68. Schein RM, Schmeler MR, Brienza D, et al. Development of a service delivery protocol used for remote wheelchair consultation via telerehabilitation. Telemed J E Health. 2008;14:932–8.

69. Schmeler M, Schein R, McCue M, et al. Telerehabilitation clinical and vocational applications for assistive technology: research, opportunities, and challenges. Int J Telerehabil. 2008;1:12–24.

70. Simmons S, Alverson D, Poropatich R, et al. Applying telehealth in natural and anthropogenic disasters. Telemed J E Health. 2008;14:968–71.

71. Slootmaker SM, Chinapaw MJ, Seidell JC, et al. Accelerometers and internet for physical activity promotion in youth? Feasibility and effectiveness of a minimal intervention. Prev Med. 2010;51(1):31–6.

72. Soopramanien A, Pain H, Stainthrope A, et al. Using telemedicine to provide post-discharge support for patients with spinal cord injuries. J Telemed Telecare. 2005;11 Suppl 1:68–70.

73. Suter P, Suter WN, Johnston D. Theory-based telehealth and patient empowerment. Popul Health Manag. 2011;14(2):87–92. doi:10.1089/pop.2010.0013.

74. Tam SF, Man WK, Hui-Chan CW, et al. Evaluating the efficacy of Tele-cognitive rehabilitation for functional performance in three case studies. Occup Ther Int. 2003;10(1):20–38.

75. Taylor D, Cameron J, Walch L, et al. Exploring the feasibility of videoconference delivery of a self-management program to rural participants with stroke. Telemed J E Health. 2009;15:646–54. doi:10.1089/tmj.2008.0165.

76. Tsuchisawa K, Ono K, Kanda T. Japanese occupational therapy in community mental health and telehealth. J Telemed Telecare. 2000;6 Suppl 2:79–80.

77. Tuerk PW, Yoder M, Ruggiero KJ, et al. A pilot study of prolonged exposure therapy for post-traumatic stress disorder delivered via telehealth technology. J Trauma Stress. 2010;23(1):116–23.

78. Wu G, Keyes LM. Group Tele-exercise for improving balance in elders. Telemed J E Health. 2006;12:561–70.

79. Vismara L, Young G, Stahmer A, et al. Dissemination of evidence-based practice: can we train therapists from a distance? J Autism Dev Disord. 2009;39:1636–51.

80. Wise M, Gustafson DH, Sorkness CA, et al. Internet telehealth for pediatric asthma case management: integrating computerized and case manager features for tailoring a web-based asthma education program. Health Promot Pract. 2007;8:282–91.

81. World Health Organization & World Bank. World report on disability. 2011. Retrieved from: http://whqlibdoc.who.int/publications/2011/9789240685215_eng.pdf Accessed Feb 9, 2012

Additional Resources

American Physical Therapy Association. Position on telehealth. Available at: http://www.apta.org/AM/Template.cfm?Section=Home&CONTENTID=67435&TEMPLATE=/CM/ContentDisplay.cfm.

American Occupational Therapy Association. Position paper on telerehabilitation. Available at: http://media.americantelemed.org/ICOT/AOTA%20telereh05.pdf.

American Speech-Language-Hearing Association. Position statement on telepractice. Available at: http://www.asha.org/docs/html/PS2005-00116.html.

American Telemedicine Association. Available at: http://www.americantelemed.org.

American Telemedicine Association. A blueprint for telerehabilitation guidelines. Available at: http://www.americantelemed.org/files/public/standards/ATA%20Telerehab%20Guidelines%20v1%20(2).pdf; also available at: http://telerehab.pitt.edu/ojs/index.php/Telerehab/article/view/6063/6293.

Association of Telemedicine Service Providers. Available at: http://www.atsp.org/.

Center for Telehealth and E-Health Law (CTel). Available at: http://www.telehealthlawcenter.org/.

Center for Telemedicine Law. Available at: http://ctl.org/.

Federal Telemedicine Gateway. Available at: http://tmgateway.org/.

International Journal of Telerehabilitation. Available at: http://telerehab.pitt.edu/ojs/index.php/telerehab.

Journal of Telemedicine and Telecare. Available at: http://jtt.rsmjournals.com/.

Rehabilitation Engineering Research Center for Telerehabilitation. Available at: http://www.rerctr.pitt.edu/.

Telemedicine and e-Health. Available at: www.liebertpub.com/TMJ.

UC Davis Telemedicine Program. Available at: http://www.telemedicine.ucdmc.ucdavis.edu/.

Chapter 11
Tele-Ergonomics

Nancy A. Baker and Karen Jacobs

Abstract Ergonomics is a scientific discipline that examines the fit between the demands of the task and the capabilities of the users, and provides interventions to improve that fit. Typically, ergonomic interventions and education are performed onsite, and involve the assessment of the person/environment fit, followed by the collaborative development and implementation of plans based on ergonomic principles. While ergonomic interventions have been shown to be effective methods to improve workers' health and productivity, limited access to ergonomic professionals restricts the use ergonomic interventions in the workplace. This chapter discusses methods to apply telerehabilitation delivery methods to ergonomic interventions, a process we are calling tele-ergonomics.

11.1 Introduction

Imagine the following scenario:

It is 7:30 AM; you are starting your work day with a second cup of green tea while reviewing your schedule for the day. It is a snowy Boston morning and you have a busy day—there are four ergonomic jobsite analyses, two life-coaching sessions, a conference call with your department chairperson, a 45-min introduction to ergonomics to students in Arkansas, and three educational sessions on proper body

N.A. Baker (✉)
Department of Occupational Therapy, School of Health and Rehabilitation Sciences,
University of Pittsburgh, 6070 Forbes Tower (Suite 6065), 3600 Forbes Avenue,
Pittsburgh, PA 15260, USA
e-mail: nab36@pitt.edu

K. Jacobs
Department of Occupational Therapy, College of Health and Rehabilitation Sciences:
Sargent College, Boston University, 635 Commonwealth Avenue – Room 511A,
Boston, MA 02215, USA

S. Kumar, E.R. Cohn (eds.), *Telerehabilitation*, Health Informatics,
DOI 10.1007/978-1-4471-4198-3_11, © Springer-Verlag London 2013

mechanics with a food service company in Florida. You turn on your computer, log onto the Internet, and smile into your web camera as you greet your first client for her ergonomic jobsite analysis in a rural area of Pennsylvania. This client has rheumatoid arthritis and, until today, has been unable to find an ergonomic professional to conduct an analysis of her computer workstation. During the 2-h interaction, she revealed that she was pleased that the virtual evaluation was not intrusive, so she did not have to disclose to her employer that she had rheumatoid arthritis. You conclude your evaluation by scheduling a follow-up meeting on Skype in 2 weeks. Before calling your next client during his lunch break for his weekly 30-min life-coaching session, you take a 15-min stretch break, trying to apply ergonomic principles to your own work routine. Your day continues with each service being delivered effectively and on time, without leaving your home office.

This scenario highlights the advantages of using the principles of telerehabilitation to conduct worksite evaluation, intervention, and prevention activities—a process we are calling *tele-ergonomics*. In this chapter, we will discuss the discipline of ergonomics and how it can be adapted to remote delivery methods.

11.2 Ergonomics

Ergonomics is "the scientific discipline concerned with the understanding of interactions among humans and other elements of a system, and the profession that applies theory, principles, data, and methods to design in order to optimize human well-being and overall system performance" [14]. Ergonomics covers a very broad field that examines the fit between the demands of the task, such as environmental, cognitive, organizational, and physical [14], and the capabilities of the users, and provides interventions to improve that fit.

A broad variety of professionals engage in the delivery of ergonomic services, including ergonomists, engineers, human factors personnel, industrial hygienists, occupational therapists, and physical therapists. Their focus can be as broad as redesigning a US Air Force plane cockpit to improve combat performance or designing playgrounds to encourage universal play; or as narrow as adapting a computer workstation to facilitate a worker with a disability to complete job tasks successfully.

Many ergonomic professionals address population-level design, developing systems that can facilitate human performance for a broad range of people (population-wide-ergonomics). Other ergonomic professionals, particularly occupational and physical therapists, may design environments that meet the needs of individuals with unique challenges, often due to a disability (ergonomics-for-one) [18]. In whatever capacity the environment/person fit is evaluated and redesign is addressed, there must be a cooperative interaction between the ergonomic professional assisting with the design of the environment, the people who function within the environment, and the environment itself (Fig. 11.1).

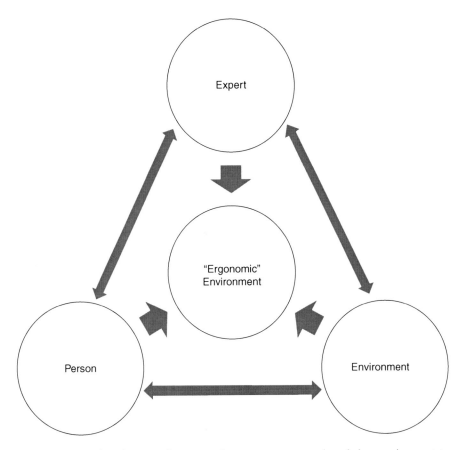

Fig. 11.1 Interactions between the ergonomics expert, person, and workplace environment to develop an "ergonomic environment"

Very often ergonomics is considered in context with work and the working environment, as this is frequently an area where a mismatch exists between the person and the environment, and this mismatch can have significant effects on worker health [20]. Ergonomic assessments and interventions have been shown to be effective in reducing illnesses and injuries in the workplace [7, 23]. This chapter primarily considers ergonomics as it applies to the workplace and workers' health, although the principles can be applied to home environments as well.

11.3 Ergonomic Intervention

The general stages of ergonomic intervention in the workplace are fairly standard [7] and are summed up in Fig. 11.2. Although these stages represent best practice, there are variations on these steps depending on the type and complexity of job

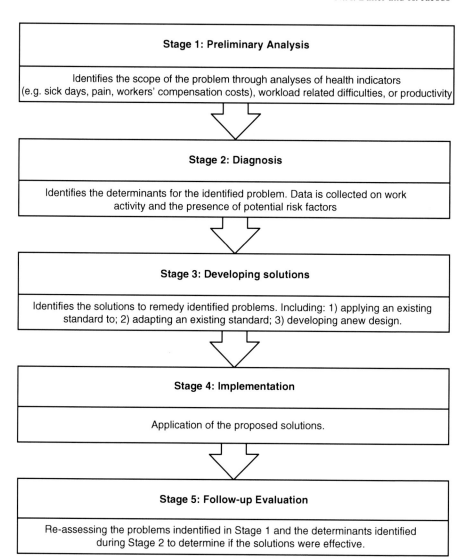

Fig. 11.2 Stages of ergonomic intervention in the workplace

being analyzed, the current guidelines of the most effective intervention, and the type and number of workers involved [7]. The extent to which the worker is included in these stages, a process called participatory ergonomics (PE), is an important consideration. A recent review by Rivilis et al. [23] indicated that interventions that were based on the principles of PE demonstrated positive reductions in musculoskeletal symptoms, injuries, workers' compensation claims, and lost days from work.

11.3.1 Participatory Ergonomics

Although a single guiding framework for conducting PE interventions is still evolving, and the definition of the term varies depending on the source, the fundamental principle of PE is that workers are involved in "planning and controlling a significant amount of their own work activities, with sufficient knowledge and power to influence both processes and outcomes in order to achieve desirable goals" [13, p. 200]. The components of PE vary, but generally the following are included:

1. A core PE "team" needs to be set up that can include workers, management, health and safety personnel, and ergonomic professionals.
2. The PE team receives training on ergonomics, typically from the ergonomic professional.
3. The team devises PE interventions that are tailored to the workplace demands [17].

The findings of a comprehensive review by Hignett and colleagues [13] suggest that the decision-making process between the ergonomic professional and the worker is the most important aspect of PE interventions.

11.3.2 Ergonomic Workstation Assessment and Interventions

The typical mechanism for conducting an ergonomic workstation assessment and intervention is face to face. That is, the ergonomic professional goes to the workplace and evaluates the workstation. This is problematic because many workers do not have easy access to ergonomic assessments and modifications [26], and therefore have to rely on self-analysis or untrained personnel to identify problems and accommodations. There are many online sites that provide the basics of ergonomic assessment and intervention [6, 8, 9, 19, 21]. While these sites provide methods to identify and intervene in problem area, self-assessment may not be adequate to help untrained personnel reduce workstation risks [25, 26]. Workers may not be able to identify risky postures correctly, particularly as people with pain or disorders may have decreased position sense [4, 15]. They may not be able to identify the appropriate workstation accommodation, such as whether to reposition existing equipment or buy new equipment [25, 27]. They may be unable to afford new equipment, and be unaware of legislations, such as the Americans with Disability Act (ADA), that can be used to assist with obtaining reasonable accommodations [12]. Thus, the ability to have a workstation assessed by an ergonomic professional may be necessary to reduce workstation risk adequately or identify the necessary modifications to allow a worker with a disability to work comfortably. Although many health professions are involved in ergonomic assessments and interventions, still a limited number of ergonomic professionals perform these evaluations. These leaves many workers without access to the experts they need.

The problem of access to ergonomic professionals is exacerbated when addressing the unique workplace challenges experienced by workers with disabilities. Conducting an ergonomic assessment to provide workstation redesign for individual workers with disabilities adds an additional degree of specialized knowledge. An ergonomic assessment for a worker with a disability requires an understanding of not only the universal principles of design, but also the effect that a disease process has on the biomechanical, cognitive, social, and sensory systems. In addition, the ergonomic professional needs to know about the availability of assistive technology. This specialized knowledge means that there are few ergonomic professionals with the necessary skills to perform ergonomic assessments of workplaces for those with special needs. This is particularly true in underserved populations, such as minorities, and rural communities.

In particular, because of the limited number of rehabilitation professionals with expertise in ergonomics, many physicians, the gatekeepers of most treatment/intervention, do not realize that ergonomic assessments can be done, and do not refer their clients for evaluations [10]. Since clients also do not realize that this service exists and can be used to help them remain in work, they rarely receive ergonomic assessments [16]. Costs can be prohibitive, if the ergonomic professional has to commute a distance to the site. This also tends to prevent follow-up visits to monitor processes and refine interventions. All these issues, access, cost, and availability, can effectively be addressed, as in our case scenario, by tele-ergonomics.

11.4   Telerehabilitation Meets Ergonomics

Although ergonomic evaluations, interventions, and education are routinely performed live, telerehabilitation methods appear to hold great opportunity for these services to be provided virtually. Telerehabilitation involves the use of technology to assess, evaluate, teach, diagnose, treat, and monitor the rehabilitative process remotely [24]. These same principles can be applied to the ergonomic process and can complement in-person services.

11.4.1   Tele-Ergonomics

Tele-ergonomics has many potential benefits to the field of ergonomics:

(a) It can reduce inequities in access to health resources by bringing ergonomic professionals remotely to underserved areas.
(b) It can improve efficiency in delivery of ergonomic services by eliminating travel time, providing instantaneous access, and improving the coordination of care.
(c) It can reduce the costs of ergonomic assessments, interventions, and education.

(d) It can promote client-centered care, since ergonomic professionals can observe clients in their own work environment.

(e) It can be used to provide onsite education on healthy work practices such as body mechanics, proper lifting techniques, energy conservation strategies, or exercises [2, 22].

One of the primary uses of telerehabilitation is to compensate for the lack of availability of experts [3]. Tele-ergonomics has the potential to revolutionize the delivery of ergonomic services, as it allows ergonomic professionals to interact with any worker at any distance, increasing the impact that they can have on the working population, as exemplified in our case scenario. The ergonomic professional was able to reach a client (ergonomics-for-one) in a remote rural area; provided the day's services (assessment, education, and intervention) in a timely, nonintrusive, and coordinated manner to an individual with a disability and to a population of workers (population-wide-ergonomics) and students (population-wide-ergonomics); and eliminated the additional costs that would have been incurred if she had to commute to reach these clients.

Although the use of telerehabilitation technologies is expanding quickly as a viable method of service delivery, it has not, to our knowledge, been used for ergonomic assessments. However, there have been descriptions of elements of tele-ergonomics used in two studies. Bruce and Sanford [5] described the use of teleconferencing to complete remote assessments. Their paper discussed the need for a highly structured and comprehensive assessment tool to be able to complete remote assessments. They did not describe their methodology but, instead, discussed a conceptual framework for developing a remote assessment tool. Backman and her colleagues [1] developed the ergonomic assessment tool for arthritis (EATA) to evaluate the workplace for people with arthritis. As many workers with arthritis do not wish to disclose that they have the disease, they often do not want an ergonomic professional to visit the workplace. Backman et al. [1], therefore, developed the EATA so that workers could gather the data for the assessment, without the professional visiting the workplace. Pilot testing of the method indicated that workers could successfully gather the appropriate information for appropriate intervention identification.

11.4.2   Tele-Ergonomic Technology

A wide range of technology can be used in tele-ergonomics. Asynchronous communication can be facilitated through instructional audio tools and posting in online discussion areas. The use of web cameras can facilitate real-time (synchronous) video interactions between the worker(s) and the ergonomic professional. These synchronous interactions promote PE through collaborative workstation design/ redesign. Videoconferencing allows clients to send real-time images of problems, and ergonomic professionals can respond quickly and effectively to address these problems. The use of social networking group sites such as on *Facebook* or *LinkedIn* can facilitate sharing suggestions about solutions or support workers' efforts to improve their work environment.

Monitoring of adherence to an intervention can be incorporated into tele-ergonomics through telemonitoring (i.e., using self-monitoring analysis and reporting technology (SMART) to monitor performance remotely). Handheld technology such as smart phones or personal digital assistants (PDAs) can be used by workers on the job to rate productions unobtrusively and quickly, identify symptoms, or provide real-time information about the job tasks. For example, workers could receive text messages at set times during the day to complete a quick feedback form and e-mail photographs of problem areas in the workplace via their smart phones or web cameras to ergonomic professionals to analyze. In addition, since notebook computers are ubiquitous and access to the web is easy, remote methods can be brought outside of the office and to any location where the workers work.

Virtual reality options can be used effectively with tele-ergonomics. For example, using three-dimensional constructions of the architectural features of the work environment can be used to determine accessibility. This approach would be appropriate for a client with a disability where accessibility may be an issue in the workplace. For example, Harrison and his colleagues [11] used a virtual environment as part of the assessment and training for inexperienced, powered-wheelchair users.

In a population-wide ergonomic intervention, the initial phase is to identify the problem [7] and its prevalence and incidence within the company (Fig. 11.2). As many workplace records are digital, it would be feasible to access them via Internet or e-mail. For example, many forms can be completed via online surveys, such as Survey Monkey or Zoomerang. As these forms are already in database format, it is easy to use database management software such as Excel or Access, or statistical software such as SPSS or SAT, to analyze and extract data that will help describe the extent and type of problems. The second aspect of ergonomic assessment is to identify specific problem areas, for both population-wide-ergonomics and ergonomics-for-one (Fig. 11.2). Typically, this aspect of assessment relies heavily on video technology and digital photography. These technologies can be used effectively with workers with unusual body types, such as those with rheumatoid arthritis. As described in our case scenario, the ergonomic professional videotaped her client typing on the computer during the assessment and then reviewed the videotape at another time to identify how the workstation could be modified to fit her specific needs. Additional enhancements over typical ergonomic interventions are the ability to synchronize all aspects of the assessment simultaneously in one place. Using an open source platform such as Moodle, all information needed to conduct a tele-ergonomic assessment can be situated in one accessible remote location. Developing and implementing tele-ergonomic interventions (Stages 3 and 4) can easily be accomplished using free high-quality video chat and videoconferencing resources, such as Skype or ooVoo, for synchronous discussions.

For management activities such as holding a meeting where working on a shared document promotes efficiency of time and resources, there are interactive technologies such as a Wiki or Googledoc. In our case scenario, the ergonomic professional had a meeting with her department chairperson to go over a manuscript they were coauthoring. They placed the manuscript on a virtual Wikispaces site and worked simultaneously to edit the manuscript. Although both these individuals have busy schedules, they were able to arrange for their appointment by using the free scheduling software, Doodle®. If opinions by multiple individuals need to be polled, Doodle® has this free feature too.

Tele-ergonomics can exceed a typical ergonomic program through its ability to provide real-time monitoring and feedback of ergonomic interventions. Workers can be provided with smart phones or other handheld devices to document, in real time, pro and con outcomes. Electronic monitoring devices, such as computer keystroke monitors, can stream productivity information directly to assessors. For ergonomic-for-one individuals who need feedback on performance or help to monitor ability, smart phones could be used for one-on-one on the job mentoring, reminders, or positive feedback. This would particularly be useful for workers with cognitive or emotional impairments that may respond best to instantaneous and focused feedback. Using this remote technology, one professional could monitor several workers at different job sites simultaneously and be ready for real-time instantaneous feedback.

Tele-ergonomics can also provide enhanced teaching opportunities through web-based applications or smart phone applications (apps). Video-based interactive technologies such as kinetics could be used to provide body mechanics training, with the opportunities for immediate and concrete feedback about performance. These technologies could also be used to provide onsite exercise programs to promote healthy behaviors.

11.4.3 Advantages of Tele-Ergonomics

There are many benefits to tele-ergonomics as a method to deliver ergonomic services. For example, since tele-ergonomics relies on low-visibility, commercially available web cameras, it can reduce the potential intrusiveness of an ergonomic assessment (as described in our case scenario), intervention, and education. Studies have suggested that even with the initial cost of equipment, telerehabilitation is very cost effective: one estimate reported that the United States could save $4.3 billion a year if it implemented telehealth in emergency rooms, prisons, nursing homes, and physician offices alone [22]. On the societal level, the tele-ergonomics has the potential to reduce the overall economic burden associated with musculoskeletal discomfort in the workplace. On the personal level, tele-ergonomics has the potential to reduce the personal cost of obtaining expert ergonomic assessments, interventions, and education. For ergonomic professionals, tele-ergonomics can provide an evidence-based and systematic program for ergonomic assessments, intervention, and education. It can broaden their client base, allowing them access to individuals and populations from a distance without geographic limitations. In our case scenario, the ergonomic expert was able to broaden her client base in California, Florida, Arkansas, and Pennsylvania without leaving Boston.

11.5   Additional Considerations

As all forms of telerehabilitation evolve, we must be mindful of ongoing issues that need to be addressed, such as the development of evidence-based guidelines for use, reimbursement, and legal and ethical ramifications [24]. Standardized methods need to be developed to create the optimal, best-practice method of using tele-ergonomics, and research will need to be conducted to ascertain its effectiveness. The good news is that there are many resources, such as this textbook, journals such as *International Journal of Telerehabilitation* and *Journal of Telemedicine and Telecare*, national and state associations, and telerehabilitation organizations to help mentor ergonomic professionals interested in telerehabilitation methods.

11.6   Conclusion

Using tele-ergonomics to identify and intervene in the workplace is really only limited by the imagination of ergonomic professionals and their access and understanding of technology. Obviously, not all ergonomic professionals will feel comfortable using all potential aspects of tele-ergonomics; however, much of the hardware, software, and other elements of the telerehabilitation technology are readily and easily available, even to novices. In the long run, tele-ergonomics has the potential to provide workers with enhanced access to ergonomic professionals, as it allows those with skills in ergonomics to interact with any worker at any distance. Tele-ergonomics will increase the impact that ergonomic professionals can have on the working population, and allow for the more efficient delivery of ergonomic services nationally and globally.

Summary

- Ergonomics is "the scientific discipline concerned with the understanding of interactions among humans and other elements of a system, and the profession that applies theory, principles, data, and methods to design in order to optimize human well-being and overall system performance."
- Although ergonomic evaluations, interventions, and education are routinely performed live, telerehabilitation methods appear to hold great opportunity for these services to be provided virtually.
- Tele-ergonomics has the potential to revolutionize the delivery of ergonomic services, as it allows ergonomic professionals to interact with any worker at any distance, increasing the impact that they can have on the working population.
- Although ergonomic interventions have been shown to be effective in improving workers' health and productivity, limited access to ergonomic professionals restricts the use ergonomic interventions in the workplace.

- Standardized methods need to be developed to create the optimal, best-practice method of using tele-ergonomics, and research will need to be conducted to ascertain its effectiveness.

Abbreviations/Acronyms

EATA   Ergonomic assessment tool for arthritis
PDA   Personal digital assistant
PE   Participatory ergonomics
SMART   Self-monitoring analysis and reporting technology

References

1. Backman CL, Village J, Lacaille D. The ergonomic assessment tool for arthritis: development and pilot testing. Arthritis Rheum. 2008;59:1495–503.
2. Bashur RL, Shannon GW. National telemedicine initiatives: essential to healthcare reform. Telemed J E Health. 2009;15:600–10.
3. Brecht RM, Barrett JE. Telemedicine in the United States. In: Viegas SF, Dunn K, editors. Telemedicine, practicing in the information age. Philadelphia: Lippincott-Raven; 1998.
4. Brouwer B, Mazzoni C, Pearce GW. Tracking ability in subjects symptomatic of cumulative trauma disorder: does it relate to disability? Ergonomics. 2001;44:443–56.
5. Bruce C, Sanford JA. Development of an evidence-based conceptual framework for workplace assessment. Work. 2006;27:381–9.
6. Cal/OSHA Consultation Service Research and Education Unit. Easy ergonomics for desktop computer users. 2005. Available at: http://www.dir.ca.gov/dosh/dosh_publications/ComputerErgo.pdf. Accessed 25 Feb 2010.
7. Denis D, St-Vincent M, Imbeau D, et al. Intervention practices in musculoskeletal disorder prevention: a critical literature review. Appl Ergon. 2008;39:1–14.
8. Division of Occupational Health and Safety (DOHS). Ergonomics for computer workstations. N.D. Available at: http://dohs.ors.od.nih.gov/ergo_computers.htm. Accessed 25 Feb 2010.
9. Ergonomics Working Group. Creating the ideal computer workstation: a step-by-step guide. 2002. Available at: http://www.ergoworkinggroup.org/ewgweb/SubPages/ProgramTools/Publications/Workstation_Guide_Web.pdf. Accessed 25 Feb 2010.
10. Gilworth G, Haigh R, Tennant A. Do rheumatologists recognize their patients' work-related problems. Rheumatology. 2001;l40:1206–10.
11. Harrison A, Derwent G, Enticknap A, et al. The role of virtual reality technology in the assessment and training of inexperienced powered wheelchair users. Dis Rehabil. 2002;24:599–606.
12. Hernandez B, Keys C, Balcazar F. The Americans with disabilities act knowledge survey: strong psychometrics and weak knowledge. Rehabil Psychol. 2003;48:93–9.
13. Hignett S, Wilson JR, Morris W. Finding ergonomic solutions – participatory approaches. Occup Med. 2005;55:200–7.
14. International Ergonomics Association. What is ergonomics. 2000. Available at: http://www.iea.cc/01_what/What%20is%20Ergonomics.html. Accessed 12 Jan 2011.
15. Juul-Kristensen B, Lund H, Hansen K, et al. Poorer elbow proprioception in patients with lateral epicondylitis than in healthy controls: a cross-sectional study. J Shoulder Elbow Surg. 2008;17:72S–81.

16. Lacaille D, White MA, Backman CL, et al. Problems faced at work due to inflammatory arthritis: new insights gained from understanding patients' perspective. Arthritis Care Res. 2007;57:1269–79.
17. Loisel P, Gosselin L, Durand P, et al. Implementation of a participatory ergonomics program in the rehabilitation of workers suffering from subacute back pain. Appl Ergon. 2001; 32:53–60.
18. McQuistion L. Ergonomics-for-one: an introduction. In: Berg Rice VJ, editor. Ergonomics in health care and rehabilitation. Boston: Butterworth-Heinemann; 1998.
19. National Institute for Occupational Safety and Health. Ergonomics and musculoskeletal disorders. N.D. Available at: http://www.cdc.gov/niosh/topics/ergonomics/. Accessed 2 Feb 2011.
20. National Research Council and the Institute of Medicine. Musculoskeletal disorders and the workplace: low back and upper extremity. Washington, D.C.: National Academy Press; 2001.
21. Occupational Safety & Health Administration. eTool – computer workstations. N.D. Available at: http://www.osha.gov/SLTC/etools/computerworkstations/index.html. Accessed 25 Feb 2010.
22. Pan E, Cusack C, Hook J, et al. The value of provider to provide telehealth. Telemed J E Health. 2008;14:446–53.
23. Rivilis I, van Eerd D, Cullen K, et al. Effectiveness of participatory ergonomic interventions on health outcomes: a systematic review. Appl Ergon. 2008;39:342–58.
24. Schmeler MR, Schein RM, Fairman A, et al. Telerehabilitation position paper: American occupational therapy association. AJOT. 2010;64:S92–102.
25. Schreuer N, Myhill WN, Aratan-Bergman T, et al. Workplace accommodations: occupational therapists as mediators in the interactive process. Work. 2009;34:149–60.
26. Shaw WS, Feuerstein M. Generating workplace accommodations: lessons learned from the integrated case management study. J Occup Rehabil. 2004;14:207–16.
27. Shaw W, Hong QN, Pransky G, et al. A literature review describing the role of return-to-work coordinators in trial programs and interventions designed to prevent workplace disability. J Occup Rehabil. 2008;18:2–15.

Chapter 12
Electronic Record and Telerehabilitation

Valerie J.M. Watzlaf and Sohrab Moeini

Abstract A health information explosion is upon us. This explosion beckons which methods should be used to store, retrieve, process, mine, and compute health information. Most health information is now stored in an electronic form, such as an electronic medical record (EMR), which is then cultivated and exchanged across health-care facilities into the electronic health record (EHR). Telerehabilitation (TR) sessions include a wealth of vital health information that is necessary for the rehabilitation professional to use to properly treat and manage their client's care. How are TR sessions stored, accessed, and used within the EMR or EHR? What are the best TR systems to use and what is the best method to use to link the TR session to the EMR or EHR? This chapter will discuss the relationship between the electronic record and TR as well as the most appropriate methods to use when integrating both systems in the provision of rehabilitation therapy.

12.1 Introduction

In 2009, the U.S. government enacted the American Recovery and Reinvestment Act (ARRA). Part of this initiative, known as the Health Information Technology for Economic and Clinical Health Act (HITECH), sets forth the necessary ground work for proper health IT adoption [4]. Most hospital systems are beginning the transition toward an electronic medium, and in the next decade a large shift toward electronic health record (EHR) interoperability will be seen. The ability to share,

V.J.M. Watzlaf (✉)
Department of Health Information Management,
School of Health and Rehabilitation Sciences, University of Pittsburgh,
6030 Forbes Tower, 3600 Forbes Avenue, Pittsburgh 15260, PA, USA
e-mail: valgeo@pitt.edu

S. Moeini
Systems Analyst, UPMC
Pittsburgh, PA
e-mail: ssm145@gmail.com

S. Kumar, E.R. Cohn (eds.), *Telerehabilitation*, Health Informatics,
DOI 10.1007/978-1-4471-4198-3_12, © Springer-Verlag London 2013

securely, electronic health documents across health-care facilities and other health-care entities is an essential goal of any health-care provider, consumer, or facility. Another piece of essential health information that may also be included in this digital space is a telerehabilitation (TR) session. The TR session may be recorded, saved, and linked to the EHR as a video or audio format, which can be accessed as necessary by a team of rehabilitation providers. Again, for this seamless transition to occur, various systems, such as a common standard for communication, are necessary so that a TR session on one system can easily integrate with an EHR on another system. To enable the integration between the EHR and the TR session, several components within both systems are necessary and will be explained throughout this chapter.

12.2 Definition of Electronic Record

Several different terms are used for different types of electronic records in health care:

- Electronic health record (EHR)
- Computer-based patient record (CPR)
- Electronic medical record (EMR)
- Electronic patient record (EPR)
- Personal health record (PHR)

Over the years, different health-care associations have defined them differently and several of the terms are not in use very much today (CPR, EPR). The term EMR refers to a legal record created in a specific health-care environment. This record is the result of data gathered into the clinical data repository (CDR) by the various EMR solutions [computerized provider order entry (CPOE), picture archiving and communication systems (PACS), etc.] within the hospital. The biggest difference between the EMR and EHR is that the EMR is usually made up of health information from one health-care facility, whereas the EHR encompasses health information across several health-care facilities. Many times, these terms are used interchangeably in the health-care industry and outside of it. Hospital systems must build and strengthen their EMR solutions if they want to realize a fully functional EHR. So, the EHR becomes the overarching collection of various EMRs at different institutions, now connected and interoperable. The road to adoption and implementation of an EMR is difficult, as each hospital system is different having varying views on technology implementations, processes, information flow, and management structures. EMRs must meet these challenges by focusing on the most important task that needs to be completed by clinicians and hospital staff, which is providing quality patient care. Another type of health record is the PHR, which is usually developed by the patient or client based on documentation that the patient has collected as well as current health record information the patient may have received from their physician or health-care facility. Each patient is encouraged to keep a PHR, not only on themselves but also on their children, parents, or other family members. Retaining a PHR is becoming increasingly important as patients collect and record their blood pressure, weight, blood sugar, etc. at home. Also, as TR sessions are conducted and clients are asked to keep a diary of certain tasks and exercises, the PHR becomes a very accurate and important document to link with the EMR/EHR for use by healthcare providers.

12.3   Definition of TR

According to the Telerehabilitation Special Interest Group of the American Telemedicine Association [1], TR refers to the delivery of rehabilitation services through communication and information technologies that encompass a range of clinical assessments, such as rehabilitation monitoring, prevention, intervention, supervision, education, consultation, and counseling. The TR services are provided by qualified professionals such as physical and occupational therapists, as along with assistance from family members and caregivers. The TR service can be provided in medical settings and schools, and, of course, at home. Credentialing, accountability, billing and coding, quality documentation, privacy and confidentiality, storage, retrieval and security of client records, client access of health information via tele-health technologies, use of proper equipment and safety issues, as well as quality management systems are all necessary when providing TR services. These issues and their relationship with the EHR will be expanded on throughout this chapter.

12.4   Background of the Electronic Record

Since 2006, we are slowly realizing the realities of a fully capable EHR system. According to the HealthCare Information and Management Systems Society (HIMSS), the U.S. utilization of an EMR is growing. Figure 12.1 shows a graph

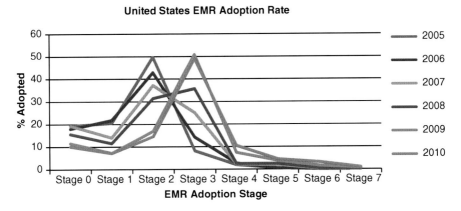

Fig. 12.1 Stages of EMR adoption in the United States by year

depicting the eight stages of EMR adoption in the United States by year. It ranges from Stage 0, which may include some clinical automation, to Stage 7, which encompasses a full paperless EMR environment with health information exchange (HIE) across the full continuum of care and the use of data mining and analytics to extract data for use in patient care and research. Based on the data collected and analyzed from the HIMSS Analytics website, one can see that the EMR is peaking around Stages 3 and 4, which include first- and second-level clinical decision support, some level of PACS, clinical documentation, and some level of CPOE. Moving toward a totally paperless electronic record environment in which HIE is second nature is not an easy task, but one in which health-care facilities are striving to meet [6].

12.5   EHR and TR

An EHR system is a large body of information. To access an EHR system, an application is built within the EHR or, a connection is achieved via various web technologies. The EHR framework endorsed by HIMSS is discussed below [6]. It contains various core system components to drive internal hospital/ambulatory data collection. This system is also connected to various other subsystems that serve to generate and gather data about a patient.

Figure 12.2 depicts a traditional EHR conceptual model with the core EMR components in blue. The core features built into an EMR system include CPOE, point of care charting systems (POC), and electronic medication administration record (EMAR). The CPOE is used by physicians and other hospital staff to enter order information directly into the system. The POC is used during bedside care to gather more information about the patient, and the EMAR is used to automate many medication administrative tasks within the hospital system. From the outside, various departmental source systems flow (radiology, laboratory, pharmacy, etc.) into the CDR, and this is the starting point of the detailed data that eventually work up to the clinical data warehouse (CDW) for a highly summarized view of the data. In the

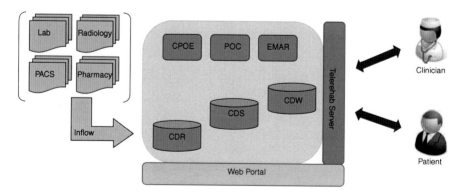

Fig. 12.2 Conceptual model of EHR with TR environment

middle is the clinical decision support system (CDS), which serves to send alerts and reminders to CPOE and EMAR systems. The CDR, CDS, and CDW are core database components of any EHR system. Without these data stores, an EHR could quickly lose its value. One of the last applications to be incorporated into the overall picture of an EHR is a web portal to connect to other EHRs and third-party applications. Also incorporated into this specific EHR model is the TR server from which the TR application will maintain sessions from clients to the server; hence, a client–server architecture can be deployed. The clients connect to the server using standard protocols such as TCP/IP. This allows them to connect not only to each other but also to the EHR database. The TR application is not a core EMR application; rather it serves as a subsystem within the overall encompassing EHR system.

12.6   Certification

The Certification Commission on Health Information Technology (CCHIT) provides criteria that vendors and other developers of health information technology products, such as the EHR, must meet to become certified. The Department of Health and Human Services (DHHS) at the Office of the National Coordinator for Health Information Technology (ONC) has recognized CCHIT as an Authorized Testing and Certification Body (ONC-ATCB) so that EHRs certified by CCHIT are capable of meeting the meaningful use (MU) criteria established by the HHS-ONC. CCHIT develops criteria for several types of EHRs such as emergency, ambulatory, inpatient, behavioral health, long-term and post-acute care, and ePrescribing. The criteria are extensive and include the following major categories [3]:

Long-term and post-acute care example of CCHIT criteria major categories:

1. Patient record and demographics
2. Problem list
3. Medication list
4. Allergy and adverse reaction list
5. Patient history
6. Patient views
7. Clinical documents and notes (e.g., document multidisciplinary case conferences)
8. External clinical notes
9. Patient instructions
10. General ordering requirements
11. Medication prescribing and ordering
12. Drug interaction
13. Medication reconciliation
14. Order diagnostic tests
15. Referral management
16. Order sets
17. Specimen collection

18. Results
19. Consents and authorizations
20. Patient advance directives
21. Care plans, guidelines, and protocols
22. Medication administration
23. Immunization management
24. Blood administration
25. Disease management, preventive services, and wellness
26. Clinical task management
27. Interprovider communication
28. Provider information
29. Medical equipment
30. Instrument assessment
31. Report generation
32. Health record output
33. Clinical research
34. Administrative
35. Clinical decision support administration
36. Confidentiality
37. Data retention, availability, and destruction
38. Concurrent use
39. ePrescribing
40. Clinical documentation
41. Access control
42. Audits
43. Authentication
44. Documentation related to system installation, etc.
45. Technical services
46. Backup/recovery
47. Interdomain (communicate identity information across domains)

Limited information is included on how TR services should be stored or documented. There was some guidance on recording case conferences, but more guidance on how TR sessions should be made an essential part of the EHR is needed within any EHR standard.

12.7 Coding and Reimbursement

If health-care facilities become certified and contain all the criteria required by CCHIT, the EHR will store a wealth of health information. As documentation within the EHR is enhanced by both structured and free text, more specificity in documentation will be seen, which may lead to improved coding and accurate

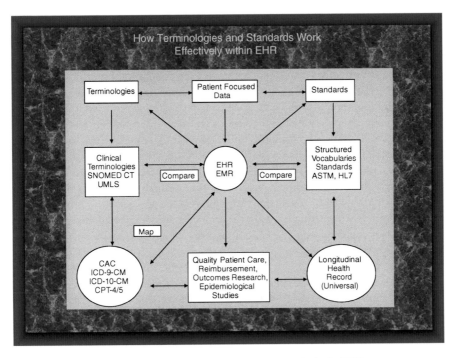

Fig. 12.3 Terminologies, classification systems, and standards within the EHR

reimbursement. On October 1, 2014, a new coding system, ICD-10-CM, will emerge. It has over 68,000 new codes compared to approximately 14,000 in ICD-9-CM. Therefore, increased documentation specificity will be necessary for accurate coding and reimbursement. Rehabilitation professionals should educate themselves on the new ICD-10-CM coding system as well as hire certified coders and include computer-assisted coding (CAC) systems within their EHR systems. Figure 12.3 demonstrates how clinical terminologies such as SNOMED will link clinical terms within the EHR to a classification system such as ICD-10-CM, which will then be linked to a diagnosis-related group (DRG) that will link to payment. A major advantage of the CAC system is that it can read, through natural language processing (NLP), the structured and free text within an EHR and then automatically provide possible ICD-10-CM codes that match the text. A coder is still needed to make sure that these codes are correct, but it provides an essential step that will be very necessary as classification systems become larger and more complex. TR documentation is essential if proper coding and reimbursement is to transpire. Speech recognition software can also be used to automatically document TR sessions as they occur so that every essential element of the session is documented. This will enhance not only the coding and reimbursement, but also the quality of documentation within the EHR, which will improve communication among health-care providers.

12.8 Education and Training on EHR and TR Use

Many EHR software companies and health-care facilities are not always certain about the most effective way to educate and train rehabilitation professionals on the use of the EHR. Also, rehabilitation professionals need education and training that is specific to their discipline and needs. Effective education and training of all EHR users are necessary and should be included in the planning phase of every EHR and TR system. The training and education of any user can be a difficult task. Some common pitfalls in EHR and TR implementation and training may include not planning on and allowing enough time for adequate and effective training, not providing training outside of the clinical setting, not providing a training room for staff to practice, not appointing a superuser, miscommunication between trainers when using the train-the-trainer method, not evaluating the staff's readiness for implementing the system, and not delaying implementation if staff are not prepared [10].

With the development of MU criteria and the EHR, effective and efficient training methods are of paramount importance in any setting. Some authors do agree that training is important and, according to Robert Lowe, training is the key to EMR success [8]. However, the types of training, the length of time to train, who to train, and when to train tend to be inconsistent. According to Capanna et al. [2], several different training methods are necessary to engage the user fully into using not only the EHR but also other telehealth technologies such as TR services. Table 12.1 describes some of these training techniques. A combination of all techniques is needed, based on individual learning preferences.

12.9 Quality Management Systems

With the establishment of several different governing agencies, such as the Centers for Medicare and Medicaid (CMS), The Joint Commission, and State Departments of Health requiring the collection, analysis, and reporting of core quality measures, many health-care entities are developing a systematic quality

Table 12.1 EHR education and training methods

Training method	Advantages	Disadvantages
In classroom training/ scenario training	Real-life examples, able to ask trainer questions	Too structured, does not show issues that are out of the box
Onsite	Uses application on real patients	Adds time to client visit, can fumble around application in front of client
Online courses	Gets to see application	Cannot interact with course or ask trainer questions
Reference materials	Visual pictures and screenshots	Not able to ask questions—no trainer present

improvement process that automatically secures this type of information. Health-care entities will want to make sure that this information is accurate because a comparison of how they meet these measures will be made available to the public. With advancements in EHR and TR systems, much of the core measure documentation is already available. The ability to extract these data so that it meets the core measures require not only a certified EHR but also health-care professionals who know how to extract, tabulate, and report this type of information. The EHR and TR information are just tools that will aid in these requirements. However, knowing the best possible technologies to use to enhance this process is essential and needed when playing a role in the development and use of the EHR and TR systems.

12.10   Privacy and Security in TR

One of the most important topics in the area of TR is addressing privacy and security. Brennan et al. [1] present technical guidelines for TR, which address areas in privacy and security. Watzlaf et al. [11] also go further in addressing TR privacy and security by presenting a checklist for ensuring proper TR implementation. A TR session presents new topics in patient security that is just beginning to be addressed. Moving away from the traditional textual information to audio and video, as the patient is being assessed, brings with it many different concerns from a privacy and security prospective, and detailed attention must be paid in ensuring this security. So how do we protect a TR session and the data it generates? It would be naïve to say that the minimum security protocols will completely safeguard this data. All systems have flaws and they can be exploited given time and skill. However, there are steps that can be taken to minimize privacy attacks and security failures. The checklist, adapted from the article by Watzlaf et al. [11], details some of the most important points to implement.

1. Form a team of health and legal professionals that will examine TR software systems to determine if it meets federal (HIPAA), state, local, and facility-wide privacy and security regulations. Also, federal and state policies change frequently, so again the team must ensure that someone is on top of these changes. The team may consist of the health-care facility attorney, risk management personnel, health information administrator/privacy officer, security officer (IT), and representative therapists (e.g., occupational therapist, physical therapist, and speech-language pathologist).
2. Educate and train therapists and other rehabilitation personnel who use TR software applications for videoconferencing on all aspects of privacy and security issues related to videoconferencing as well as exchange of other protected health information (PHI). Awareness training on all aspects of HIPAA security rules in relation to TR and software use, spyware, password security, and encryption should be emphasized in relation to videoconferencing.

Education and training should emphasize what therapists should look for when considering use of certain software applications for video therapy in relation to privacy and security as well as quality and reliability. Many times, the privacy and security of a system are overlooked because of how well it can provide a TR service.

3. Develop an informed consent that patients sign; it should explain the TR therapy that will be provided, how the technology software will be used and why, the benefits of the TR and the use of videoconferencing communication, as well as the risks related to privacy and security. Have the team attorney review the informed consent to make sure that it meets all federal (HIPAA), state, and local regulations.

4. Incident response is necessary and should include documentation regarding the incident, the response to the incident, any effects of the incident, as well as policies and procedures that were followed in response to the incident. If policies and procedures are not in place for incident response, then these should be developed with the security and privacy officers.

5. Use the HIPAA compliance checklist or purchase HIPAA compliance software specific to TR systems that will walk you through each piece of the HIPAA legislation to make it certain that the software is private and secure.

6. Follow all applicable security safeguards when using TR systems, such as those recommended by the Garfinkel [5] and NIST [7]. These include not using the username and password for anything else but videoconferencing, changing it frequently, and not making it easy to identify; not having viruses on the computer used for videoconferencing; never using it for emergency services; and consistently authenticating who you are communicating with, especially when used for teletherapy video sessions.

7. Provide audit controls for using software applications so that they are secure and private. Focus on the transmission of data through videoconferencing, how that data are made private and secure during the telecommunication, and also how privately and securely the data are stored and released to internal and outside entities.

To address the ATA technical guidelines [1] and work done by Watzlaf et al. [11], a TR implementation should include the following:

Physical security policy: Implement up-to-date firewall and antivirus software on the server. When accessing the server, provide the users/employees with a level of access appropriate to their job function. Employ network procedures such as disabling port mirroring on switch/router. Disabling port mirroring can help lessen the chance that packets on one port are copied on another by an unauthorized party.

Dedicated server: This will completely eliminate non-TR-related computer activity that could leave the system open to virus, Trojans, worms, logic bombs, etc.

Strong encryption method for transferring data: Audio and video must be encrypted to ensure security in transmission. For example, real-time transport protocol (RTP) is used heavily in streaming video and videoconferencing today. Because TR deals with confidential, patient-sensitive data, something different must be employed requiring authentication. Two subsets of RTP are secure real-time transport protocol (SRTP) and secure real-time control protocol (SRTCP), which use encryption, message authentication, and integrity within each packet. Using these types of methods will help ensure further security for patient data.

Two-factor authentication: The users connecting to the system must be legitimate users, in this case clinicians. Implementing this type of protocol will ensure that if a password is stolen then there is another layer of defense in unauthorized access. Also implement policy to change passwords frequently.

12.11 VISYTER: A Model for TR Therapy

In this brief case study, a software platform known as VISYTER (Versatile and Integrated System for Telerehabilitation) is described [9]. VISYTER is a software platform for building TR-related applications. The implementation costs of VISYTER are fairly low, needing only a web cam and a modern PC; everything else is handled via the software client. This also lends nicely to ease of use, as setup of the client is seamless once the PC and web cam are running. The VISYTER architecture consists of client software, a server, and hardware equipment. One or more clients connect to each other via the client software and the server. VISYTER also employs authentication, authorization, and encryption protocols to make sure that only valid users are able to connect for each session [9]. VISYTER can be further outfitted with various hardware accessories such as a teleprompter, a stylus, and a tablet for specific TR exercises. VISYTER's architecture is divided into three main layers: interface, application, and transport. The application layer allows the ability for EHR access [9]. Furthermore, one of the strengths of VISYTER is that it allows the clinician to connect to an EHR system allowing for seamless integration of the rehabilitation session and also the patients' medical information. Over a 2-year period, VISYTER was implemented in a wheelchair mobility program in rural areas of western Pennsylvania. The TR assessment was initiated by expert wheelchair practitioners at the University of Pittsburgh Medical Center (UPMC) in conjunction with therapists in each rural clinic. Overall, the assessment was a success showing positive feedback with above average scores on a TR survey [9]. This is just one of the many interventions that are beginning to shape the field of TR. Figure 12.4 shows the benefits of this TR application. In relation to our EHR model, Fig. 12.5 shows how VISYTER would work with the model. In Fig. 12.5, VISYTER is an outside system, independent of the EHR model, connecting to the web portal to access the EHR data.

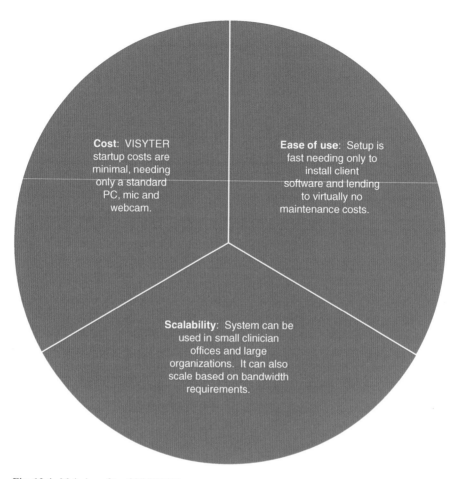

Cost: VISYTER startup costs are minimal, needing only a standard PC, mic and webcam.

Ease of use: Setup is fast needing only to install client software and lending to virtually no maintenance costs.

Scalability: System can be used in small clinician offices and large organizations. It can also scale based on bandwidth requirements.

Fig. 12.4 Main benefits of VISYTER

12.12   Conclusion

A realization of much of the work that has gone into designing a fully operational EHR system has begun to emerge. One of the keys to the successful growth of EHR systems is interoperability. Along this bridge of interoperability come TR and its connection with the EHR. If the EHR is to serve as the digital blueprint of a client, then surely TR will help facilitate this idea by connecting clinicians to clients and to further contribute to the client record. However, there are also administrative, clinical, and technical guidelines to follow when implementing a TR solution, and each plays a role in protecting the privacy and security of the patient.

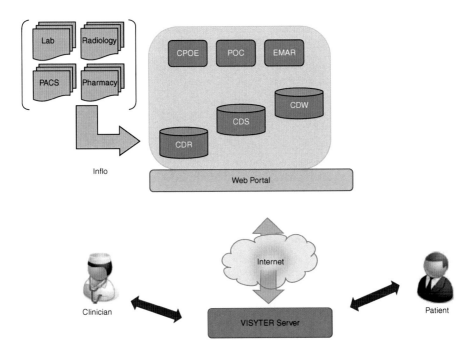

Fig. 12.5 VISYTER as an outside system connecting via web portal

Summary

- Most health information is now stored in an electronic form, such as an electronic medical record (EMR), which is then cultivated and exchanged across health-care facilities into the electronic health record (EHR). EMR is usually made up of health information from one health-care facility, whereas the EHR encompasses health information across several health-care facilities.
- Telerehabilitation refers to the delivery of rehabilitation services through communication and information technologies that encompass a range of clinical assessments, such as rehabilitation monitoring, prevention, intervention, supervision, education, consultation, and counseling.
- A telerehabilitation session may be recorded, saved, and linked to the EHR as a video or audio format, which can be accessed as necessary by a rehabilitation team of providers.
- Effective education and training of all EHR users are necessary and should be included in the planning phase of every EHR and telerehabilitation system.
- Addressing the issue of privacy and security is very important in telerehabilitation. Moving away from the traditional textual information to audio and video, as the patient is being assessed, brings with it many different concerns that require detailed attention in ensuring privacy and security.

Abbreviations/Acronyms

ARRA	American Recovery and Reinvestment Act
ATA	American Telemedicine Association
CAC	Computer-assisted coding
CCHIT	Certification Commission on Health Information Technology
CDR	Clinical data repository
CDS	Clinical decision support system
CDW	Clinical data warehouse
CMS	Centers for Medicare and Medicaid
CPOE	Computerized Provider Order Entry
CPR	Computer-based patient record
DHHS	Department of Health and Human Services
DRG	Diagnosis-related group
EHR	Electronic health record
EMAR	Electronic medication administration record
EMR	Electronic medical record
EPR	Electronic patient record
HIE	Health information exchange
HIMSS	HealthCare Information and Management Systems Society
HITECH	Health Information Technology for Economic and Clinical Health Act
MU	Meaningful use
NLP	Natural language processing
ONC	Office of the National Coordinator for Health Information Technology
ONC-ATCB	Authorized Testing and Certification Body of ONC
PACS	Picture Archiving and Communication Systems
PHI	Protected health information
PHR	Personal health record
POC	Point of care charting systems
RTP	Real-time transport protocol
SRTCP	Secure real-time control protocol
SRTP	Secure real-time transport protocol
TR	Telerehabilitation
UPMC	University of Pittsburgh Medical Center
VISYTER	Versatile and Integrated System for Telerehabilitation

References

1. Brennan D, Tindall L, Theodoros D, et al. A blueprint for telerehabilitation guidelines. Int J Telerehabil. 2010;2(2):31–4. doi:10.5195/ijt.2010.6063.
2. Capanna A, Watzlaf V. Lessons learned during ambulatory electronic health record (EHR) implementation and training. In: Proceedings of the AHIMA convention, Orlando, Oct 2010.

3. CCHIT website. Available at: http://www.cchit.org/sites/all/files/CCHIT%20Certified%20 2011%20LTPAC%20Criteria%20FINAL%2020100726.pdf. Accessed 1 Feb 2011.

4. Department of Health and Human Services, Office of the National Coordinator for Health Information Technology. Health information technology: initial set of standards, implementation specifications, and certification criteria for electronic health record technology: interim final rule. Federal Register/Vol 75, No 8, Pages 2013–2047. 13, Jan. 2010.

5. Garfinkel S. VoIP and skype security. Skype security overview – Rev 1.6. 2005. Available at: http://www.tacticaltech.org/files/tacticaltech/Skype_Security.pdf. Accessed 11 July 2010.

6. HIMSS data analytics website. Available at: http://www.himssanalytics.org/. Accessed 1 Feb 2011.

7. Kuhn D, Walsh T, Fries S. Security considerations for voice over IP systems: recommendations of the National Institute of Standards and Technology (NIST). Technology Administration, U.S. Department of Commerce Special Publication; Gaithersburg, MD. 2005. p. 800–58.

8. Lowe R. EMR success: training is the key. Med Econ. 2004;81:TCP11.

9. Parmanto B, Saptono A, Pramana G, et al. VISYTER: versatile and integrated system for telerehabilitation. Telemed J E Health. 2010;16(9):939–44. Epub 2010 Oct 29.

10. Pennell U, Fishman E. Known pitfalls and proven methods for a successful EMR implementation, EMR consultant: the physician's guide to EMR solutions. 2010. Available at: http://www.emrconsultant.com/emr_pitfalls.php. Accessed 27 May 2010.

11. Watzlaf V, Moeini S, Firouzan P. Int J Telerehabil. VOIP for Telerehabilitation: A Risk Analysis for Privacy, Security, and HIPAA Compliance. 2010;2:3–10. doi: 10.5195/ijt.2010.6056. Available at: http://telerehab.pitt.ed.

Chapter 13
Health Information Management and Rehabilitation: Moving Toward an Adequate Ethical Framework for Telerehabilitation

Katherine D. Seelman

Abstract With information and communications technology as its backbone, the electronic health information system has become an increasingly important component of telerehabilitation (TR) service delivery. The purpose of this chapter is to examine ethical responsibility for resolution of issues emerging within the intersection of the fields of rehabilitation and health information management (HIM). These issues involve areas of clinical competencies and user accessibility that might further inform the development of codes of ethics and other guidance for HIM and TR practice. Case studies anchor the narrative in actual problem-solving situations. Bioethics and practice documents are used to illustrate existing guidance. Conclusions and recommendations present interdisciplinary examples of research problems and best-practice initiatives, and also touch upon the ethical dilemma of the ethical vacuum when no human agent can be identified due to the complexity of the information environment.

13.1 Introduction

The introduction of technological innovation, such as information and communications technology (ICT), into health care can change practice and challenge values [17, 24, 26]. With ICT as its backbone, the electronic health information system is an increasingly important component of telerehabilitation (TR) service delivery. The purpose of this chapter is to examine ethical responsibility for resolution of issues emerging within the intersection of the fields of rehabilitation and health

K.D. Seelman
Department of Rehabilitation Science and Disorders,
School of Health and Rehabilitation Sciences, University of Pittsburgh,
3600 Forbes Avenue, 5036 Forbes Tower, Pittsburgh, PA 15260, USA
e-mail: kds31@pitt.edu

S. Kumar, E.R. Cohn (eds.), *Telerehabilitation*, Health Informatics,
DOI 10.1007/978-1-4471-4198-3_13, © Springer-Verlag London 2013

information management (HIM) [2]. These issues involve areas of clinical practice and user accessibility that might further inform development of codes of ethics and other guidance for HIM and TR practice.

The constitution of the World Health Organization (WHO) states: "enjoyment of the highest attainable standard of health is one of the fundamental rights of every human being" [61]. In turn, ethicists generally view justice as the guiding principle in the distribution of the benefits and risks of health care, which may now include broadband availability [28, 39]. Laws can be neutral or they can be used to endorse ethics. In the United States, 2010 Patient Protection and Affordable Care Act generally endorses the WHO's ethical norm of health as a human right by extending availability of health care to most Americans. The Health Insurance Portability and Accountability Act (HIPAA) of 1996 endorses the notion that protection of privacy and security of electronic health information is necessary to fulfill clinical responsibilities for respect for a person, a basic ethical tenet. The 21st-Century Communications and Video Accessibility Act of 2010 endorses the notion that meeting a standard of equitable distribution of resources requires access to next-generation Internet-based and digital communication technologies.

Health information technology (HIT) is a relative newcomer in the health field and brings with it computer science, informatics, and HIM personnel. The application of ethical principles and tenets to HIT to meet the needs of users, such as those with disabilities, and rehabilitation practitioners has not yet been endorsed in law. The Health Information Technology for Economic and Clinical Health Act (HITECH Act) is part of the American Recovery and Reinvestment Act (ARRA) of 2009. ARRA contains general incentives related to HIT such as building a national health-care infrastructure and specific incentives designed to accelerate the adoption of electronic health record (EHR) systems among providers. Accessibility of HIT is at the policy discussion stage [59].

Rehabilitation involves a broad range of fields such as audiology and speech pathology, engineering and assistive technology, physical and occupational therapy, and psychology and counseling. While practice traditions and clinical needs differ, the intersection of clinical practice and HIM for TR has created the potential for complementary roles for clinicians and HIM personnel across practice areas [13]. HIM personnel design information systems and manage data and processes for systems used by clinicians [63]. HIM professionals are also partners with computer scientists within the field of informatics and with a wide range of health information users, prompting consideration of the adequacy of computer science ethical codes to drive accessibility and usability. As clinical case studies presented later show, HIT has generated problems of an ethical nature. For example, should a clinician simply accept the design of a health system he/she will use for a clinical assessment? Should health intake forms be designed to meet the communication and information accessibility needs of users with disabilities? Who is responsible? Attributing ethical responsibility in this complex information environment is an ever-increasing challenge for all users.

13.1.1   Challenges and Opportunities

TR, like other telehealth applications, is being introduced into health care at the same time as it is being evaluated for safety, efficacy, and cost effectiveness. Standardization of technology and management are evolving. Policy guidance and regulatory constraints are at a nascent stage, and professional oversight is uneven across HIM and rehabilitation practice areas. Ethical dilemmas are generated both by the impact on users of uncertainties inherent in the rollout stage itself and by the many challenges and opportunities of remote delivery of service. Challenges exist in assigning and distributing ethical responsibility [29] for system failures within a system with multiple technical, corporate, government, and professional jurisdictions. Nonetheless, opportunities abound. Many rehabilitation services are uniquely suited for remote delivery [50, 55]. TR has the potential to reach underserved populations worldwide and to extend the benefits of rehabilitation to a burgeoning population of older disabled adults as well as those under 65 [35, 49, 58]. According to the National Council on Disability, in the United States, people with disabilities experience more problems accessing health care than other groups, and these difficulties increase for those with the most significant disabilities and who are in the poorest health [56]. Moreover, lack of access to health care has been associated with increased risk for secondary conditions for people with significant disabilities.

13.1.2   Chapter Organization

The chapter introduction is followed by a discussion of Fig. 13.1—the telehealth system. Figure 13.1 illustrates system components as well as introduces a standard for HIT system design, a universal design, which, in turn, introduces consideration of ethical responsibility [28] for accessibility and usability. The ethical significance of system components is anchored in a series of TR clinical case studies of rehabilitation and HIM professionals interacting with each other and with clients. The case studies provide examples of TR and HIM in a shared practice context and illustrate the tasks involved in interactive problem solving. The next section briefly introduces theories and principles in bioethics, which form the basis for HIM and rehabilitation practice codes of ethics. This section also introduces additional ethical issues relevant to TR that are derived from rehabilitation, computer, and information ethics literature. The adequacy of traditional ethical theories to guide practitioners toward solutions for some of these issues is a consideration in this section.

TR practice models and guidance are examined in the next section. Documents from the American Telemedicine Association (ATA), such as *Core Standards for Telemedicine* [7], and ATA's TR special interest group's (SIG's) a *Blueprint for Telerehabilitation Guidelines* [1] are examined to determine sensitivity to ethical

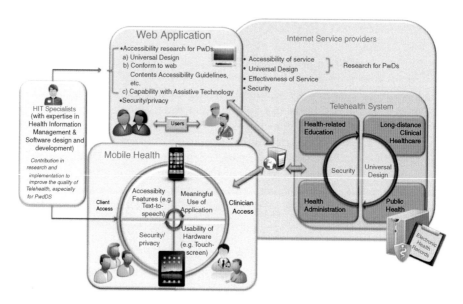

Fig. 13.1 Telehealth system and TR (Y. Daihua, personal communication 2009)

issues introduced in previous sections. Documents from some of the rehabilitation practice professional organizations and from HIM are also examined. Commonalities across practice areas are among the considerations in this section. Section 13.5 lays out recommendations that might strengthen ethical guidance and proposes research to support development of recommendations.

13.2 The Telehealth and TR System

Figure 13.1 presents components of a telehealth system with accessibility support. ICT and the Internet form the backbone of and environment for the telehealth system, of which HIT is an increasingly important part. The telehealth medical system itself provides the umbrella framework for comprehensive management of health information, including the electronic medical record, and secure exchange of information between consumers, providers, government and quality entities, and insurers. This information exchange includes the health record, medical/health evidence base, and provider guidance for patient care. The system is also responsible for disposal of health information.

In Fig. 13.1, the telehealth system focuses on three major components. The first component is the Internet telephone provider (ITP), (e.g., companies such as Verizon and AT&T), which delivers broadband, a signaling method capable of increased information-carrying capacity necessary for TR services. ITP providers may or may not be within the jurisdiction of medical telehealth systems and HIPAA. Title III of the HiTech

Act extends the complete privacy and security provisions of HIPAA to business associates of covered entities [30, 31]. In any case, an ITP service provider must fulfill federal public interest responsibilities for secure and reliable transmission [20]. ITP practices and processes for data collection and use are not transparent; companies are not required to disclose policies and practices for information collection and use. Federal Communication Commission (FCC) oversight of ITPs is a gray area of regulation.

The second component of the telehealth system is the medical telehealth system itself. This system delivers services in two ways: using the Internet and mobile health technology. Ideally, supported by HIM skills in design, the system will meet the standard of universal design. Universal design is a widely recognized approach for satisfying the technology accessibility requirements for just distribution of health care to users. More realistically, barriers exist. For the Internet, barriers include problems related to web page design and web navigation experienced by blind users as well as more general concerns such as availability and affordability. Mobile health devices and transmission may create barriers because of inaccessible and unusable hardware design, software design, and reliability. Diagnostic equipment, such as videofluoroscopy and video otoscopy [40] in the case of speech-language pathology, must be compatible with the HIT system that, in turn, must process the resulting clinical data accurately. Decisions about allocations of resources and personnel to solve accessibility problems involve organizational ethics. Decisional responsibility is within the purview of the health-care organization. Thus, Fig. 13.1 locates universal design within the responsibility of the telehealth medical system. Nonetheless, requirements for HIT compliance with the Americans with Disabilities Act, Section 504 of the Rehabilitation Act, and other laws are only in the planning stage. The telehealth system is, of course, subject to HIPAA privacy and security rules. To ensure security of health data and privacy of patient information, HIPAA requires implementation of standards for the electronic exchange of health-care information between health-care providers, suppliers, insurers, and other entities that handle health-care records.

HIPAA standards have considerable impact on the behavior of rehabilitation practitioners working in the medical telehealth system. However, clinicians are the product of a professional infrastructure that provides oversight throughout their careers. Practice-related accreditation bodies certify their educational programs. Professional organizations for each practice area provide oversight over their behavior, using codes of ethics and other guidance. Other organizations assure their competencies by executing a rigorous certification process. Finally, practice acts, often within the jurisdiction of states rather than the federal government, set out the rights and responsibilities of licensees and, in varying degrees of specificity, state what they are authorized to do in their professional roles. Professions vary as to whether or not their academic curricula and ethics codes address remote delivery of TR services such as teleconsultation, telehomecare, telemonitoring, and teletherapy services [43]. Nonetheless, all TR professions recognize that individual practitioners must provide services that respect the patient, and do them good, or at least no harm, with benefits and risks distributed equitably.

The third component of the telehealth and TR system is HIM. HIM serves as the responsible conduit, if not the designer of interfaces between the IT provider and the client. As Fig. 13.1 indicates HIM professionals often serve in bridge roles in tele-health medical systems, connecting clinical, operational, and administrative functions. Therefore, HIM personnel may affect the quality of patient information and patient care at every touch point in the health-care delivery cycle. They design and manage HIT systems and EHRs. The determine information to be collected, which must meet best practice and regulatory standards. They design the way the information is presented to the user. They also design system software. When interacting with practitioners and clients, they provide support in design, testing system hardware and software, training, and ongoing problem solving.

Like rehabilitation professions, HIM is constrained by professional oversight and government regulation, in particular HIPAA. HIM personnel graduate from professionally accredited academic programs. Their competency as professionals is reflected in successfully achieving a credential, and like most clinical practice areas, a code of ethics guides the practice. The degree of involvement of HIM personnel with TR practitioners may vary according to factors such as complexity of the technology, the intricacies of clinical interventions, and accessibility and usability [54]. The case studies discussed below illustrate various points of intersection between HIM personnel, rehabilitation practitioners, and clients. They also present examples of disconnects between client and clinician needs and system responses.

13.2.1 TR Case Study Examples Showing Interaction Between End Users and the Telehealth System

13.2.1.1 Client Teleassessed for Autism Spectrum Disorders by a Rehabilitation Counselor

Using a teleportal within the medical system's HIT, the clinician delivers a standardized diagnostic assessment to evaluate a person for autism [46]. The clinician needs a system that can deliver assessment with the same validity as an assessment delivered face to face. Because evaluating eye contact is important in the diagnosis of autism, a teleprompter may be used to stimulate direct eye contact. The counselor is also interested in assessing the social interaction of the client. Therefore, a tablet is used to display the visual stimuli, usually pictures, so the clinician can evaluate whether or not the client engages the clinicians in their responses to the stimuli. The teleprompter and tablet products were identified and integrated into the videoconferencing and documentation system by HIM professionals. The practitioner did extensive education on autism with the HIM personnel to sensitize them to the needs of both the client and the clinician. The client needed to have a system design that was streamlined and that would not distract him/her from carrying out the assessment. The clinician needed the ability to see multiple views of the client and to manipulate those views. The scoring forms are integrated into the system. The clinician needed an electronic means of documenting client responses and the ability to reference those notes when completing the scoring form. HIM is trying to make the system as usable as possible for clinicians. The system may eventually be marketed to clinicians.

13.2.1.2   People Who Are Deaf and Design of Health Forms

A person who is deaf wants a sign-language interpreter to be available when communicating with a health professional in person or remotely, using a video telephone relay system or telecommunication devices for the deaf (TDD). These special needs must appear on the intake health form, but often either this information is not requested or the form cannot accommodate it. HIM personnel are not familiar with the communication needs of deaf users and do not include mode of communication in the list of necessary items in the design of health intake forms. In the medical telehealth system, form design for telehealth system is executed in an office of health medical records.

13.2.1.3   Client with Lymphedema and Telehomecare

A client has limited mobility because her lymphedema causes chronic swelling of her lower limbs [47]. She has difficulty walking and prefers not to travel. As a subject in a research project, she has been introduced to TR services. Inexpensive yet high-quality desktop videoconferencing equipment has been installed in her home and connected to a teleportal. She needs training to operate the equipment that will be provided by the clinician or an HIM specialist. Using this equipment, the client has downloaded a training video that provides her with introductory instructions on how to manage her treatment and execute appropriate therapeutic exercise. Using interactive videoconferencing, she will be trained to perform certain hand movements to do direct lymphatic massage. She will be remotely monitored, and outcomes of the training and interventions will be evaluated. High-speed video broadband captures clear images of hands at various stages and locations during the massage. With a single image, the rehabilitation practitioner can see only limited hand movement, but fast speed allows true technique to be revealed. Speeding up an image is within the expertise of the HIM specialist. With a smartphone, using wireless broadband, the client can execute prevention strategies by sending information, including images of skin wounds, to her provider. Again, the high-speed broadband connection provides a clear image for the doctor who can then communicate with the local caregiver and the patient. The images will be integrated into the patient's electronic record by the HIM personnel.

13.2.1.4   Client Who Is Blind and Telemonitoring

A physical therapist is working with patients having retinopathy second to diabetes. The clinician needs to train her retinopathy/diabetes patients to examine their feet to determine skin breakdown as an important step to prevent amputation. She also needs to have her patient take and send images to medical personnel. She must work with an HIM expert to design interfaces for technology that will measure temperature and other skin variables and is usable by the blind client—akin to a talking glucometer. The therapist will also work with HIM personnel to assure that the images are part of a provider electronic record.

13.2.1.5   Wheelchair User with Quadriplegia Who Participates in Many Activities Using a Smartphone for Task Execution

A person with a wheelchair that is equipped with many smart functions, including a robotic arm, goes to a coffee shop and wishes to refill his coffee cup at a coffee dispenser. He has worked with an HIM to design an interface on his mobile phone to accommodate his usability needs. Using high-speed broadband, he can press a quick key and dial a remote assistant to work cooperatively to perform the task. The broadband signal is dropped out and the task is interrupted. The wheelchair will be transitioned to a safety state, and will resume operation after the broadband connection is re-established.

13.2.2   Discussion

As these case studies show, the impact of ICT innovation and HIT on practice has created situations that may differ from those in conventional practice and, in turn, generate questions about the locus of ethical responsibility and the nature of ethical behavior. In the case of autism, the clinician could have simply accepted the system as designed and the HIM personnel could have resisted system adjustments. Instead, they worked together to adjust the design to meet a standard for scientific validity, thus also meeting their ethical responsibilities to do their duty as scientist and designers. In the case of the HIM professional, he/she was meeting the requirements of the code of ethics for interdisciplinary collaboration [3]. However, the scope of a clinician's ethical responsibility for competency in using and adjusting the equipment is unclear, as is the HIM professional's responsibility for competency in autism. In the case of the patient with lymphedema, the clinician also called for telehealth system adjustments to speed up the images. The clinician did her duty by meeting a standard of quality for training and monitoring. In both cases, the HIM professional has a role in integrating the information about the intervention into the EHR.

In the case of the deaf individual and the medical record, the locus of the ethical responsibility shifts from the individual to the organization and organizational ethics. Administrators are responsible for fostering a culture of accessibility for all users, which, in turn, will improve the quality of decisions about information access that are made by staff [12]. However, they need model technical and corporate standards and case studies to guide their decisions about distribution of resources among all system users. The case of the blind individual's need for accessible diagnostic equipment may be resolved if the locus of the problem is in interface design and, as in all cases involving HIM personnel, the telehealth system or insurance will cover the cost of design adaptations. If the locus of the problem is with diagnostic equipment manufacturers, then solutions may require legal and regulatory change. In all cases, diagnostic equipment must be compatible with HIT, which exchanges data with different information technology systems, software applications, and networks in various settings, while preserving the original purpose of the data [2].

The case involving Wi-Fi system failure for a wheelchair user also poses considerable challenges in determining the locus of ethical responsibility. Should Wi-Fi providers and mobile phone manufacturer be held to a standard of reliability and performance that is like that imposed by the Food and Drug Administration for medical devices? In all cases on the individual level, decision-making capability would be enhanced by a shared knowledge base about the needs of clients and rehabilitation practitioners and the capabilities of HIM. Administrators, managers, and HIM and rehabilitation professionals would benefit from information about the laws and regulations that inform service delivery, including the Americans with Disabilities Act, Section 504 of the Rehabilitation Act, the 21stCentury Communications Video Accessibility Act and, of course, HIPAA [15]. Barriers to TR practice such as lack of reimbursement and state-based licensure requirements are clearly within the proper activities of professional practice organization that educate and lobby. Finally, some problems of attribution of responsibility have no easy solution in a system characterized by the movement of complex chains of information such as clinical evidence that is not necessarily generated by the clinician who must communicate it to a trusting client. The literature of bioethics, organizational ethics, computer ethics, and information ethics is populated by these problems.

13.3 Bioethics, Rehabilitation and HIM, Computer Ethics, and Information Ethics

13.3.1 *Bioethics, Organizational and Business Ethics*

Commonalities can be found between the ethical foundations of HIM and rehabilitation. The codes of ethics for HIM [3] and rehabilitation professional practice areas are based on theories and principles derived from bioethics. These theories and principles routinely use as their unit of analysis either the individual as an agent or the individual's action. Therefore, the individual is the locus of ethical responsibility. Some of the most commonly used ethical theories and principles are presented in Table 13.1. Theories such as virtue ethics are strongly associated with health practice. Individual agents act in "a good way" [42]. Virtue ethics emphasizes the

Table 13.1 Normative ethical theories [23, 27, 37, 41]

Theory	Source	Description
Virtue ethics	Roots in Plato (427–347 BCE) and Aristotle (384–322 BCE)	Key idea is to find proper end for humans and to seek that end. People seek perfection/excellence and seek to live virtuous lives. What sort of person should I be? Contributes to the understanding of professional ethics and in the training necessary to produce ethical professionals
Deontological theories	Immanuel Kan (1724–1804)	Deon (deontological) means duty in Greek; science of doing our duty. Thus, doing the right thing might not always lead to an increase in the good
Teleology/consequentialism	Utilitarianism (Jeremy Bentham,1748–1834, and John Stuart Mill, 1806–1873)	Maximize the good of situation; the greatest good to the greatest number; make a decision dependent on consequences of an action
Caring ethics	Feminist ethics	Raises questions about relationships and other factors in the context of doing health care; recognizes the impact of the uneven distribution of power on ability to make autonomous decisions

role of character and virtue, as in whistle blowing in the case of billing fraud, dishonesty in describing an error to a patient, or inaccessible medical forms [51]. Other bioethical theory is concerned with the analysis and evaluation of volitional action, with what makes a chosen action right or wrong, good or bad, whether in terms of intentions and obligations as in deontological theory or in terms of outcomes of good for the greatest numbers as in consequentialism. Duty ethics might motivate a rehabilitation practitioner to take a course in HIM , to develop better skills and competency in HIT. Consequentialist ethics might drive professional organizations to educate and lobby for any number of issues such as HIT accessibility and usability, to extend beneficial outcomes to the greatest number. Caring ethics focuses on the relationship between the clinician and the client. A clinician motivated by caring ethics may place greater value on the perceived trust developed in face-to-face interventions and regard remote delivery as less ethical in most situations.

Rehabilitation practice and HIM have also been influenced by a "principles approach" [10, 11]. The principles are respect for autonomy (respect the decision-making capacities of autonomous persons), non-malfeasance (avoid causing harm), beneficence (provide benefits and balance benefits against risks), and justice (fairness in the distribution of benefits and risks). These principles can serve as an ethical framework and the basis for legal requirements for design and management of health information systems [25]. For example, the patient may be the final stop in a chain of information. To maintain trust between the clinician and the patient and meet the duty of care, the clinician must trust the information that he/she provides for a patient. Each link on the chain has responsibility for adhering to these four principles. However, while these principles can be assigned, the relevant jurisdictions, whether manufacturer, supplier, designer, or manager, would have to voluntarily sign on laws and regulations enacted.

The context in which clinicians do their work has become increasingly complex so that organizations often shape individual behavior [38, 48]. Bioethical principles, such as autonomy, non-malfeasance, beneficence, and justice, may not be sufficient to address ethical issues that arise [64]. The locus of ethical responsibility for delivery of TR may then expand or shift beyond the individual to the organization. Principles in organizational and business ethics then become useful. They include stewardship, fidelity, trust and honesty, and corporate social responsibility. As the clinical case study about the deaf user and medical records suggests, a corporate culture of accessibility for all users affects individual behavior in assuring that people with disabilities are included. A corporate culture that is supportive of a team composed of consumer, clinical, and HIM members may advance the needs of all users.

13.3.2   Rehabilitation, Computer, and Informatics Ethics

The introduction of ICT and HIT into rehabilitation has also ushered in new areas of ethics, such as information ethics [32, 34] and computer ethics [18], while not diminishing the importance of bioethics. TR researchers and practitioners have recognized that issues of privacy and security are central to meeting their ethical responsibilities to their research subjects and clients. Rehabilitation research has been second to none in linking research and development (R&D) to ethical principles of autonomy and justice. R&D, in particular in engineering, has produced universally designed medical equipment, information and communications products, processes, and systems to advance desired outcomes of inclusion and participation of people with disabilities in society and to advance practice [14, 44, 57]. Nonetheless, both rehabilitation research and practice and HIM have been slow in conducting R&D on accessible HIT and protocols that delineate the roles and tasks of involved professionals. Engineers, computer scientists, psychologists, and other clinicians have joined forces in a modest but important research engineering center in TR [45]. The clinical case study on autism presented earlier is an example of a product of their partnership.

HIM professionals work closely with those in technical fields such as computer science that provides the theoretical knowledge base for HIT. Information and computer ethicists have introduced a range of relevant ethical issues for the TR practice mix. Like rehabilitation, information and computer ethicists recognize the centrality of issues such as privacy and security of data, but they are also sensitive to societal, structural, and policy dilemmas. They see a need for balancing concern for privacy and security against the desirability of linking disparate sources of information. Clearly, the operationalization of global health-care data exchange [4] would serve justice if the number of underserved people in health care were diminished. Nonetheless, data exchanges are not without related ethical dilemmas. While there has been continuing progress in the development of standards for delivery of quality and secure accurate health data, privacy, security, and accuracy of data are matters of concern [21].

Computer and information ethicists also share with individuals related to the field of rehabilitation a concern for design, often within the context of obligations of designers [36, 62]. Some ethicists have expressed concern about design of direct computer interfaces (DCIs) in which, unlike TR, some of the intellectual tasks of the clinician are taken over by the computer [22]. DCIs collect patient data, draw inferences from the data, and respond back to the patient. Ethicists question whether traditional bioethics is sufficient to address the full range of concerns generated by the complex contexts of ICT [19, 33, 52]. Bioethics focuses on discrete actions and identifiable agents and outcomes. As information and computer technology becomes increasingly networked and integrated, often without transparency, it becomes difficult to identify individual agents that can be considered morally responsible for system impacts, which result from the interaction of many different agents.

13.4 Grounding TR and HIM Ethics in Professional Standards, Guidance, and Codes

13.4.1 Standards, Guidance, and Codes

Standards, guidance, and codes for telepractice that directly address HIT are the exception, not the rule, perhaps because HIT is a recent addition to the TR mix [60]. Nonetheless, telepractice standards, guidance, and codes have been evolving over a decade or more. In 2000, a proposal for an ethical code in telemedicine was introduced [53]. The code was based on virtue ethics. In Chap. 19 of this book, Janet Brown describes guidance on the use of TR issued by rehabilitation professional organizations—dating back to 1997 in the case of the American Speech and Language-Hearing Association (ASHA). In 2008, the ATA released its *Core Standards for Telemedicine* [7]. Based primarily on the ATA's Core Standards for Telemedicine operations, the ATA's TR SIG released *A Blueprint for Telerehabilitation Guidelines* in 2010 [1]. These documents do not apply to specific clinical practices. ASHA, American Physical Therapy Association (APTA), American Occupational Therapy Association (AOTA), and the Commission on Rehabilitation Counselor Certification (CCRC), among others, have issued guidance on telepractice. The American Health Information Management Association (AHIMA) has recognized the need for collaboration with telepractice in its code of ethics [3].

The ATA's Core Standards for Telemedicine are comprehensive in distribution of responsibility. This document recognizes both individual practitioners and organizations as agents responsible for implementation of standards. Separate standards address administration, health professionals, telemedicine ethics, and clinical and technical components. Using a search tool, HIT appeared once in the ATA's Core

Standards, in the glossary of terms; a search for accessibility and usability did not produce any examples. A search of the text of *A Blueprint for Telerehabilitation Guidelines* produced one reference to HIT and one reference, located in the technical section, to accessibility (physical accessibility of the treatment space) and usability of equipment (clients have a variety of impairments).

Rehabilitation practice areas have addressed quality, competencies, and skills in telepractice and, to a limited extent, in equipment and systems. ASHA and APTA guidance for telepractice adopts the principle of equivalency for the quality of face-to-face and remote delivery of services [6, 9]. ASHA requires that practitioners be competent in delivering services in an electronic communications environment, including the calibration and maintenance of clinical instruments and telehealth equipment in accordance with standard operating procedures. APTA provides guidance on quality of the electronic communication devices and systems and consideration of scope of personal competence, expertise, and skills with electronic communications when choosing to engage in telehealth [5]. ASHA's code of ethics permits the delegation of services to technicians and support personnel under certain circumstances, but the certified clinician maintains responsibility for the welfare of the client. The clinician also has responsibility to maintain the equipment used in practice so that it is in working order and calibrated [8]. The ASHA, APTA, and AOTA codes of ethics do not specifically address accessibility, but the AOTA code does refer to its commitment to support participation of clients in society.

The CCRC Code of Professional Ethics for Rehabilitation Counselors, like other rehabilitation organizations, adheres to an equivalency rule of behavior and competence for telepractice [16]. The CCRC Code contains a section on technology and distance counseling, and addresses accessibility as well as a separate section on advocacy and accessibility. The code acknowledges behavioral differences with the use of the Internet and recognizes issues around electronic records, data storage and disposal, and validity of information on the Internet. The AHIMA Code of Ethics does not specifically address accessibility. The code does contain a section entitled "Facilitate interdisciplinary collaboration in situations supporting health information practice," which is as follows:

> 10.1. Participate in and contribute to decisions that affect the well-being of patients by drawing on the perspectives, values, and experiences of those involved in decisions related to patients. Professional and ethical obligations of the interdisciplinary team as a whole and of its individual members should be clearly established [3].

13.5   Conclusions and Recommendations

The purpose of this chapter was to examine ethical issues in TR emerging within the intersection of the fields of rehabilitation and HIM, especially those issues specific to clinical practice and user accessibility. An examination of these issues has produced examples that can lead to further development of codes of ethics and other guidance for HIM and TR practice.

In the process of chapter development, the need to more rigorously distinguish between telecommunications (ICT) as the backbone for HIT and HIT itself has become evident in order to identify issues specifically related to HIT. Most practitioners have used the Internet and mobile phones to send and receive information using ITPs. Many practitioners use and are comfortable with diagnostic and assessment equipment when used in-person but perhaps not in telepractice. Rehabilitation is sensitive to the accessibility needs of clients and has developed guidelines, including telepractice guidelines in the ATA SIG document *A Blueprint for Telerehabilitation Guidelines*. However, few clinicians have delivered services within an information environment increasingly dominated by HIT.

The clinical case studies, guided by bioethics, suggest a need to ask basic questions at both the individual practitioner and the organizational levels. Should clinicians ask and be able to respond to the question: Is this information system designed to meet my needs in assessing, monitoring or treating a client? Or, in the case of HIM personnel: Should I be able to design a system that corresponds with a profile of a particular medical condition? If so, are educational tools and competency guidelines in place to provide professionals with the necessary analytic, content, and skills to respond? When complex telemonitoring of exercise regimes require interdisciplinary input, are markers in place to distinguish the role of the clinical from the role of the HIM professional? Should rehabilitation professionals work with HIM professionals on work flow charts for joint projects, on system adjustments, and on securely transferring medical images and treatment documentation and their integration into medical records? The intersection of rehabilitation and HIM in TR seems to suggest the need for more interdisciplinary collaboration.

13.5.1 Interdisciplinary Collaboration

Challenges in interdisciplinary collaboration may be eased because both HIM and rehabilitation have common roots in bioethics which protects human rights, a commitment shared by both fields. Ethics provide guidance on "right" behavior, duty, consequences of actions, and reminders that the ethics of care may reject substitution of technology for human beings. Bioethics also recognizes the usefulness of principles derived from organizational and business to provide guidance on problems that are not easily resolved on the individual level, such as the need for a culture of accessibility for all users. Further, HIM has close association with computer and informatics ethics, which is futuristic in its concern for ethical design. Some health systems have no identifiable human agent. In this case, health technology may be guided by algorithms designed by humans that instruct the technology to carry out functions that were once performed by human beings. HIM's code of ethics is also strong in interdisciplinary collaboration. Perhaps most important to interdisciplinary problem solving, many rehabilitation professions have joined together under the umbrella of ATA to produce *A Blueprint for Telerehabilitation Guidelines*. However, future efforts may need to involve the HIM profession.

13.5.2 Research, Best Practices, and System Design

Research has a primary role to play in continuing to generate evidence of the equivalency of face-to-face and remote delivery of care. Case studies of clinicians functioning within the information environment in collaboration with HIM personnel will illustrate real examples of specific tasks, overlap in task execution, and harmonization in integration of information into the EHRs, and best practices will be developed. Case studies involving compatibility of diagnostic equipment with HIT will contribute to standards development. Designers should test their HIT system designs for accessibility at the development/prototype stage. In a concluding note, many of the problems emerging in HIT are profound, rooted in questions of human responsibility and the ethical vacuum when none can be identified.

Summary

- Ethics provide guidance on "right" behavior, duty, consequences of actions, and reminders that the ethics of care may reject substitution of technology for human beings.
- With electronic health information system becoming an increasingly important component of TR service, the resolution of issues related to clinical practice and user accessibility might require development of codes of ethics and other guidance for HIM and TR practice.
- TR has the potential to reach underserved populations worldwide and to extend the benefits of rehabilitation to a burgeoning population of older disabled adults as well as those under 65 years of age.
- However, TR is being introduced into health care at the same time as it is being evaluated for safety, efficacy, and cost effectiveness. Ethical dilemmas are generated both by the impact on users of uncertainties inherent in the rollout stage itself and by the many challenges and opportunities of remote delivery of service.
- The context in which clinicians do their work has become increasingly complex, so bioethical principles (autonomy, non-malfeasance, beneficence, and justice) may not be sufficient to address ethical issues that arise. The locus of ethical responsibility for delivery of TR may then expand or shift beyond the individual to the organization.
- TR researchers and practitioners have recognized that issues of privacy and security are central to meeting their ethical responsibilities to their research subjects and clients.

Abbreviations/Acronyms

AHIMA	American Health Information Management Association
AOTA	American Occupational Therapy Association
APTA	American Physical Therapy Association
ARRA	American Recovery and Reinvestment Act
ASHA	American Speech and Language-Hearing Association

ATA	American Telemedicine Association
CCRC	Commission on Rehabilitation Counselor Certification
DCI	Direct computer interface
EHR	Electronic health record
FCC	Federal Communication Commission
HIM	Health information management
HIPAA	Health Insurance Portability and Accountability Act of 1996
HIT	Health information technology
HITECH Act	Health Information Technology for Economic and Clinical Health Act
ICT	Information and communications technology
ITP	Internet telephone provider
R&D	Research and development
SIG	Special interest group
TDD	Telecommunication devices for the deaf
TR	Telerehabilitation
WHO	World Health Organization

Acknowledgements The authors thank Mervat Abdelhak, Ph.D., Chair of the Department of Health Information Management, School of Health and Rehabilitation Sciences; Joan Rogers, Ph.D., Chair of the Department of Occupational Therapy; and two exceptional doctoral students, Daihua Yu, Health Information Management, and Jamie Schutte, Rehabilitation Sciences and Technology Counseling for their invaluable advice and assistance. Any inaccuracies are solely the responsibility of the author.

References

1. A blueprint for telerehabilitation guidelines. 2010. Available at: http://www.americantelemed.org/files/public/standards/ATA%20Telerehab%20Guidelines%20v1%20(2).pdf. Accessed Apr 2011.
2. Abdelhak M, Grostick S, Hanken MA. Health information management of a strategic resource. St. Louis: Elsevier; 2012.
3. AHIMA code of ethics. Available at: http://library.ahima.org/xpedio/groups/public/documents/ahima/bok1_024277.hcsp?dDocName=bok1_024277. Accessed May 2011.
4. AHIMA. HIM principles in health information exchange (practice brief). Available at: http://perspectives.ahima.org/index.php?view=article&id=147:redefining-the-roles-of-health-information-management-professionals-in-health-information-technology&option=com_content&Itemid=84. Accessed May 2011.
5. American Physical Therapy Association (2010). 1111 North Fairfax Street, Alexandria, VA 22314-1488. Telehealth. BOD PO3-06-10-20.
6. American Physical Therapy Association (2009). 1111 North Fairfax Street, Alexandria, VA 22314-1488. Telehealth–definitions and guidelines BOD GO3-0609-19.
7. American Telemedicine Core Standards for Telemedicine Operations. 2007. Available at: http://www.americantelemed.org/files/public/standards/CoreStandards_withCOVER.pdf. Accessed Apr 2011.
8. ASHA code of ethics. 2009. Available at: http://www.asha.org/Practice/ethics/EthicsCode Revision/. Accessed May 2011.
9. ASHA professional issues in telepractice for speech-language pathologists. Available at: http://www.asha.org/docs/html/PI2010-00315.html. Accessed May 2011.
10. Beauchamp TL. Methods and principles in biomedical ethics. 2011. Available at: http://jme.bmj.com/content/29/5/269.long. Accessed May 2011.

11. Beauchamp TL, Childress JF. Principles of biomedical ethics. Oxford: Oxford University Press; 2001.
12. Boyle PJ, DuBose ER, Ellingson SJ, et al. Organizational ethics in health care: principles, cases, and practical solutions. New York: Jossey-Bass; 2001.
13. Brennan D, Tindall L, Theodoros D, et al. A blueprint for telerehabilitation guidelines. Int J Telerehabil. Available at: http://telerehab.pitt.edu/ojs/index.php/Telerehab/article/view/6063. (SIG ATA).
14. Center for Universal Design in the Built Environment. Available at: http://www.buffalo.edu/news/11804. Accessed May 2011.
15. Coalition of organizations for accessible technology. Available at: http://www.coataccess.org/node/2. Accessed May 2011.
16. Code of Professional Ethics for Rehabilitation Counselors. 2009. Available at: http://www.crccertification.com/pages/crc_ccrc_code_of_ethics/10.php. Accessed May 2011.
17. Committee on Planning a Continuing Health Profession Education Institute, Institutes of Medicine. Redesigning continuing education in the health professions. Washington, D.C.: National Academies Press; 2010.
18. Computer and information ethics. Available at: http://plato.stanford.edu/entries/ethics-computer/. Accessed May 2011.
19. vand der Velden, M. Design for a common world: On ethical agency and cognitive justice. Ethics Info Technol. 2009;11(1): 37–47. doi 10.1007/s10676-008-9178-2. Available at: http://philpapers.org/rec/VANDFA. Accessed 28 Mar 2012.
20. Detailed summary of FERC'S standard market design NOPR. Available at: http://library.findlaw.com/2002/Jun/25/132372.html. Accessed May 2011.
21. Ethical challenges of telemedicine and telehealth. Available at: http://www.uapd.com/wp-content/uploads/Ethical-Challenges-of-Telemedicine-and-Telehealth1.pdf. Accessed May 2011.
22. Ethics in e-trust and e-trustworthiness: the case of direct computer-patient interfaces. Available at: http://www.springerlink.com/content/h6g65035l4411068/. Accessed May 2011.
23. Gabard DL, Martin MW. Physical therapy ethics. Philadelphia: F.A. Davis Co; 2003.
24. Goodman KW, editor. Ethics, computing and medicine: informatics and the transformation of health care. Cambridge: Cambridge University Press; 1998.
25. Green A. Chains of trust and duty in health information management. 2009. Available at: http://www.bepress.com/selt/vol3/iss1/art7/. Accessed May 2011.
26. Greiner AC, Knebel E, editors. Health professions education: a bridge to quality. Committee on the health professions education summit. Washington, D.C.: National Academies Press; 2003.
27. Harman LB. Ethical challenges in the management of health information. 2nd ed. Gaithersburg: Aspen Publishers; 2004.
28. Hastings Center. Connecting American values with health reform. Available at: http://www.thehastingscenter.org/Publications/SpecialReports/Detail.aspx?id=3528&terms=Connecting+American+Values+with+Health+Reform+and+%23filename+*.html. Accessed May 2011.
29. Hastings Institute. Connecting American values with health reform. Available at: http://www.thehastingscenter.org/Publications/SpecialReports/Detail.aspx?id=3528&terms=Connecting+American+Values+with+Health+Reform+and+%23filename+*.html. Accessed May 2011.
30. Health Insurance Portability and Accountability Act. Available at: http://en.wikipedia.org/wiki/Health_Insurance_Portability_and_Accountability_Act. Accessed May 2011.
31. HIE Management and Operational Considerations (Updated). . J AHIMA. 2011. Available at: http://library.ahima.org/xpedio/idcplg?IdcService=GET_HIGHLIGHT_INFO&QueryText=xPublishSite+%3Csubstring%3E+%60BoK%60+%3CAND%3E+(xSource+%3Csubstring%3E+%60AHIMA+Practice+Brief%60+%3CNOT%3E+xSource+%3Csubstring%3E+%60AHIMA+Practice+Brief+attachment%60)&SortField=xPubDate&SortOrder=Desc&dDocName=bok1_048938&HighlightType=HtmlHighlight&dWebExtension=hcsp. Accessed May 2011.
32. Information ethics. Available at: http://en.wikipedia.org/wiki/Information_ethics. Accessed May 2011.
33. Information technologies and the tragedy of the good will. Available at: http://portal.acm.org/citation.cfm?id=1188145. Accessed May 2011.
34. Institute for Information Ethics and Policy. Available at: http://www.sis.pitt.edu/~ethics/. Accessed May 2011.

35. International Telecommunications Union. Available at: http://www.itu.int/themes/accessibility/dc/. Accessed May 2011.
36. Is there an ethics of algorithms? Available at: http://www.ethicsandtechnology.eu/news/comments/colloquium_is_there_an_ethics_of_algorithms/. Accessed May 2011.
37. Kornblau BL, Starling SP. Ethics in rehabilitation: a clinical perspective. Thorofare: Slack; 2000.
38. Managing for organizational integrity. Available at: http://organizacionysistemas.com/ARTICULOS/oi.pdf. Accessed May 2011.
39. Mapping the Way Forward: NTIA Releases Interactive Broadband Map. 2011. Available at: http://broadbandandsocialjustice.org/2011/02/mapping-the-way-forward-ntia-releases-interactive-broadband-map/. Accessed May 2011.
40. Mars BO, Russo M, Barajas I, et al. Telehealth in audiology: the need and potential to reach underserved communities. Int J Audiol. 2010;49(3):195–202.
41. Morrison EE. Health care ethics. Critical issues for the 21st century. Sudbury: Bartlett Publishers; 2009.
42. Oakley J, Cocking D. Virtue ethics and professional roles. Cambridge: Cambridge University Press; 2006.
43. Parmanto B, Saptono A. Telerehabilitation state of the art from an informatics perspective. Int J Telerehabil. 2011. Available at: http://telerehab.pitt.edu/ojs/index.php/Telerehab/search/authors/view?firstName=Bambang&middleName=&lastName=Parmanto&affiliation=University%20of%20Pittsburgh%2C%20Pittsburgh%2C%20PA&country=US. Accessed May 2011.
44. R.S. Mace. Universal Design Institute. Available at: http://www.udinstitute.org/history.php. Accessed May 2011.
45. Rehabilitation Engineering Research Center on Telerehabilitation. Available at: http://www.rerctr.pitt.edu/. Accessed May 2011.
46. Schutte JL, McCue M, Parmanto MB. Usability, reliability, and validity of remote autism diagnostic observation schedule module 4 administration. Telemed E Health. 2011;17(S1):A-57.
47. Seelman KD. Panel: furthering national purposes and people with disabilities (National Broadband Policy). Washington, D.C.: Federal Communications Commission; 2009. 20.
48. Solomon RC. Business ethics. In: Singer P, editor. A companion to ethics. Oxford: Blackwell Publishing; 1991.
49. Successful strategies from AHRQ Health Care Innovations. Available at: http://www.ahrq.gov/qual/nhdr10/nhdr10key.pdf. Accessed May 2011.
50. Swanepoel S, Clark JL, Koekemoer D, et al. Telehealth in audiology: the need and potential to reach underserved communities. Int J Audiol. 2010;49(3):195–202.
51. Teaching and learning ethics: practical virtue ethics: healthcare whistleblowing and portable digital technology. Available at: http://www.ncbi.nlm.nih.gov/pmc/articles/PMC1734023/pdf/v031p00612.pdf. Accessed May 2011.
52. Technology as empowerment: a capability approach to computer ethics. Available at: http://www.springerlink.com/content/v71020650653u56w/. Accessed May 2011.
53. Telemedicine: a proposal for an ethical code. Available at: http://journals.cambridge.org/action/displayFulltext?type=1&fid=45980&jid=CQH&volumeId=9&issueId=03&aid=45979. Accessed May 2011.
54. Telerehabilitation technologies: accessibility and usability. Available at: http://telerehab.pitt.edu/ojs/index.php/Telerehab/article/view/6016/6195. Accessed May 2011.
55. Telerehabilitation: state-of-the-art from an informatics perspective. Available at: http://telerehab.pitt.edu/ojs/index.php/Telerehab/article/view/6015/6194. Accessed May 2011.
56. The current state of health care for people with disabilities. Available at: http://www.ncd.gov/newsroom/publications/2009/HealthCare/HealthCare.html. Accessed May 2001.
57. Trace Institute. Available at: http://trace.wisc.edu/. Accessed May 2011.
58. U.S. Department of Health and Human Services, Office of Asst. Secretary for Planning and Evaluation. Available at: http://aspe.hhs.gov/sp/reports/2009/underserved/report.pdf.

59. U.S. Department of Health and Human Services, Office of the National Coordinator for Health Information Technology (ONC) (2011–2015). Federal strategy plan, Federal health information technology strategic plan, p. 39.
60. Veatch RM, Flack HE. Case studies in allied health ethics. Upper Saddle River: Prentice Hall; 1997.
61. WHO Health and Human Rights. Available at: http://www.who.int/hhr/en/. Accessed May 2011.
62. Why values I design? The challenge of incorporating moral values in design. Available at: http://www.ncbi.nlm.nih.gov/pubmed/20224927. Accessed May 2011.
63. Zeng X, Reynolds R, Sharp M. Redefining the roles of health information management professionals in health information technology. Perspect Health Inf Manag. 2009;6:1f.
64. Zoubul C. Healthcare institutional ethics; broader than clinical ethics. In: Morrison E, editor. Health care ethics. 2nd ed. Boston: Jones and Bartlett Publishers; 2009.

Chapter 14
Remote Accessibility Assessment System

Jongbae Kim

Abstract While home modification has come to be recognized as an important intervention strategy for the quality of life of people with disabilities, the availability of skilled professionals with experience in home modifications for accessibility is limited. A remote accessibility assessment system (RAAS) could enable clinicians to assess the wheelchair accessibility of users' homes from a remote location. There have been many attempts to develop an effective RAAS. In this chapter, several approaches will be introduced, including the use of a survey instrument, videoconference system, 3D reconstruction system, robot motion planning technique, probabilistic roadmap planner, laser scanner, and quantitative measurement of accessibility. The RAAS could be applied to home and workplace, especially in underserved locations such as rural areas and islands. Research that applied several RAASs to diverse areas will be reviewed.

14.1 Introduction

The number of wheelchair users aged 18 years or older is estimated at more than 2.3 million in the United States [13]. An important trend in usage of wheeled mobility devices is that the number of people using wheelchairs is increasing yearly; thus, the demand for wheelchairs is likely to grow in the foreseeable future [3].

For any limitation in function, the amount of disability an individual experiences will depend on the quality of the social and physical environments [1]. Consideration of the built environment is especially critical for wheelchair users given the potential limitations that environment can impose. The most effective rehabilitation outcomes are realized when programs consider both functional restoration and

J. Kim
National Rehabilitation Center Research Institute,
Seoul, South Korea
e-mail: jbkim@pitt.edu

S. Kumar, E.R. Cohn (eds.), *Telerehabilitation*, Health Informatics,
DOI 10.1007/978-1-4471-4198-3_14, © Springer-Verlag London 2013

environmental modification [1]. Most importantly, for mobility devices to be used effectively, the environments in which they are used must be physically accessible [8]. The 1995 American Housing Survey (AHS) investigated whether members of households had permanent physical activity limitations and, if so, whether home modifications had been performed. Based on the survey, approximately 5.1 million (57.4 %) of the households in which a member had an activity limitation had no home modification [23].

The home environment introduces new considerations related primarily to the safety and the performance of basic living activities [15]. Home modification has come to be recognized as an important intervention strategy to manage health-care conditions, maintain or improve functioning, ensure safety, and reduce the wheelchair user's dependency on others [20]. Effective home modification requires consultation with skilled professionals capable of assessing the home environment and identifying any changes necessary to meet the wheelchair user's needs. While many building and remodeling contractors are able to perform the modifications, the availability of skilled professionals with experience in home modifications for accessibility is limited. Providing services in rural areas is particularly difficult. Such service requires lengthy travel times that increase cost and consume the limited time of skilled professionals. Even if a specialist is willing to travel a long distance, travel cost is too high relative to the fee for modification. Previously, even a specialist could not accurately assess the environment's accessibility without visiting the site.

A system that enables accurate remote assessments would be an important tool to improve the ability to perform home assessments more easily and at a decreased cost. Therefore, several efforts were undertaken to develop a remote accessibility assessment system (RAAS). In this chapter, several approaches will be introduced, including the use of a survey instrument, videoconference system, 3D reconstruction system, robot motion planning techniques, probabilistic roadmap planner, laser scanner, and quantitative measurement of accessibility. The RAAS could be applied to home and workplace, especially to underserved locations such as rural areas and islands. Research that applied several RAASs to diverse areas will also be reviewed.

14.2 Development Works

14.2.1 RAAS Using Survey Tool

An effort was undertaken by Extended Home Living Services in Wheeling, Illinois, which developed a remote assessment protocol using a survey instrument, the Comprehensive Assessment Survey Process for Aging Residents (CASPAR™). The CASPAR instrument can be mailed to residents in remote areas to obtain information about consumers' priorities, their activities of daily living, their ability to participate in home-specific occupations, and the space, layout, and design of their residences, so that home modifications can be recommended [17, 20]. The CASPAR has a significant limitation: with no 3D view of the structure of the built environment, it depends upon photographs taken by consumers,

14.2.2   RAAS Using Quantitative Measurement Tool

Lim et al. [12] proposed a quantitative formula for measuring wheelchair accessibility in homes. The motivation of this research is to provide clinicians, rehabilitation professionals, and architects with objective, quantitative measures in home adaptation for improving accessibility in homes. When there are specific measurement methods of wheelchair accessibility before home adaptation, wheelchair users will have an opportunity to verify areas in their homes that require adaptation to improve wheelchair accessibility. A real-world implication of this method will be a cost-effective method for measuring accessibility, as well as a way to determine to what extent modifications are needed in the home. The proposed formula can be used with individuals who are nondisabled as well as disabled, and also provides a simple, logical way to compare their relative accessibilities:

$$\text{Accessibility} = \sum_{1}^{J}\left(\frac{\text{Distance} * \text{Time}}{\text{Routes}}\right) \tag{14.1}$$

$$\textit{Relative Accessibility}\ (\textbf{of A to B}) = (\text{Accessibility}_A / \text{Accessibility}_B) \tag{14.2}$$

14.2.3   RAAS Using Videoconference System

Some developmental work has been done using a remote assessment system in rural or underserved areas. A team of clinicians at the Shepherd Center (Atlanta, GA) performed a case study of remote home modification evaluation using a videoconference system with a video telephone [2, 19]. They demonstrated that remote telerehabilitation assessments have the potential to enable specialists to diagnose potential accessibility problems in home environments and to prescribe appropriate modifications regardless of the location of the client, home, or specialist. The Shepherd Center's research team used a low-bandwidth Plain Old Telephone System (POTS)-based videoconferencing system. However, the POTS line could not provide sufficient resolution to discern the physical objects in detail. Moreover, in addition to the services of a home modification specialist, the study required a technician skilled at operating video equipment who would be paid as much for travel and labor as the home modification specialist. This additional expense might threaten the cost effectiveness of the intervention.

14.2.4 RAAS Using Motion Planning

Han et al. developed a hybrid approach, using encoding, prescriptive-based provisions supplemented by performance-based methods to support compliance and usability analysis for accessibility. They developed an online code-checking program that automated generation of an IFC (industry foundation classes) project model and automated ADAAG code compliance checking. After the prescriptive-based provisions are used to check for compliance, performance-based methods directly test the design intent for usability of a facility by executing simulation of a wheelchair moving through space in the 3D virtualized environment [5].

A team of Israeli researchers developed and evaluated an interactive living environment model that will facilitate the planning, design, and assessment of optimal home and work settings for people with physical disabilities. This interactive model was implemented via an immersive virtual reality (VR) system that displays 3D renderings of specific environments, and responds to user-driven manipulations such as navigation within the environment and alteration of its design [14].

The study by Han et al. made as significant contribution to VR accessibility assessment by adapting the automated ADAAG code-checking system and simulation of wheelchair maneuvering in the built environment. The Israeli team's study also presented a good tool to enable an optimal fit between the individual and the environmental setting by using VR and simulation technology. However, both studies assumed that the layout of the target built environment is obtainable. For the purposes of simulating wheelchair maneuvering in the built environment to evaluate accessibility, it can be very difficult to acquire the accurate dimension of the target's physical environment.

14.2.5 RAAS Using Laser Scanner

For 3D reconstruction of indoor environments, Sequeira et al. [22] presented a new 3D scene analysis system that automatically reconstructs the 3D model of real-world scenes from multiple range images acquired by a laser range finder aboard a mobile robot. Although active methods such as range finding or laser scanning are accurate, they require specially trained operators [10] as well as expensive laser scanning systems such as the Leica Geosystems HDS ranging system. Even if a company like Quantapoint provides as-built documentation using laser scanning technologies [18], this service is too expensive for practical application to individuals' homes [7].

14.2.6 RAAS Using Virtual Reality and Telerehabilitation System

University of Pittsburgh researchers developed a RAAS using VR technology and telerehabilitation concepts to mitigate the limitations of previous RAAS development efforts. They named it "Virtual Reality Telerehabilitation System (VRTS)."

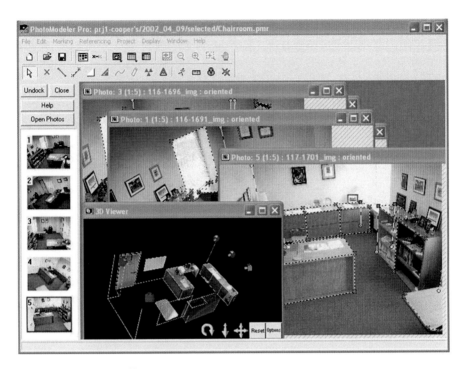

Fig. 14.1 Photomodeler Pro

The system was designed to evaluate the accessibility of physical environments of wheelchair users, employing a virtualized 3D model. VRST took advantage of state-of-the-art digital imaging, 3D reconstruction, and photogrammetry technologies.

While active methods such as range finding or laser striping are accurate, they require expensive equipment. The problem of cost has motivated work toward the implementation of passive techniques that seek to infer 3D depth information from one or more 2D intensity images [16]. Photogrammetry, which loosely translates from the Greek as "light drawn to measure," is a cost-effective technique that can obtain measurements from photographs. The use of engineering photogrammetry to achieve extremely accurate 3D models has become affordable and convenient with improvements in the processing power of desktop computers and the ready availability of inexpensive, user-friendly packages for image processing. The researchers chose Photomodeler Pro 4.0 for use in the VRTS for the following reasons: accuracy is the most important factor in 3D reconstruction; its 3D reconstruction features best fit the requirements of their system; it provides many easy-to-use tools; and several studies support its value (Fig. 14.1).

Based on the results of camera comparison study, a consumer-level digital camera was chosen as a reasonable instrument for this system. It is very important to take good-quality 2D photographs to make 3D models of the home environment efficiently and accurately. As the client and/or his/her helpers will likely not be familiar with the kinds of pictures needed for the 3D modeling process, the researchers developed a comprehensive manual that provides instructions on how to take good pictures. The researchers also created a survey form to gather information about each client's diagnosis, mobility aids, and home environment by referring to the CASPAR, adapting some of the tasks of the CASPAR as checklist items. They also developed an evaluation form for systemic and objective assessment of the accessibility of a wheelchair user's built environment. In addition to the tasks of the CASPAR, they added some features necessary to wheelchair users, such as whether enough space exists to build a ramp or to install a stair glide or a lift.

VRTS provides an accurate measurement tool and allows the evaluation specialist, architect, or rehabilitation engineer to see the space in 3D scenes. It can produce better results than previous studies because specialists can evaluate the environment with more realistic, visual information beyond numeric data. Nevertheless, accuracy remains a critical concern in the virtualized environment [4] and usability is a primary concern for the telerehabilitation system [9]. They conducted research to determine the value of the RAAS in assessing a built environment's accessibility by calculating the congruence level between the VRTS and the conventional in-person (CIP) method. The results showed that the proportion of overall agreement was high at 94.1 %, and the overall sensitivity and specificity were 95.6 and 90.3 %, respectively [6].

14.3   Enhanced VRTS Using State-of-the-Art Technologies

Although the previous version of VRTS showed its potential value through field trials, it had following limitations: (a) it was difficult for a novice photographer to take good pictures for 3D reconstruction; (b) there was no way to communicate efficiently and sufficiently between evaluator and consumer; (c) 3D models of only subparts of the whole home environment were created; and (d) it took time to create the 3D model by marking and referencing the shared points in each photo [6]. The University of Pittsburgh research team improved the system by overcoming the above limitations through the following developmental works: a remote imaging system using an IP camera; an improved 3D reconstruction protocol; a web-based decision-supporting system via house model online delivery; and a simulated wheelchair maneuvering system via dynamic VRML control.

14.3.1   Teleimaging

In the previous version of VRTS, researchers deployed an undergraduate student with a digital camera and instructions on how to take good pictures of a client's home environment. However, it was not easy for a novice photographer to take 2D photos that were of sufficient quality to support the creation of 3D models – since novice photographers do not typically grasp the 3D reconstruction concepts. Researchers therefore developed a remote imaging system through which a 3D reconstruction technician can take pictures of the client's home environment from a distance.

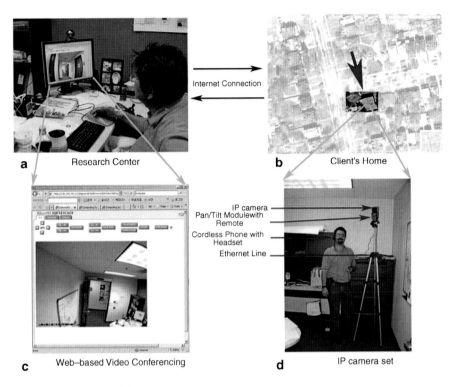

Fig. 14.2 Web-based teleimaging system

In the updated protocol, an undergraduate student was sent to the client's home at the remote location with an IP camera. The research center and client's home were connected via a high-speed Internet connection (cable modem or DSL); the IP camera showed the remote home environment. A technician from the remote research center directed the student (via the phone) to move, pan, and tilt the camera to an appropriate angle to take a good 2D photo. Figure 14.2 shows the client's side where a part-time undergraduate student wears a cordless phone and a headset and holds a remote of pan–tilt module under the camera. It also shows the technician's side where a technician looks at the remote site of the client's home at high frame rate via the videoconferencing program provided by the camera company and an FTP program through which the technician can see the pictures, taken and transferred, at almost real time.

14.3.2 Three-Dimensional Reconstruction of the Whole House Model

The research team took advantage of commercial photogrammetry software, Photomodeler Pro (EOS LTD) as a 3D reconstruction tool. When they developed the previous version of VRTS, they used Photomodeler 4.0, in which a 3D model could be created for each subpart of the home environment such as the bathroom, bedroom, hallway, entrance, etc.; however, there was no function to incorporate subparts into an integrated 3D home model.

In this study, they created a 3D model of the client's entire home by using the "Open Merged Project" function which was added in Photomodeler Pro 5.0. By defining points within each room that are shared with the adjacent rooms, the software was able to merge the separate room models into one overall house model.

14.3.3   Web-Based Decision-Supporting System via House Model Online Delivery

The house model delivery is an important part of this research for data sharing among stakeholders. A web portal environment is used to store and share documents, and each house assessment project is hosted in an individual subportal. The reconstructed 3D house models are posted on the subportal, and are accessible only for the home owner and the professionals involved in the project so that the privacy of the home owner as well as the security of the house can be protected. The Microsoft Office SharePoint Portal Server 2003 served as the platform of the web portal with which the telerehabilitation portal infrastructure was built as a development task of the Rehabilitation Engineering Research Center (RERC) on telerehabilitation [21].

14.3.4   Simulated Wheelchair-Maneuvering System via Dynamic VRML Control

The VRML 3D simulation environment was created by combining a reconstructed house model and a dynamically controlled wheelchair with two sets of navigation controls. As shown in Fig. 14.3, three black arrows are to rotate and move the wheelchair in a normal mode and three red ones are to rotate and move in a faster mode. Navigation controls move along with the wheelchair to ensure that they are always accessible by users throughout the 3D simulation.

The dimensions of the individual wheelchair that a client uses in the target environment can be used for their VR wheelchair. Through this simulation system, the wheelchair users and other project members can, from any location, drive their wheelchair through the target environment. This can be helpful especially to a new wheelchair user who has recently suffered a spinal cord injury and is still recovering in a rehabilitation hospital. They can attempt to drive the VR wheelchair through their VR home and decide which parts of the home should be modified for their return. This simulation system provides an intuitive way for both the novice and the professional evaluator to make accessibility assessments. The system can be available via the Internet anytime and everywhere.

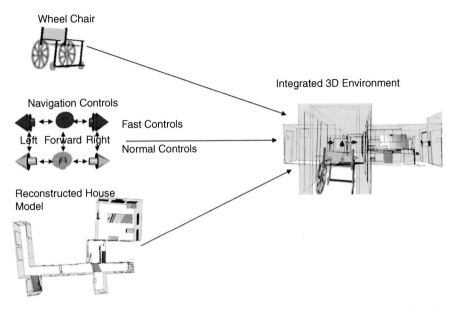

Fig. 14.3 The integrated 3D environment from reconstructed house model and wheelchair with dynamic controls for virtual accessibility assessment

14.3.5   Distance Measurement Based on 3D Models

In addition to the interactive simulation within the web-based 3D environment, the actual distances within the physical built environment will also need to be measured for the assessment. Regular VRML plug-in software does not provide a measurement function. Therefore, commercial 3D visualization software VCollab® with distance measurement capability was developed. It supports VRML visualization as well as 3D distance measurement from VRML models. As shown in Fig. 14.4, a VRML model is read and displayed in VCollab and the distance of the doorway is measured.

14.4   Research

14.4.1   Effectiveness of VRTS

The University of Pittsburgh research team evaluated the value of the RRAS in assessing a built environment's accessibility by calculating the congruence level between the RAAS and the CIP methods [6]. The proportion of overall agreement was high at 94.1 %, and the overall sensitivity and specificity were 95.6 and 90.3 %, respectively. As a significant kappa coefficient of 0.857 and the 95 % confidence interval of odds ratio of [104.062, 404.921] were calculated, a high level of overall

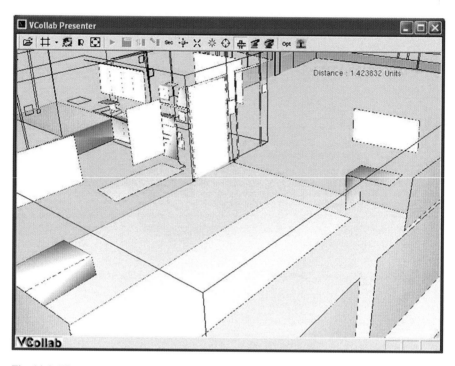

Fig. 14.4 Distance measurement based on 3D models

agreement rate was shown. A high *p*-value (0.868) of the McNamar test implied that there was no marginal homogeneity, that is, no tendency to identify the task incorrectly in the positive or negative direction. This system proved that VR and 3D reconstruction technology may provide an effective means to investigate the architectural features of a built environment without an expert's visit to the site. This system can become an efficient tool for the service provider and provide expert service to underserved clients that would otherwise be unavailable.

14.4.2 Application to Hawaiian Islanders

The enhanced VRTS was applied to workplaces of people with disabilities in Hawaii. The research team wanted to ensure that the RAAS is effective and robust in remote and underserved areas in Hawaii and, likewise, in other such areas across the nation and throughout the world. Thus, this study will help to reduce geographical limitations on services to beneficiaries. This research project was supported by the NEC Foundation of America. The proportion of overall agreement was high at 97.3 %, and the overall sensitivity and specificity were reported as 25.0 and 98.4 %, respectively.

Given the results of this study, one can say that the RAAS method can be used to evaluate the accessibility of remote workplaces. The RAAS method has many advantages, such as reducing travel expenses, manpower, and evaluation time. In this study, the RAAS evaluator performed the assessment from Korea. The evaluator spent only 3 h analyzing the physical structure and evaluating the accessibility of three workplaces in Hawaii with 3D models and 2D photos on the office desk in Seoul, Korea. Through this study, it was anticipated that the RAAS method could be used to assess the accessibility of remote workplaces in underserved areas, such as the Pacific islands. Moreover, the funds and time needed by accessibility professionals to conduct accessibility evaluations could be reduced.

14.4.3   Application to the Workplace Assessment

The Workplace Rehabilitation Engineering Research Center (Work-RERC) at the Georgia Institute of Technology, and the Telerehabilitation Rehabilitation Engineering Research Center (RERC-TR) at the University of Pittsburgh, are collaborating to develop a workplace remote assessment to allow employees in a wider geographic area access to workplace assessments in a timely, efficient, and cost-effective manner. The Workplace Remote Assessment Protocol (WRAP) is being developed based on a prior analysis of a number of assessment tools that resulted in a conceptual framework to guide the process [11]. The WRAP system adopted a concept of "points of interest" that allows engineers who use a 3D modeling tool, (i.e., Photomodeler) to create 3D models of the points of interest from photo images that will correspond to a list of measurable items in the workplace assessment table (Fig. 14.5). For further study, they will need to review the photo-taking rules to specify an optimum number of photos to increase the usability ratio in 3D modeling.

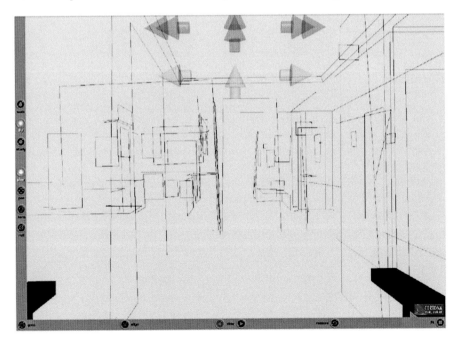

Fig. 14.5 Wheelchair simulation in 3D model

14.5   Discussion

The study by Han et al. provided valuable contributions to VR accessibility assessment by adapting the automated ADAAG code-checking system and simulating wheelchair maneuvering in the built environment. The Israeli team's study also presented a good tool to enable an optimal fit between the individual and the environmental setting by using VR and simulation technology. If the automated ADAAG code-checking system and the wheelchair-maneuvering simulation system can be integrated in the VRTS, the performance of the system should be improved remarkably. One might also consider developing a video-based 3D reconstruction system to easily construct accurate 3D models. This should be an automatic system, so that only a video need be taken with a digital camcorder.

14.6   Conclusion

Several development efforts presented the possibility of the real-world application of the RAAS, and some research studies showed that the RAAS may provide an effective means to investigate the architectural features of a built environment without an expert visiting the site. The RAAS can become an efficient tool for the service provider and provide expert service to underserved clients that would otherwise be unavailable. As the IT technologies evolve rapidly, what was impossible will become possible. Likely, future advancements in IT technologies will make it easier to give body to the RAAS.

Summary

- For the most effective rehabilitation outcomes, both functional restoration and environmental modification need to be considered. For mobility devices to be used effectively, the environments in which they are used must be physically accessible.
- Although home modification has been recognized as an important intervention strategy for the quality of life of people with disabilities, the availability of skilled professionals with experience in home modifications for accessibility is limited.
- Several efforts were undertaken to develop a RAAS—a system that helps perform home assessments more easily and at a decreased cost.
- University of Pittsburgh researchers developed VRTS that combines VR technology and telerehabilitation concepts to mitigate limitations of previous RAAS development efforts. It was designed to evaluate the accessibility of physical environments of wheelchair users, employing state-of-the-art digital imaging, 3D reconstruction, and photogrammetry technologies.

- With the rapid evolution of IT technologies, RAAS will fast gain popularity worldwide.

Abbreviations/Acronyms

ADA	Americans with Disabilities Act (ADA) of 1990
ADAAG ADA	Accessibility Guidelines for Buildings and Facilities
AHS	American Housing Survey
CASPAR	Comprehensive Assessment Survey Process for Aging Residents
CIP	Conventional in-person
DSL	Digital subscriber line
FTP	File transfer protocol
IFC	Industry foundation classes
IP	Internet protocol
POTS	Plain Old Telephone System
RAAS	Remote accessibility assessment system
RERC	Rehabilitation Engineering Research Center
RERC-TR	Telerehabilitation RERC
VR	Virtual reality
VRML	Virtual reality modeling language
VRTS	Virtual Reality Telerehabilitation System
Work RERC	Workplace Rehabilitation Engineering Research Center
WRAP	Workplace Remote Assessment Protocol

References

1. Brandt Jr E, Pope A, editors. Enabling America. Washington, D.C.: National Academy Press; 1997.
2. Burns RB, Crislip D, Daviou P, et al. Using telerehabilitation to support assistive technology. Assist Technol. 1998;10(2):126–33.
3. Cooper RA, Cooper R. Trends and issues in wheeled mobility technologies. Presented at the international workshop on space requirements for wheeled mobility, Buffalo, 9–11 Oct 2003. www.ap.buffalo.edu/ideaproto/space%20workshop/Papers/WEB%20-%20Trends_Iss_WC%20(Cooper).htm. Accessed on 15 Feb 2012.
4. Durlach NI, Mavor AM, editors. Virtual reality: scientific and technological challenges, chapter 8. In: Computer science and telecommunications board. Washington, D.C.: National Academy Press; 1994. p. 247–303.
5. Han CS, Kunz JC, Law KH. Compliance analysis for disabled access. In: Space requirements for wheeled mobility, an international workshop. 2001. Available at: http://www.ap.buffalo.edu/idea/space%20workshop/.
6. Kim J, Brienza DM, Lynch RD, et al. Effectiveness evaluation of a remote accessibility assessment system for wheelchair users using virtualized reality. Arch Phys Med Rehabil. 2008;89:470–9.
7. Laiserinm J. High tech for old house. Old House J. 2001. Available at: http://www.oldhouse-journal.com/magazine/2001/sep_oct/high_tech.shtml. Accessed Oct 2001.

8. LaPlante LM. Demographics of wheeled mobility device users. In: Requirements for wheeled mobility, an international workshop. 2002. Availability at: http://www.ap.buffalo.edu/idea/space%20workshop/.

9. Lathan CE, Kinsella A, Rosen MJ, et al. Aspects of human factors engineering in home telemedicine and telerehabilitation systems. Telemed J. 1999;5:169–75.

10. Leica Geosystems HDS LLC. Leica Geosystems HDS. Available at: http://hds.leica-geosystems.com/index.html. Accessed 15 Feb 2012.

11. Lim S, Kim J, Brienza DM, et al. Time and cost effectiveness of workplace assessment for individuals with disabilities. In: Proceedings of RESNA, Toronto, June 2011.

12. Lim S, Kim J, Ikpeama U, et al. Quantitative approach of remote accessibility assessment system (RAAS) in telerehabilitation. In: Proceedings of the 8th international conference on smart homes and health telematics (ICOST 2010), Seoul, 22–24 June 2010.

13. McNeil JM. Americans with disabilities: 1997 U.S. Department of Commerce, Economics and Statistics Administration, Bureau of the Census, Washington, D.C.; 2001.

14. Palmon O, Oxman R, Shahar M, et al. Virtual environments as an aid to the design and evaluation of home and work settings for people with physical disabilities. In: Proceedings of the 5th international conference on disability, virtual reality and associated technologies, Oxford, 2004. p. 119–24.

15. Pope MA, Tarlov AR. Disability in America: toward a national agenda for prevention. Washington, D.C.: National Academy Press; 1991. p. 233.

16. Pratt T. From photo to 3D model. IEE Rev. 2000;46(1):9–12.

17. Pynoos J, Sanford J, Rosenfelt TA. Team approach for home modification. OT Pract. 2002;7(7): 15–9.

18. Quantapoint Inc. Quantapoint. Available at: http://www.quantapoint.com/index.shtm.

19. Sanford JA, Jones M, Daviou P. Using telerehabilitation to identify home modification needs. Assist Technol. 2004;16(1):43–53.

20. Sanford JA, Pynoos J, Tejral A, et al. Development of comprehensive assessment for delivery of home modifications. Phys Occup Ther Geriatr. 2002;20(2):43–55.

21. Saptono A, Parmanto B. An integrated telerehabilitation infrastructure to support speech-language therapy. In: Technology and telecommunications of the ATA2007 12th annual meeting of the American telemedicine association, Nashville, 13–15 May 2007. Abstract published in: Telemed e-Health. 2007;13(2):167–201.

22. Sequeira V, Goncalves JGM, Ribeiro MI. 3D reconstruction of indoor environments. In: Proceedings, international conference on image processing, Lausanne, 1996, vol. 2, p. 405–8.

23. U.S. Department of Housing and Urban Development, U.S. Census Bureau. American housing survey for the United States, supplement, current housing reports, series H151/95. Washington, D.C.: U.S. Government Printing Office; 1995.

Chapter 15
TeleAbilitation: GameAbilitation

Anthony L. Brooks

Abstract This chapter presents the TeleAbilitation concept and describes the potential of contemporary video game gesture controllers in rehabilitation and therapy via their online connectivity. It reflects on the author's previous work focusing on ability rather than on impairment. A novel sensor-based prototype enabling control of multimedia (e.g., games, music, and painting) was used to investigate development of a product for brain-injured patient-to-clinic remote interactions to supplement traditional therapeutic and rehabilitation training methods. At the core of this work is a focus on creativity, challenge/success, and motivated play, all too often ignored aspects of rehabilitation. The potentials from advances in Internet speed and multi-touch interface potentials (e.g., iPad) in the field are also presented.

15.1 Introduction

TeleAbilitation is a concept emerging from the author's body of research called "SoundScapes," originating around 1985. "TeleAbilitation" rather than "telerehabilitation" is selected through SoundScapes' focus on ability rather than on impairment where alternative sensing channels of end-user development are targeted through interactive activities with tailored digital media. It was designed to augment quality of life by motivating engagement through fun experiences via creative expression (i.e., music or painting) or through video game playing.

A.L. Brooks, Ph.D.
Director SensoramaLab, AD:MT, School of ICT, Aalborg University Esbjerg,
Niels Bohrsvej 8, 6700 Esbjerg, Denmark
e-mail: tb@create.aau.dk

S. Kumar, E.R. Cohn (eds.), *Telerehabilitation*, Health Informatics,
DOI 10.1007/978-1-4471-4198-3_15, © Springer-Verlag London 2013

The research is responsible for a family of patent publications[1] that details use of the Internet. Following 3 years of preliminary studies using a self-created prototype gesture-control device with leading brain injury clinics, a feasibility study to develop a product began in 2000. The study was originally reported in the *International Conference for Disability, Virtual Reality, and Associated Technologies (ICDVRAT 2004)*.

Such sensor-based technologies that are invisible to the naked eye enable unfettered gesture control. An affordable home-based self-training system was designed as shown in Fig. 15.1. A marketable product where gesture data are communicated to a health-care facility for case-assigned professionals to monitor progress/regression and conduct remote therapy was envisaged.

15.2 Project

Control of responsive multimedia via gesture offers significant potential for therapy and rehabilitation. This chapter refers to a project funded by the Danish government to develop a marketable product for clinical dissemination [2].

Problems with the commercial partner employed to develop the product resulted in limitations and constraints in the developed apparatus; the connectivity aspect of the prototype was never realized. Therefore, the content of this chapter is reflective of the concept (rather than a report of the study) as there are compelling positive potentials of the original concept design relative to the emergence of gesture controllers in the game industry over the last decade. The contemporary controllers, namely the Sony Playstation EyeToy/MOVE, Nintendo Wii, and Microsoft X-Box Kinect, all have online connectivity. The controllers are also affordable due to the size of the game market. This is important for the concept of original design that targeted wide utilization and differentiated from the commercial company's strategy that aimed for market monopolization and thus control of price. This also means that the TeleAbilitation concept, as presented herein and in the patents (see footnote 1), is now feasible with adaptation of commercially affordable devices. However, problems are still evident as described in the rest of this chapter.

The original project, titled Humanics (phase 1: feasibility testing of existing, and phase 2: follow-on prototype/product development), was built upon the author's prior research across a range of impairment. The project work was carried out at the Centre for Rehabilitation for Brain Injury (CRBI), which is located adjacent to the University of Copenhagen, Denmark. This leading, self-contained clinic has been granted special institute status since 1993. The clinic trains adults through holistic and individual treatment with a main focus on return to work and/or improved quality of life. Research and education programs are also conducted at

---

[1] Patent family # EP 1279092 (B1) # WO 0186406 (A1) # US 6893407 (B1) # DE 60115876 (T2) # AU 5822101 (A) # AT 313111 (T).

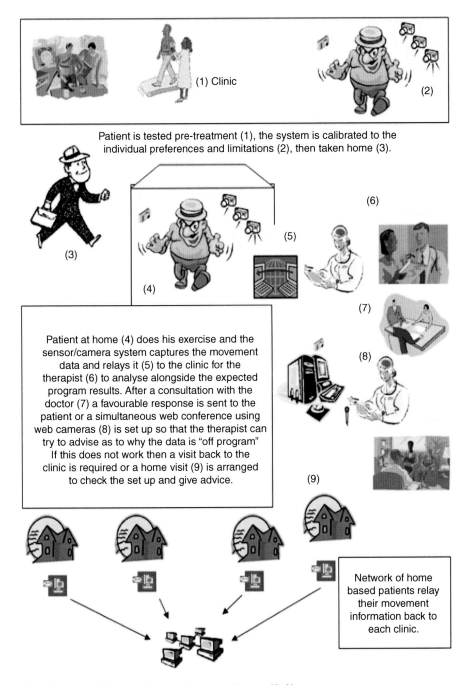

Fig. 15.1 TeleAbilitation (Humanics) concept diagram [2, 3]

the clinic. The clinic is highly respected in the field and considered one of the top European centers, with the team consisting of psychologists, physiotherapists, neurologists, and speech therapists. The mission of the clinic is to facilitate integration through training, and awareness of psychological and physical deficits and strengths through insight and compensatory techniques. The director of CRBI became aware of the research when the author presented *SoundScapes and TeleAbilitation at the 1997 Year of the Brain Conference* in Aalborg, Denmark. The research was conducted for 3 years at two leading institutes: one in Aarhus and one in Copenhagen.

15.3   SoundScapes Concept

A whole-person, nontherapist approach evolved the research from its conception around 1985. Instead of concentrating on specific dysfunction, alternative sensory channels are targeted as a means to stimulate the brain's ability to adapt and, thus, to contribute to development, learning, and/or habilitation. Self-responsibility of training at home with an affordable system that is connected to a health-care clinic via the Internet was a main aspect of the development. Video camera recordings of sessions played a main role in the concept and system evaluations. The camera is positioned to assess and correlate human input data to responsive game/art content and sequential affect. Triangulated session data (e.g., interviews, questionnaires, etc.) supplement the video recordings. The intervention targets longevity and transfer to ADL rather than spontaneous symptom improvement. In many cases, (e.g., persons with profound disabilities), family members, health care professionals, and others close to the end-user assisted with the assessments through their input.

The concept reflects that most people joyously appreciate moving or dancing to music. The prototype sensor system enabled the manipulation of multimedia, (e.g., the creation of music, control of robotic devices, and/or the manipulation of images), all via gross or fine gesture. Such empowerment augments the participants' joy.

Traditional physical rehabilitation after sustained brain injury is often an enduring and cumbersome task for the patient who is encouraged only when a feeling of progression is present. The SoundScapes-empowered activity engenders game playing and creativity. Each interaction can be programmed according to participant profiles so that end-users experience feelings of progression. The actions thus become the unit of analysis. The data resulting from the actions are available for transmitting via the system connectivity to the clinic. The data are monitored by the clinic's health-care professional who matches the data to a planned progression program drawn up by the therapist. If there is any deviation from the predicted program data, the therapist is consulted and a review of interactions ensues to ensure that the setup corresponds to the initial clinical calibration and protocol.

Usually a facilitator leads the initial calibration sessions in the clinic so that the feeling of progression is "trained." This gives an opportunity for the system to be optimized. Subsequent sessions reduce the facilitator input so that the responsibility for training is transferred to the participant. Once achieved, this self-driven motivation transfers to the home-based system.

This work supplements feelings of progression and has the potential to "be the progression" rather than solely a representation of the progress. In this way, physical rehabilitation might be a different, more exciting, and inspiring part of life after sustained brain injury. This hypothesis has grown in strength since the Humanics project with the recent advent of contemporary commercial sensor-based gesture perceptual controllers that replace traditional video game interfaces, e.g. Sony Playstation EyeToy (1 and 2 including MOVE), Nintendo Wiimote (including Motionplus, Nunchuk, and Balance Board), and Microsoft Kinect. Each of these controllers has a different sensitizing profile based on a combination of integrated sensors. Selection of controller can be matched to variance of intervention use within the rehabilitation field. Such gaming platform systems embody responsive multimedia content that is engaging and fun such that the playing through motion is motivational enough to encourage a patient to self-drive his/her own training. Since creativity, challenge/success, and motivated play are at the core of the original system, the work also focuses on these (all too often ignored) aspects of rehabilitation. From this perspective, these foci potentially can affect the creativity and motivation with which the patient meets everyday tasks.

Figure 15.1 illustrates the concept. The upper segment of Fig. 15.1 (image segments 1 and 2) shows the patient being tested in the clinic with "the system." As outlined above, advances in motion-based game controllers offer wider choices for intervention tools to be matched to a patient's profile of need for motion rehabilitation such that a more meaningful rehabilitation program can be planned. Thus, "the system" takes on more varied form compared to the Humanics study wherein the infrared prototype was researched. After the system is set up and calibrated, the patient takes the system home, and trains with family support and without the stress and costs involved in having to report physically to the clinic daily or weekly (Fig. 15.1—image segment 3). The progress of the patient's home training (Fig. 15.1—image segments 1–4) is sent automatically via the Internet to the clinic for monitoring (Fig. 15.1—image segments 1–5), fine-tuning, and feedback via web cam and e-mails (Fig. 15.1—image segments 1–8). In cases where distant monitoring could not realign any discrepancy in training, a local consultation was arranged to examine what went wrong (Fig. 15.1—image segments 1–9). In this way, the concept is inclusive so that more patients could network with the clinic. Benefits for patients include therapy that is both economical and time saving, and a methodology that enables families to participate and provide support (Fig. 15.1 lower segment). The conceptual benefit for health-care professionals is that the technical TeleAbilitation system improves time management and thus can contribute to the predicted future service industry shortages to address imminent social demographics.

15.4   The Intervention Triangle

The SoundScapes concept of intervention primarily involves a triad of (a) a participant/patient/client, or end-user; (b) a facilitator/therapist/carer/family, also known as the "significant other," especially in cases of profound and multiple learning disability (PMLD); and (c) a responsive environment content, i.e. a technical interactive multimedia system that is responsive to the participant input data. This "intervention triangle" is established to stimulate inter- and intra-subjective interaction and communication without defining transmitter, receiver, and other components. Gestural translations, and resulting interpretation and response of and to the interactions are present in all elements (a)–(c). They include conscious, subconscious, and/or machine—in other words, (a) relative to (b) and (c), (b) relevant to (a) and (c), and (c) relevant to (a). The relationship between (b) and (c) differs in that the facilitator can increase the parameters of (c) or decrease the interaction challenge/task. It may be reflected that (b) can, in a related way, manipulate (a); however, this can be through physical intervention, (e.g., physically moving the limbs so that the participant receives stimuli to augment awareness of the activity space). It can also be through manipulation of the interactive environment through parameter change, either hardware or software. The facilitator goal is to become increasingly transparent such that the participant is self-driven. In the near future, machine intelligence will be more autonomous through an innate design parameter in line with Dynamic game difficulty balancing, also known as dynamic difficulty adjustment (DDA) or dynamic game balancing (DGB) - (in gaming often referred to as the 'rubber band effect') – to adapt (c) directly and immediately to the input from (a) to optimise the experience [6].

TeleAbilitation, under the SoundScapes Humanics concept (2), extends this intervention triangle through home to clinic connectivity with an embedded content management system (CMS) [7].

The participant is central to the concept such that the intervention change parameters are (a) adaptation of facilitator in-action activity and/or (b) system setup. Early intervention, (e.g., with a new participant), involved the design of intervention/system being determined by information given on participant ability. The first session often involves much experimentation and improvisation by the facilitator as the change parameters are tuned to the participant. Often, a physical action, where the facilitator guides the participant physically to gain awareness of the active sensing space, is required irrespective of the impairment. Once awareness is evident by the participant's actions relative to the active sensing space, the facilitator's goal evolves to allow the participant freedom to explore and learn the space through his or her own actions. Mirroring evolves from being between (a) and (b) where physical gestures of the facilitator (a) are copied by (b) resulting in a (c) digital output that stimulates and motivates the physical interaction - to a (c) mediated mirroring where the facilitator steps back to monitor and interpret a (b) to (b) interaction loop where (b)'s gestures are digitally mirrored directly and immediately (approximately 1ms), which motivates and stimulates the afferent efferent process so that self-driven therapy training results. This can then be managed via the CMS from the distant clinic assigned facilitator.

15.5   Development

This form of learning according to intervention parameter change relates to participant "microdevelopment" profiling of engagement, (i.e., progress and regression through incremented challenge). Learning is also evident for the facilitator—primarily of the participant's needs, desires, and preferences, and the matching of system parameters to a current state with a view to the subsequent changes to incremented challenges related to the microdevelopment. In line with this, Brooks [4] describes a next-generation system where parameter adaptation is autonomous such that change decisions are supported and implemented via an artificial intelligence (AI) engine that "learns" according to participant input and predefined profile. Whether such a system can replace affective human intervention fully is doubtful; however, much activity within affective computing suggests that a potential for supporting future service needs in the field may not be too far away and a virtual therapist [3] may soon be a reality.

15.6   Extending the Intervention Triangle

The SoundScapes TeleAbilitation concept is further described in this chapter. Thus, extension of the "intervention triangle" from a local situation, where the facilitator intervention evolves from physical guidance actions, to observed (i.e., nonphysical) supportive actions is realized by utilizing the exchange of data remotely via the Internet. The inter-subjective aspects are focused upon the home-based participant interaction with the local system. The intra-subjective aspects are in line with subliminal cognitive/motor learning. The system is fine-tuned to the participant such that afferent efferent neural feedback loop closure is achieved to stimulate the inter- and intra-aspects of interaction where the microdevelopment is conceptualized as occurring.

The removal of the facilitator to a remote location from where the intervention is monitored according to a time management program of scheduled observation times considers the future challenges of the service industry. In this way, many more participants should be able to be effectively and efficiently served without diminishing the support for their rehabilitation. The concept has an expectation for the participant to exercise self-responsibility for his or her training. There is also expectation for the family of the participant to provide support by playing the games and creating the music/paintings available on the system.

15.7   Acquired Brain Injury

Essentially, the distinguishing aspect between acquired brain injury rehabilitation needs and others with physical impairment such as spinal cord, or amputees, is that for the former, damage transpires in the brain such that cognitive, emotional, and behavioral processes are permanently altered. Training a person who has acquired brain injury rehabilitation is an enduring process, especially as only limited recovery is acknowledged.

Training often requires travel to a clinic, which involves certain stressful situations for the participant such as public–environment interaction that is challenging, meeting of public–private transportation schedules to be able to attend specific training time, and economic considerations. For the clinic there are management challenges, especially those related to acquired brain injury.

A system design where private individuals could be motivated to train at home and, utilizing the Internet, send their progress information to the clinic therapist for management was novel and judicious. Furthermore, the essential support from family members could provide added motivation, as all are capable of "playing" together with the system in the home setting. The question was asked, however, whether a generic system could be created that would be "user friendly" and efficient across age groups and ability groups, and have continued worth over novelty value as is often seen in similar "tools."

15.8   Creativity and Motivation

Creativity seems to defy definition, and along with motivation is often overlooked in rehabilitation. This means that it is often dismissed as a parameter when trying to define measurable goals in rehabilitation (and in many other areas). Yet we know that the feeling of creating something unique or personal is often a source of satisfaction. Thus, creativity may well be a source for motivation. In rehabilitation, it is clearly apparent that focusing on improvement promotes motivation for the patient to exercise. With use of feedback to movement of the whole body as well as parts thereof, the project used concepts of music and dance as well as games, tasks, and challenges to keep patient's motivation high when "working out." A main idea relative to the brain injury participants is to be able to "hear the way you move" toward an improved proprioception of sense of motion through auditory or visual channels as opposed to traditional proprioception. This is proposed in line with brain plasticity. Thus, Brooks, under his evolving SoundScapes concept, explores Digital Media Plasticity applied to affect Human Performance Plasticity.

15.9   Gesture-Control Rehabilitation

"Motion capture" or "motion tracking" is about capturing human movement and translating it into knowledge about movement efficiency. It is used, for example, in sports, film animation, and rehabilitation. Several different approaches have been used ranging from expensive multi-tracking camera systems (Vicon, Qualisys, and

SIMI) to more low-cost "wearable systems" (DIEM and Troika). Such camera systems involve "expert knowledge and training" for operation and are typically located at institutes that either are funded accordingly or charge high rates for use of the systems. The advent of gesture controllers in video games has changed the need for such specialist setups. However, to be clear, this chapter does not suggest that the commercial game controllers will replace systems that are able to capture and provide advanced data for assessment. It is rather envisaged that the game controllers will supplement by enabling home training; thus, we anticipate that side-by-side training and evaluations will be more accessible in the future. New test batteries are predicted to emerge through such system cooperation [5].

While this work reflects on people with impairment, specifically those with brain injuries, an adaptation of the work includes the aged as this group has the highest prevalence of impairment. Also, as demographic trends indicate increased demands on the future service industries that will cater for increased numbers of older people and people who are impaired, there is envisioned an increased demand for technical systems to support the health-care industries personnel in their intervention.

15.10   Denmark: An Example

This research is based in Denmark.

Denmark has a population of 5.5 million; about 10 % of this is directly affected by functional disability, a percentage that is still increasing. The growing numbers of elderly people result in an increased demand, and an analysis of the demographic development shows that this is an upward trend. In Denmark, the public sector is the largest buyer of assistive technology. From 1999 to 2006, the public expenditure for assistive technology increased by approximately 40 %. In 1999, the total costs for assistive technology amounted to approximately 2.5 billion DKK compared with 3.5 billion DKK in 2005.

In 2005, the total costs for the social sector amounted to about 176 billion DKK, corresponding to a little more than 21 % of the total public expenditure (Eurostats[2]).

In line with the above is the fact that Denmark is highly regarded with respect to innovation (see "Denmark considered 'Innovation Leader' by European Commission"— http://en.vtu.dk/press/2011/denmark-considered-innovation-leader-by-european-commission).

Advances in online speed complement the TeleAbilitation concept in Denmark. The change from dial-up to broadband connections led to online video, cloud computing, and countless other applications. Now we are seeing ultra-high-speed fiber connectivity and Danish Government activities to utilize this as optimally as possible

---

[2] epp.eurostat.ec.europa.eu/.

within many fields. For example, recently the Danish Ministry of Science, Technology, and Innovation focused on the practical applications of photonics. Currently, the high-speed connectivity is provided by fiber optics and Danish researchers are working to develop wireless fiber-optic connections for even faster data transfer. The Danish Government has an objective of making high-speed Internet accessible to all Danes by 2020, giving Denmark the best conditions for knowledge and communication in the future.[3]

Contemporary game systems enable data to be exchanged via Internet between a person's home and a health-care clinic. However, there are still some unanswered questions such as how the raw data can be meaningful to a health-care professional's evaluation of a patient's progression, and how the progression that needs to be "experienced" can be presented, (especially as acquired brain injury rehabilitation entails a long and enduring process toward training the individual to a realization of potentials so as to be able to live a life with optimal quality following injury). Training often requires travel to a clinic, which involves certain stressful situations, economic considerations, as well as environmental consequences. A system design where private individuals could be motivated to train at home and, utilizing the Internet, send their progress information to the clinic therapist for management was novel and judicious. Furthermore, the all-essential support from family members could provide added motivation, as all are capable of "playing" together with the system in the home setting. The question was asked, however, whether a generic system could be created that would be "user friendly" and efficient across age groups and ability groups, and have continued worth over novelty value as is often seen in similar "tools."

This chapter reflects mostly upon the research that was based upon the author's concept, which was established as a feasibility study to ascertain if members of the target group could benefit from such a product, and to receive their input. While all were positive about the concept, there were milestones and deliverables that were not achieved. Even so, the work was foundational and served to advance the philosophies involved.

15.11   The SoundScapes Studio, Café and Spa Day, and Residential Training Center

The research has evolved a consultancy and training facility where day and residential weekends are established for interested parties in advances in the field of perceptual controllers for rehabilitation and therapy. The wheelchair-accessible studio, café, and spa environment host parents, teachers, therapists, as well as end-users.

---

[3] en.vtu.dk.

The TeleAbilitation concept is an integral part of the overall strategy and international clients are anticipated.

15.12   Synopsis

Each of the game controllers uses a camera. Access to the camera-sourced motion data is limited when using the perceptual controller with the platform games. It has not been possible to get a secondary stream of Bluetooth information to monitor and archive motion apart from the game control data stream. Thus, position of the camera for assessment is usually adjacent to the perceptual controller.

Non-game platform data are available from both the Wii and Kinect systems, (i.e., controller motion data). The Wii data can be sourced via software such as Glovepie[4] on PC and OSCulator[5] on Macintosh computers. The MOVE controllers can be tracked in camera-based systems such as Eyesweb.

Game playing mapping of end-user motion data to non-game platform content is often problematic, as the meaningfulness needs to be evident to stimulate interactions to optimize the engagement and motivation of the participant. In the Humanics study, simple games created in Macromedia Flash were used. The simple games and mapping were satisfactory as motion dynamic could be matched to the screen content. However, beyond an initial curiosity (and sometimes interest) the games lacked the narrative or incremental challenge that is common to the commercial game platforms. The intervention in such instances of using a noncommercial game platform requires the facilitator to monitor and change interaction parameters of sensitizing and response of hardware/software.

As well as game playing, SoundScapes uses nongame platform content to stimulate participant's creative expressivity. Early manipulation via the prototype gesture controller was solely auditory feedback, a sort of "gestural disk jockey." Later, around 1993, gesture control of lighting was added via a MIDI-to-DMX translator of the dynamic motion data. The advent of the video jockey (VJ) who uses images to stimulate the audience response to music being played uses similar techniques and mappings for abstract visual output as in this research. Thus, the online activities and developments in VJ culture offers a rich resource for researchers interested in this field of rehabilitation who may not possess technical programming skills, as only basic mapping knowledge is required. Further, the field of interaction is producing numerous students and a potential job market. Such "artists" are also envisaged as a rich resource as collaborating partners within this field to work with teachers, therapists, parents, etc., who may be technophobic, and/or do not have skill in technology. A speculation is that such involvement would evolve the artist's art!

---

[4] http://glovepie.org.

[5] http://www.osculator.net.

15.13   Conclusions

Just as learning is traditionally approached via educational paradigms, rehabilitation is approached through paradigms of therapy and training. Such formalized structures tend to restrict the embedded potentials being recognized in confrontational experiences with interactive environments. A body of research (titled "SoundScapes") is referenced that crosses the borders between such frameworks. In SoundScapes, play, fun, and experiential learning and rehabilitation are intertwined to be a simple "designed doing event." An environment is created as a virtual interactive space [1] where human input is responded to by digital media. Game playing, making music, painting, and robot control are motivated. The learning that is achievable has consequences for functional and independent living. Subjects are persons with disability and older people.

With the advent of noninvasive sensors presenting new opportunities for TeleAbilitation, gesture control is also being explored on the latest touch-sensitive surfaces commonly found on mobile phones and devices such as iPad, etc. This technology offers another avenue for creative and game playing expressions that can assist in TeleAbilitation. In line with this, the concept of ArtAbilitation and GameAbilitation has evolved.

Summary

- TeleAbilitation, emerging from the author's earlier research called "SoundScapes," is designed to augment quality of life by motivating engagement through fun experiences via creative expression (e.g., music and painting) or through video game playing.
- SoundScapes targets alternative sensory channels as a means to stimulate the brain's ability to adapt and, thus, to contribute to development, learning, and/or habilitation. Self-responsibility of training at home with an affordable system that is connected to a health-care clinic via the Internet was a main aspect of the development.
- Traditional physical rehabilitation after sustained brain injury is often an enduring and cumbersome task for the patient who is encouraged only when a feeling of progression is present. The SoundScapes-empowered activity through game playing and creativity can be programmed to reflect progression.
- An environment is created as a virtual interactive space wherein human input is responded to by digital media through game playing, music, painting, and robot control. The benefits achieved include functional and independent living for people with disability and older people.
- The advent of noninvasive sensors presents new opportunities for TeleAbilitation. Gesture control is also being explored on the latest touch-sensitive surfaces commonly found on mobile phones and devices such as iPad, etc.

- SoundScapes thus acts as a catalyst in leading ongoing investigations of Digital Media Plasticity, its evolution in relation to applied practices of rehabilitation, and its affect on Human Performance Plasticity. Developing from this research are original apparatus, systems and strategies to supplement traditional methods as well as new models of intervention, assessment, and validated testing means that utilise digital media.

Abbreviations/Acronyms

ADL   Activities of Daily Living
AI   Artificial intelligence
CRBI   Centre for Rehabilitation for Brain Injury
ICDVRAT   International Conference for Disability, Virtual Reality, and Associated Technologies
PMLD   Profound and multiple learning disability
VJ   Video jockey

References

1. Brooks AL. Virtual interactive space (V.I.S.) as a movement capture interface tool giving multimedia feedback for treatment and analysis. 1999 Available at: http://sciencelinks.jp/j-east/article/200110/000020011001A0418015.php.
2. Brooks AL. Humanics 1: a feasibility study to create a home internet based telehealth product to supplement acquired brain injury therapy. In: Sharkey P, McCrindle R, Brown D (eds) The 5th international conference in disability, virtual reality and associated technologies, ICDVRAT and The University of Reading, Reading, 2004. p. 43–50.
3. Brooks AL. Robotic synchronized to human gesture as a virtual coach in rehabilitation therapy. In: 3rd international workshop on virtual rehabilitation (IWVR2004), VRlab, EPFL, Lausanne, 2004. p. 17–26.
4. Brooks AL. Intelligent decision-support in virtual reality healthcare and rehabilitation. Advanced computational intelligence paradigms in healthcare 5. Studies in computational intelligence, vol. 326. Berlin: Springer; 2011. p. 143–69.
5. Brooks A, Brooks PE. Perceptual Controllers and Fibromyalgia. In: International Conference for Disability, Virtual Reality & Associated Technologies, Laval, France, 2012.
6. Hunicke R, Chapman V. AI for Dynamic Difficulty Adjustment in Games. Challenges in Game Artificial Intelligence AAAI Workshop. San Jose, 2004. pp. 91–6.
7. Mauthe A, Thomas P. Professional Content Management Systems: Handling Digital Media Assets. John Wiley & Sons, 2004. ISBN: 978-0-470-85542-3.

Chapter 16
Virtual Reality Technologies and the Creative Arts in the Areas of Disability, Therapy, Health, and Rehabilitation

S.V.G. Cobb, Anthony L. Brooks, and Paul M. Sharkey

Abstract A key theme in the ArtAbilitation conferences is the relationship between sound, movement, and art, and how these can be used for rehabilitation and/or expression by individuals who may have limited access to conventional communication. The development of VR environments and interactive technology has led to a variety of applications that might broadly be considered as telerehabilitation, including the use of 3D space and interactive feedback for remote assistance of users in the areas of navigation and home living. These technologies can provide access to activities and communication for individuals for whom such affordances are otherwise restricted, and can make the process of rehabilitation more engaging and motivating.

16.1 Introduction

The early 1990s witnessed the birth of a number of international conferences whose focus was solely on the use of emerging interactive technologies in the areas of disability, therapy, health, and rehabilitation. The primary conference concerning the application of virtual reality (VR) technology in the wide field of medicine is

S.V.G. Cobb (✉)
Human Factors Research Group, University of Nottingham,
Room B2, ITRC Building, University Park, Nottingham NG7 2RD, UK
e-mail: sue.cobb@nottingham.ac.uk

A.L. Brooks, Ph.D.
Director SensoramaLab, AD:MT, School of ICT, Aalborg University Esbjerg,
Niels Bohrsvej 8, 6700 Esbjerg, Denmark
e-mail: tb@create.aau.dk

P.M. Sharkey
University of Reading, Reading, UK
e-mail: p.m.sharkey@reading.ac.uk

S. Kumar, E.R. Cohn (eds.), *Telerehabilitation*, Health Informatics,
DOI 10.1007/978-1-4471-4198-3_16, © Springer-Verlag London 2013

Medicine Meets Virtual Reality (MMVR). Held annually in environs of Newport Beach, California, MMVR is now in its 18th year. Strong contributions in the areas of psychology and therapy began to emerge at the early MMVR conferences and, in 1995, led to the establishment of *CyberTherapy*—a recurring theme at MMVR. In 2003, *CyberTherapy* formally separated from MMVR. Remaining in California for its first 2 years, also being held at the same time of year, from 2005, the conference series has been held in a variety of locations internationally in Europe, Asia, and the United States. CyberTherapy, currently held in June as a multi-track conference, has established itself as one of the main foci for research and development in the application of VR tools and technologies in the broad area of therapy and cyberpsychology.

In 1995, a U.K. workshop on the theme of disability and VR technology led to the launch of the biennial *International Conference (series) on Disability, Virtual Reality and Associated Technologies* (ICDVRAT) in 1996. This 3-day single-track conference, held in September, addresses issues relating to the design, development, and application of VR and emerging technologies in disabilities research and practice. The growing interest in the use of creative arts as a medium for rehabilitation and therapy gave impetus to the establishment of a forum for discussion under the title of *ArtAbilitation*.

In 2002, the first *International Workshop on Virtual Rehabilitation* was held in Lausanne, Switzerland. Changing to the *International Conference on Virtual Rehabilitation* (ICVR) in 2007, and with themes broadly similar to ICDVRAT, the 3-day annual conference is also single track, latterly held during the month of June. In 2008, the research community established a new society—the *International Society for Virtual Rehabilitation* (ISVR)—to provide "a multidisciplinary forum for engineers, scientists and clinicians who are interested in employing new technologies for physical, psychological, cognitive, and social rehabilitation applications." The society is now the formal sponsor for both ICDVRAT and ICVR series of conferences, with each conference being held in alternating years.

A key common characteristic of the community is that it is multidimensional and multifaceted, bringing together a diverse mix that has, over the years, included engineers, computer scientists, designers, psychologists, neuroscientists, medical practitioners, physical and occupational therapists, educational scientists, and, more recently, musicians, artists, and actors, all focused on the core objective to explore how these technologies can best be used to the benefit of individuals, practitioners, and carers within medical, health-care, or special educational sectors.

16.2   Terminology Versus Nomenclature

Around the world, approximately 600 million people live with disabilities. The World Health Organization [58], in issuing and reviewing the international classification of impairments, disabilities, and handicaps [28, 29] along with the international classification of functioning, disability, and health [27], acknowledged problematic referral and use of terminologies and nomenclature in the field. Nonuniformity of definitions or classifications is evident by service providers (medical, educational, social welfare, or rehabilitation services), researchers, and policy makers. This is especially prevalent in countries where direct translations can inadvertently cause problems.

Terminologies used in this research field may not be uniform across disciplines, cultures, or practices, and, depending on the reader, may not be considered politically correct or displaying knowledge of a specific medical-related domain. This is evident, for example, from the archives of various conferences in this field, where authors may be academics or scientists from various disciplines, health-care practitioners from distinct fields, or artists with various backgrounds. This wide melting pot results in differing interpretations of terminologies that further test the political correctness of the terms used for classification. No matter how much consistency and correctness are attempted, it appears evident that such diversity of definition and inherent inertia in language will remain.

16.3 Review of ICDVRAT 1996–2006

To mark the 10th anniversary of the ICDVRAT series, a comprehensive review of the conference series over the past 10 years was conducted in 2006, which identified an extensive range and variety of content in some 220 conference contributions to that date. The review paper [15] defined this diversity along three interwoven themes: technology (software, hardware, and interface components), disability (user populations for whom the technology is being developed), and application (specific nature of the research studies presented). This was not a straightforward task as many of the papers did not fit neatly into categories. For example, a paper may present a research study in which a specific user group has tested a technology application designed to support a particular aspect of learning. Another paper may focus on details of technology development for an application that may be relevant to a variety of users. One paper may describe software development only, and another may present an evaluation method with no reference to any specific technology. Yet another may focus on accessibility and interface design issues of assistive technology in general terms.

The classification method used to describe ICDVRAT papers was not exhaustive, nor was it intended to compartmentalize the community—it was merely a means to identify the range and variety of content represented in the ICDVRAT conference series. The full papers from 1996 to 2010 are available through the conference series archive [26].

In very broad terms, the following categorization system was defined:

Technology: The term virtual reality and associated technologies (VRAT) was defined to include "an 'environment,' which can be anything from the real world, through networked real world (telecommunication), 'mixed reality' environments, to non-immersive simulated virtual environments, and fully-immersive virtual environments (VEs); interaction with computers using a variety of devices such as joystick, mouse, 3D controller, gesture and body movement, gaze, and haptic interfaces; feedback from computers via visual, audio, tactile or force-feedback sensory channels; sensor technology such as motion tracking, infrared, ultrasound and camera vision; real-time software filtering to compensate for, or enhance feedback to, users with specific interaction and/or sensory requirements" [15, p. 52]. Categories generated from grouping papers included three-dimensional (3D) VEs, multimedia, multisensory and acoustic environments, interaction methods, haptic force-feedback and tactile devices, and wheelchair-mounted devices.

Disabilities: As has already been discussed in Section 2, the authors recognize that the wider terminology relating to "disability" is inconsistent and confusing, with differing terminology being applied across subject areas or between the levels of involvement. For some, the term "disability" itself carries negative connotations of labeling associated with restricted capabilities and expectations. In the ICDVRAT context, naturally this is not the intention. Rather, it is merely a means of defining and describing what emerging VRAT can offer to enhance and facilitate greater ability for individuals who may find certain tasks and activities difficult.

"As with the definition of 'virtual reality' the definition of 'disability' remains broad, and includes physical, social, cognitive and behavioural needs supported in some way by the emerging technologies in ICDVRAT. Whilst it is difficult, and perhaps inappropriate, to categorize users into single disability groups, analysis of the ICDVRAT papers revealed some sectors with whom considerable research and development work has been conducted. This does not suggest that VRAT is best applied to supporting these groups, but rather it is in these areas that we have seen progressive research studies and therefore greater maturity of technology application and outcome" [15, p. 54]. Arranging papers around the primary end-user group referred to within the papers generated the following broad categories: visual impairment, hearing impairment, cognitive impairment, motor impairment, learning disability, and mobility. An interesting outcome of this classification was the comparatively high number of research papers in the area of visual impairment, when the technology has traditionally been seen as a unique visual experience.

Research applications: "A primary focus of the research and development that emerged over the [first] decade of the conference series has been the validation of proposals for practical *application* in the real world. Many of the applications are devoted to direct care, or assessment or treatment; others include developments that will be targeted at clinicians, physiotherapists and other care providers. It is not surprising therefore that the majority of papers describe applications of VRAT and these are presented at different stages of development from conceptual, through feasibility and pilot study, to experimental and clinical testing. As in the previous sections, our categorization is not exhaustive but represents main themes described in the conference papers" [15, p. 57]. These themes were access and interaction, training and education, assessment and rehabilitation, behavior therapy and phobias, mobility aids, language and communication, technologies for professional use, and technology as design tools.

Conclusions drawn from the review of ICDVRAT conferences 1996–2006 were that, while the field is still very much in its infancy, early-stage research was showing "evidence of potential for VRAT in rehabilitation of motor control and cognitive skills development."

16.4   ArtAbilitation[1]

Even in the early 1990s, it was readily apparent that VR technologies were being employed beyond the early adopters in computer science laboratories, with many artists taking up the challenge of exploring this new medium as a new creative tool. From the first conference in 1996, papers have been presented on how "virtual art"—both visual and aural—can be used as a creatively expressive tool, as a tool to explain impairment, and as a therapeutic tool for individuals in the most challenging circumstances.

The occasional contributions to ICDVRAT in the field of creative arts coalesced in 2006 with the launch of a parallel international conference, *ArtAbilitation*. In its inaugural year, ArtAbilitation was held in Esbjerg, Denmark, alongside ICDVRAT at the *Musikhuset Esbjerg—Esbjerg Performing Arts Centre*. There were 13 presentations in the ArtAbilitation stream complementing some 40 presentations at ICDVRAT. Both conferences were supported with interactive demonstrations, posters, and exhibits by industry, students, and organizations. ArtAbilitation 2006 papers are available in full through the ICDVRAT archive [2].

In 2007, ArtAbilitation featured as a dedicated workshop held in Porto, Portugal, at the architecturally acclaimed *Casa da Música*, as a special session at the *International Computer Music Conference* (ICMC), held in Copenhagen, followed by a series of smaller workshops in Singapore and Australia, and culminating in November with the second ArtAbilitation international conference, held alongside the *17th International Conference on Artificial Reality and Telexistence, ICAT 2007*, once again in Esbjerg, Denmark.

In April of the following year, ArtAbilitation returned to Casa da Música in Porto where the second international public workshop was held. Five months later, at the same venue and jointly in the nearby city of Maia, the 7th ICDVRAT was held with ArtAbilitation 2008 as a joint plenary conference. The conference hosted an extended session on the use of music and sound in the field of disability. The conference concluded with a closing invited presentation, titled *Interpretations*, and held in the main concert hall, see Fig. 16.1. The presentation featured three pieces with the *Orquestra Nacional do Porto*, with guest conductor Luis Carvalho, where the concept of stimulating deaf audience access to classical music through alternative sensitizing channels was presented. The concept of cross-referencing audience-perceived performance motion (conductor and musicians) and performance audition (music) data and resulting visual interpretation of the music and live performance

---

[1] See Sharkey (p. 177) in Wiederhold B (2007) Virtual healers. ISBN: 0-9724067-2-7.

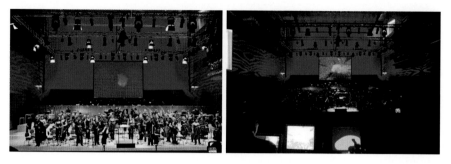

Fig. 16.1 Interpretations, at Casa da Música, Porto (Adapted from Ref. [5]. Images by Paul Sharkey)

offering stimulation was presented. The concept was previously commissioned for concerts in Aarhus, Denmark (1999), and Auckland, New Zealand (2002). The event segued to the opening of the second *Art, Brain and Languages* symposium, also held in Casa da Música.

After the comprehensive calendar of events over the previous 2–3 years, the ArtAbilitation "movement" continued with a much lowered profile in 2009, returning as a special session at ICDVRAT 2010 conference held in Chile. The relatively muted response to the calls for papers for ArtAbilitation in 2010 contrasted the interest in earlier years, although this may be explained in part by the relative challenge represented by the conference location in terms of time, cost, and uncertainty due to the 2010 earthquake.[2]

Reflecting on this, it is possible that the economic downturn played a contributory role as universities became more reluctant to support delegates to attend a relatively small specialized conference. Another reason could have been that ArtAbilitation was too widely banded and, in this way, lost its identity as initially interested networks questioned whether ArtAbilitation referred to a conference, panel, symposium, or even entertainment. Perhaps, the research community devoted to the creative arts in the areas of disability and rehabilitation and enablement has yet to reach the critical mass necessary to sustain a level of activity that was so promising between 2006 and 2008.

It should be noted that the ArtAbilitation movement was never intended to be a single-channel vehicle (i.e., solely as a conference). Rather the transdisciplinary/transindustry strategy (e.g., academia, scientists, practitioners, students, etc.) targeted presenting works via small conferences, symposia, and/or panels, while also making available more practical and inclusive and accessible (usually commissioned) workshops, seminars, and "master classes" where the audiences' application area dictated design. To date, this is what has been achieved. However, because of this disruptive strategy, it has not always been feasible to present ArtAbilitation,

---

[2] Any fears or uncertainties due to the earthquake some 6 months earlier were completely unfounded. The infrastructure in Chile is, in fact, very robust and there was little evidence of any damage in the central region between the capital, Santiago, and the coastal city of Viña del Mar where the conference was held.

and also its sibling entities "GameAbilitation" and "Ludic Engagement Designs for All" (LEDA), as self-standing "happenings" due to these being presented as embedded aspects of a greater whole where titling inclusion was impossible.

Thus, the core thread of the movement since its conception, and one that differentiates the approach taken to augment the field, is the focus on entertainment computing to supplement traditional intervention in disability, therapy, health, and rehabilitation. Thus, a focus is on means, methods, and processes toward human-attributed outcome, including creative expression, playful interactions, and fun. Such "entertainment computing" is the subject of increased investigations, research publications, and events,[3,4] albeit with delimited focus (when compared to traditional) on disability, therapy, health, and rehabilitation. In line with this, ArtAbilitation's identity increasingly becomes clearer, contributing alongside its siblings as a multifaceted entity to fill this void. Thus, in 2011, the ArtAbilitation and GameAbilitation symposiums were run alongside the third iteration of ICST/Create-Net/European Alliance for Innovation sponsored conference series "ArtsIT," this being for its inaugural exposure outside Asia,[5] previously held in Yi-Lan, Taiwan (2009), and Chong-Qing, China (2010).

16.5   Updated Review of ICDVRAT/ArtAbilitation

As may be expected, the content of any individual ICDVRAT/ArtAbilitation conference reflects the current interests of the presenting delegates attending the conference. Attendance or absence from a specific conference is determined by many factors, including the opportunity to travel and available funding. Therefore, in a conference community that is so broadly defined, paper content at different conferences can vary considerably from 1 year to the next, and so it is difficult to draw out themes and evidence of progressive development of research within the community. However, as the authors have followed the conference series from the outset, this section presents an overview of selected trends and developments that we have observed in the ICDVRAT and ArtAbilitation research communities.

A key theme in the ArtAbilitation conferences is the relationship between sound, movement, and art, and how these can be used for rehabilitation and/or expression by individuals who may have limited access to conventional communication. First presented in 2002 through the work of Brooks et al. [6], a good description of the concept is given by Lopes-dos-Santos et al. [38], which is as follows:

The concept of musical virtual space refers to an environment where human physical movements are translated into real time auditory feedback provided through appropriated stimuli for music making (e.g., percussive sounds, notes from different scales, and chords delivered by distinct "instruments"). While interacting with such

---

[3] http://www.acm.org/pubs/cie/.

[4] http://www.ace2011.org/.

[5] http://www.artsit.org.

environments, immediate "musical" responses to gestures are likely to be so pleasing that make individuals unaware of the effort involved in the generation of movement [6]. Pleasurable experiences resulting from immersion in musical virtual spaces increase the motivation to move and stimulate the performance of motor activities. On the other hand, if embedded in meaningful interpersonal contexts, movements produced in relation with technology may acquire a communicative value, developing into expressive gestures [38, p. 370].

A review of papers presented at ArtAbilitation conferences shows examples of how the array of technologies encompassed within the ArtAbilitation movement have been applied in a variety of ways to enhance learning, experience, communication, and self-expression among different groups of individuals. These are summarized under the following three headings depicting the nature of user experience offered. The review then continues with an updated summary of papers presented at the 2008 and 2010 ICDVRAT conferences.

16.5.1 Multisensory Interaction

One of the first papers presented described how the SoundScapes system previously cited [6] had been used to "empower interaction through creativity" [23]. This paper reports a single case study conducted at a special school in Sweden that featured an autistic young adult with severe physical and behavioral dysfunction, interacting within an immediately responsive multisensory active environment where nonintrusive technological interfaces (two soundbeams) were used alongside traditional switch interfaces to a great effect. A more elaborate, yet affordable, multisensory system is described in another school-based case study conducted at a school in Wales [57]. Three children with profound and multiple learning disabilities (PMLDs) created "digital art" through their physical movement. A standard video-camera-based system was used to capture images of the child to produce "digital painting" and auditory feedback in response to gestural movement, in coloring, patterning, and style. A study from Portugal presents another case example of digital painting through gesture along with auditory feedback [3]. This study reports improvements in quality of movement control, intentionality, and behavior in a child with cerebral palsy.

This concept was extended in further work conducted by research team members at the SensoramaLab complex at Aalborg University, Denmark. A rapid prototyping approach is demonstrated to facilitate gesture control of games in which control is adaptive to end-user needs, preferences, and desires by using different sensors and modalities of influence according to idiosyncratic profiles [5]. Additionally, explorations of an open online 3D virtual world where users can socialize, connect, and create are reported. Outcomes highlight how the availability of a simple prototyping platform with free games and new interfaces opens the discussion on the design of original rehabilitation and therapeutic applications. Implementation in future healthcare service needs and the use by future generations of collaborative therapist/artist/programmers are predicted.

Further examples of gesture-based interaction to control music and visual digital displays include the "CaDaReMi—educational interactive music game" [20] and the "SOUND=SPACE opera," a 14-week residency at Casa da Música in Porto, Portugal, with special-needs end-users that cumulated in public performances that showcased the results [1]. Experimental artist/author Mick Grierson [22] describes the technical and aesthetic approach used for the development of a freely available interactive audio–visual performance system designed specifically for use by children with multiple learning difficulties, including deafness and autism.

However, the HCI challenges in designing such systems can be complex and difficult, as reported in other papers [11], which describe the limitations and problems in designing a novel infrared sensor-based music and sound controller for special-needs end-users and [50] report studies that question providing disabled persons in developing countries access to computer games through a novel simple-to-manufacture and low-cost gaming input device.

16.5.2 Communication and Self-Expression

Some papers have focused on how multi- and intersensory interaction can provide a means of communication and self-expression. For example, van Leeuwen and Ellis [53] describe the iMuse project in which elderly people living in sheltered accommodation creatively express themselves through voice, microphone, and special-effect units that manipulate the output, or/and their movement via the nonintrusive sensor soundbeam with output mapped to a sound module. The study is a part of a long-term research project, and current evaluation strategies are reported. In another example, a "tangible interaction system" was demonstrated by Yau and McCrindle in 2006. A design prototype of "MusiCam" used Lego bricks as an easily manipulated colored interface that produced musical tones when presented into the field of view of a standard web camera [59].

In other studies, technology has been applied specifically as an augmentative and alternative communication (AAC) system to stimulate language and communication skills. "Explorascope" is an interactive, adaptive educational toy designed for children between 1 and 4 years of age with multiple handicaps [25]. In Japan, a talking robot that has mechanical organs like a human is used alongside an adaptive learning strategy for auditory feedback control. The robot initially learns vocalizations autonomously and then reproduces the speech articulation from auditory input. This system is used as a vocalization training system for the auditory-impaired individuals [32].

Whole-body movement is important for rehabilitation. Members of the Théâtre Aphasique Montréal in Canada describe how acquired brain damage patients diagnosed with aphasia rebuild aspects of their lives, especially communication skills, and self-esteem, with the help of a dedicated theatre situation [16]. The work is notable from the positive outcomes achieved by the team. A recent collaborative project between Tokyo University, Japan, and Monash University, Australia, shows how body-worn devices can be used to encourage participants to view and experience their bodies from alternative perspectives [55]. The researchers' intention is to provide a rich playground for self-expression, as well as learning opportunities that might be relevant for people with physical challenges and unconventional or altered abilities.

16.5.3 Exploration and Discovery

Some ArtAbilitation papers focus on the use of interactive technologies to support learning and/or discovery of the world around us. For example, a demonstration of interactive flashlights used in special needs education was given by Cobb et al. [14]. Innovative computer vision software enables the interface to "magically bring to life" objects and areas that are used for children with special needs in exploration, playing, and learning activities toward development. Torres [52] details how new mental and physical activities such as contemporary video games can be used to decrease the morbidity resulting from biopsychosocial losses associated with old age. Effects on self-concept and the quality of life are investigated.

The previous review of ICDVRAT conference papers [15] identified a significant body of research that focused on development of applications for individuals with visual impairment. Recent examples presented at ArtAbilitation demonstrate the effectiveness of 3D virtual models to communicate information. Kirner et al. [31] gave an example of an augmented reality tool to help blind people understand, describe, and convert 3D scenes into 2D embossed representations. Lahav and Levy [35] demonstrated the use of a sonified model for blind students to learn about gas particles, showing how vision-impaired students can understand complex scientific models through compensatory sensory channels.

A strong theme of the ArtAbilitation movement is that it uses technology to give a means of self-expression to individuals who have limited channels of communication. An important aspect of this is that the individuals are given freedom to control how they interact with the system. Too often, well-meaning interventions by support staff negate the intended interactions that a user wants to achieve. This is illustrated in two independent case examples in creative intervention sessions with special needs children [56]. Williams suggests that a lack of understanding of roles is evident that is inconsiderate of specific end-user needs, preferences, and desires. An inability to optimally support the end-user in processes (often hands-off) where most benefit could be gained is reported.

The final report in this section exemplifying creative works in the ArtAbilitation field is from the closing event of ICDVRAT 2008, in the main auditorium Casa da Musica, Porto, featuring *gesture and music mapped to interactive visuals and responsive tactile feedback experience* performances by the Orquestra Nacional do Porto, which many refer to as the national symphony orchestra of Portugal. The concept attempts to advance the field of visual music[6] while evolving research that bridges performance art and empowerment of people with different abilities. "Interpretations" is the title given to this event that represents the performance art perspective of a body of work titled SoundScapes. In this context, exploration of intersensory stimulus and representations that target deaf audience's appreciation of classical music live performance were investigated featuring renowned Portuguese conductor Luis Carvalho with Orquestra Nacional do Porto. In this context, the concept of cross-referencing audience-perceived performance motion (conductor and musicians) and performance audition (music) data and resulting visual interpretation of the music and live performance offering stimulation was presented. Core to the sourcing of data is an array of stage hardware that establishes numerous invisible active sensing areas referred to as virtual interactive spaces (VIS). Autonomous information is sensed and then routed to a mixer workstation. Mixing and mapping are improvised to visual representations so that (a) connections and relationships to the dynamic sourced data are made obvious, (b) a direct and immediate effect is evident that corresponds to the musical output, and (c) a correlated ambience is created as a complementary palate upon which to create and experience the more immediate dynamic interpretations. The conductor's expression is catalytically forever prevalent. The concept was previously commissioned for concerts in Aarhus, Denmark (1999), and Auckland, New Zealand (2002). Further details of this specific event that illustrated the work in progress is via a publication hosted at the website for the 7th International Conference on Disability, Virtual Reality, and Associated Technologies held alongside ArtAbilitation 2008.[7]

16.5.4 Cognitive Assessment and Rehabilitation

The first keynote paper in the 2008 conference was given by Professor Skip Rizzo from the Institute for Creative Technologies (ICT), University of Southern California [45]. This paper comments on how VR, described as a "fad technology" in 1998, has developed into a functional technology for use in clinical psychology and rehabilitation. Professor Rizzo commends the diligence of researchers in the VR community for battling through the phases of "hype" and "disillusionment," working with time-consuming, expensive, and cumbersome technology and power-hungry graphics requirements to demonstrate that, despite the fact that early VEs displayed anything but ecological validity, appropriate design of VR-based tasks was sufficient to demonstrate effective application for rehabilitation and therapy. As has already been discussed, rapid advances in computing technology over the last decade have enabled more control over the design of interactive content and faster development periods. This has brought many more researchers into the community, and we are

---

[6] For example, McDonnell (2002) Available at: http://homepage.eircom.net/~musima/visualmusic/visualmusic.htm.

[7] http://www.icdvrat.reading.ac.uk/2008/interpretations.htm.

now seeing more studies being conducted in clinical, rather than in laboratory-based, settings. As a consequence, VR-based programs are emerging among the battery of methods used in clinical assessment and rehabilitation. For example, the Virtual Reality Cognitive Performance Assessment Test (VRCPAT) is now available as a viable tool for neurological assessment [44]. The development in this field is covered extensively in the CyberPsychology literature. Examples presented at ICDVRAT include the Virtual Executive Neuropsychological Rehabilitation project, which created a series of tasks to assess and empower executive function and other cognitive skills [39]. This included the V-Store, described as a "virtual environment (internal store) in which the subject (clinical or experimental) has to solve a series of tasks ordered in six levels of increasing complexity. Tasks are designed to stress executive functions, behavioural control and programming, categorical abstraction, short-term memory and attention" [39, p. 168]. Unfortunately, this paper did not include test results. However, the work of Evelyne Klinger and colleagues at Arts et Metiers ParisTech had developed a virtual action planning supermarket (VAP-S) and found this to be an effective and viable tool for assessment of executive function skills in individuals with central nervous system (CNS) deficit [33]. In later studies, this system was used successfully to identify differential performance profiles in patients with different types of clinical diagnoses [30]. Recently, Klinger's research group demonstrated effective utility of an ecologically valid therapeutic virtual kitchen (TVK) for the assessment of executive function skills in patients with brain injury [10]. These results illustrate progressive development of a concept of VR application to rehabilitation training that began in the early 1990s. Early examples of VEs designed to emulate real-world tasks and activities (for example, the Virtual City project [7]) focused on usability and therapist acceptance of the technology (e.g., the virtual coffee-making task [17]).

16.5.5   Physical Exercise and Motor Coordination

Another significant area of research in the application of associated VR technologies has been directed toward management of physical exercise and improvement of motor coordination skills. Perhaps, this is because the repetitive nature of the exercise regimen is ideally suited to automation in some form. While it is important that such tools are not applied in an unsupervised way, the nature of the supervision becomes less intensive and, as a consequence, expertise can be delivered more widely.

There is a wealth of research in the area of robot-assisted physical therapy with many hospital based-trials having been conducted, each reporting varied success. For example, Frisoli et al. [19] tested the PERCRO L-Exos (Light-Exoskeleton) system for robot-assisted rehabilitation therapy in clinical trials with nine chronic stroke patients. The results found significant improvement on a variety of active and passive movement scales. Merians et al. [41] also found improvement in kinematic measures and upper limb stability in chronic-phase post-stroke patients

9.3.4   Synchronous Audiology Systems and Services

There are several different ways to configure audiometric equipment for audiology services. For example, a wide range of audiometric services was provided to individuals in northern California using interactive video only. A certified technician provided services at the patient site using typical audiometric equipment. A certified audiologist used the interactive video to observe clients and also to counsel the client once services were provided [2].

9.3.5   Remote Computing Audiometry

A second method in which synchronous audiology services could be provided is through the use of remote computing software to control PC-based audiometric systems. As this audiometric equipment was operated by Macintosh or Windows-based operating systems, remote computing software could be employed in conjunction with PC-based audiology systems to provide hearing tests at distant sites. The early remote computing projects described in the 1990s used this paradigm to evaluate the feasibility for programming hearing aids. In addition, researchers also used remote computing with pure-tone and OAE tests [2, 14]. Figure 9.2 shows how pure-tone testing could be conducted using remote computing software and off-the-shelf computerized audiometric equipment.

However, dedicated teleaudiology systems have been developed in the past decade. And while both off-the-shelf and dedicated systems have performed equally as well, the convenience of dedicated telehealth systems will likely encourage their adoption more so than off-the-shelf systems. One example of a dedicated teleaudiology system has been presented by Swanepoel et al. [24]. Hardware is not required at the remote site to use this system. For testing, clients at the clinical site wear both insert and circumaural headphones to reduce ambient noise. The headphones also contain microphones to monitor ambient noise levels. The client uses a gamer's control pad attached to the computer at the local site to register a response to stimuli. Use of microphones within the headphones offers a means to determine the noise floor levels and is created expressly for teleaudiology purposes.

Finally, it should be noted that web-based audiometers have been developed and are available online at modest prices. However, web-based audiometers have not been subject to vigorous validation and therefore might have validity issues. These issues include lack of calibration of headphone or earbuds, ambient noise levels at test sight, client use of these systems, and accuracy in the assessment of various kinds of ear pathology.

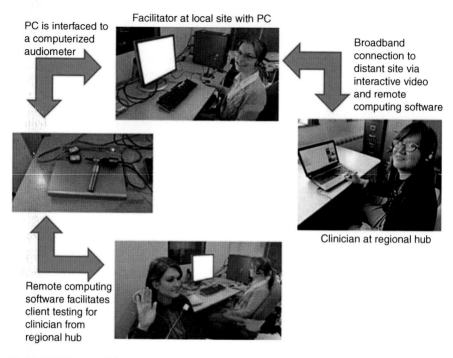

Fig. 9.2 Using an off-the-shelf computerized system, it is possible to test clients over a network or the internet. In the example provided in this figure, the audiology clinician is at a regional clinic providing hearing health care to a client at another location

9.3.6 Otoacoustic Emissions

Less information is available concerning the efficacy of important procedures that are an essential part of complete hearing evaluations. One procedure that has received only minimal validation in teleaudiology is OAE. A thesis conducted by Schmiedge [20] detailed the use of teleaudiology with an off-the-shelf OAE system made by Virtual Systems and Timbuktu remote computing software. This project appears to be the first attempt to test hearing using remote computing technology. While all 30 subjects of the study were tested within the same building in which Schmiedge was located, this proof of concept study indicated that remote computing applications was feasible. It is notable that Schmiedge was also able to use this technology to test subjects in Canada from his location in North Dakota. Replication of this work in adults was later reported by Krumm et al. [16], who used PC-based technology to test subjects over 1,000 miles away. Elangovan [7] also reported similar success with an OAE system using a dedicated interface and software to accomplish testing as a proof of concept study.

All of the published studies on OAE have been conducted with adults except in one case. Specifically, Krumm et al. [15] demonstrated that OAE testing could be conducted in newborns over a distance of 150 miles. Krumm and colleagues used who had used a VR simulation interfaced with a robotic arm for only 2 weeks of intensive training.

The use of haptic-based robot-assisted therapy allows a range of benefits from a wholly robot-guided motion in the initial phase, through an assistive phase whereby the robot only acts to guide motion where the use deviates from the required path. The robot system benefits from being able to monitor motion trajectories and thus track any improvements that have been made over time. A major disadvantage is the expense of providing such systems, even in a hospital setting. The cost of using such systems in the home environment is prohibitive. Thus, there is a good argument for other interactive sensor tools to be used in the latter stages of rehabilitation.

16.5.6 *"Virtual Reality" and Beyond*

The previous conference review paper stated that "The predominant technology applied in ICDVRAT is Virtual Reality (VR) or Virtual Environments (VE)" [15, p. 52]. Perhaps this is not surprising, given the conference title, but an interesting observation is that, only 4 years later, this is no longer the case. Noted as an emerging trend in 2006, "a recent theme has developed in the use of simple technology and widely available interfaces such as the EyeToy for rehabilitation" [15, p. 52], we are now seeing more examples of other types of interactive technologies and adaptations to off-the-shelf games applied to rehabilitation and fewer examples of "traditional" VR/VEs.

With a target audience who may have cognitive and/or motor impairments, the design of such applications and interface devices is all the more challenging. Langdon et al. [36] highlighted this issue by focusing on a user-centered design process to consider how individuals with different levels of motor and/or cognitive ability can interact with a number of reference applications, through a variety of input devices using a home-based set top box system. Meanwhile, Burke et al. [9] report on a set of identifying principles that are considered to be important in the design of serious games in the rehabilitation of upper limb rehabilitation following stroke. They report on how such principles might be implemented and include an evaluation, based on playability, usability, and engagement, of a number of games.

In 2008, Herbelin et al. [24] propose a rapid prototyping approach using various commercial devices and open source software as a path to establish a common basis for development and experimentation. By using freely available games, and extending their application to Second Life, they were able to demonstrate the flexibility of this approach across a wide target group of health-care professionals, patients, and families. Also in 2008, Vickers et al. [54] have considered the very essence of interaction in massively multiplayer online games (MOOGs) and worlds (such as World of Warcraft and Second Life), and the barriers and privacy issues encountered by participants with disability where the dexterity required of keyboard/mouse interfaces presents a severe challenge.

Flynn and Lange [18] explored, from the perspective of the users, the experience of the user participation through an online survey of more than 150 participants.

Some of the questions posed included the game play experience and interaction on a range of popular video games, but also addressed how off-the-shelf games have been used in rehabilitation and indeed how they might be improved from both leisure/pastime and rehabilitation points of view.

16.5.7 Wearable Assistive Technologies

There is a strong interest in developing wearable technologies as tools and aide memoires, or as a more persistence virtual aide de camp. Sánchez and colleagues have focused their recent attention on mobility and navigation for people with severe visual impairment or who are blind. In their 2008 paper, this was through a hand-held device, *AudioTranssantiago*, that allowed users to plan and navigate routes through the bus transportation network in the city of Santiago [47]. In 2010, they investigated a real-time audio feedback system that allowed the users to navigate through a space that had been instrumented with augmented reality markers, thus providing users with a better sense of orientation and mobility [48]. Meanwhile, Kuroda et al. [34] also presented a marker-based location system where the markers were used as aide memoires for users with memory impairment. While these devices and applications are strictly assistive in nature, it would be possible in each case to extend the functionality of the wearable devices to allow data to be reviewed by a health-care professional, or indeed, for more immediate assistance to be available. One such example is reported by McCrindle et al. [40] who introduce a wearable device to assist independent living for older people. The paper reports on the development of a wearable that monitors health status, detects potential problems, can provide activity reminders, and can also offer communication and alarm services.

16.5.8 Virtual Humans

Finally, we return to high-fidelity avatars in the research conducted at the ICT at the University of Southern California. Since 1999, ICT has been exploring how the creative talents of the games and film industry, together with leading technologists and psychologists, might be best harnessed. A number of projects, under the direction of Rizzo, have been developed in the psychology and neuroscience areas, including, for example, the use of VR in the treatment of post-traumatic stress disorder. In an interesting development, Parsons et al. [44] reported on the Virtual Patient project, where a number of advanced conversational human avatars have been applied in the psychiatric medical field as training "foils" for clinicians. Here, the trainee clinician is presented with an avatar with a particular back story, for example, a drug addict or a victim of sexual assault. By engaging with the avatar, the trainee learns the skills required to deal more effectively with real-world clients.

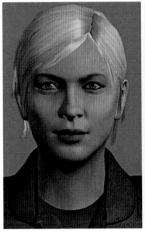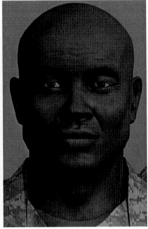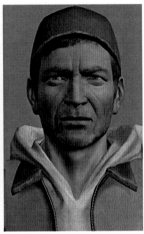

Fig. 16.2 SimCoach archetypes—female aviator, battle buddy, retired sergeant major

The technology behind the Virtual Humans project has since been adapted for use in SimCoach [46] whereby a veteran or a member of the (U.S.) armed forces in need of advice with regard to their health care may engage the help of a virtual friend to confide in and seek additional help (see Fig. 16.2). The purpose of the SimCoach is to establish an initial route into health care for individuals who might otherwise avoid seeking help

In a third project from ICT, called *Warrior's Journey*, Morie et al. [42] also tackle the issue of remote assistance for veterans by exploring how to reach recently returning veterans who are experiencing mental health problems or having difficulties adjusting to home life. The *Warrior's Journey* presents a narrative that the participant engages with to build self-esteem, allowing them to construct their own warrior's story within the application's Coming Home space.

An important and growing area of research in this field is concerned with the use of VR and associated technologies for telerehabilitation. This topic is covered widely in associated conferences as well as technology journals (e.g., *Presence, Teleoperators and Virtual Environments*) and domain-related journals. The following section presented the current state of the art in this field as reported in ICDVRAT/ArtAbilitation papers of 2008 and 2010.

16.6 Developments in Research and Application of VR for Telerehabilitation

The vision for use of VR for telerehabilitation was first proposed by Walter Greenleaf in 1997 [21]. This early concept of a "VR rehabilitation workstation," through which patients could conduct motivational functional tasks in their own home, has been difficult to realize. Only recently we have seen examples of systems successfully placed in the home through which clinicians can remotely monitor patient performance. And still these are affected by problems relating to cost and reliability of network services [43].

The development of bespoke VR environments and interactive technology has led to a variety of applications that might broadly be considered as telerehabilitation, including the use of 3D space and interactive feedback for remote assistance of users in the areas of navigation and home living. In more recent years, there has been an increasing interest in the use of standardized, off-the-shelf (and hence low cost) game-based systems, in terms of both the video content and the commercially available interface tools, or adaptations thereof, through which the patients can access content.

The question of realism versus ecological validity remains a widely debated topic. The realism with which a VE is presented is directly related to the resource that can be made available for any given project in the development phase. And, while it is true that increasingly detailed models—of the environment such as buildings, infrastructures, furniture, other general objects, as well as human avatars—are more readily available online, the expertise to general bespoke application environments remains a challenge. Conversely, it is also well documented that VR-based rehabilitation can be very effective regardless of the sophistication—or distinct lack thereof—of environments used. What remains important lies more with the design of the environments and engagement of the participant.

In 2008, Pareto et al. [43] addressed the question of "usefulness of virtual reality based rehabilitation equipment in practical therapy, by letting experienced therapists explore one such equipment during 6 months in their regular practice under natural circumstances." The authors concluded that such equipment does have benefits beyond real-life training but requires sufficient variation in content and cognitive challenge to make such a system particularly suitable. In the intervening years, this group started to test such a telehealth system in rural Sweden, as reported by Broeren et al. [4], whereby a number of stroke subjects participated. The initial findings led to clinical changes for all subjects, although some training issues were also highlighted in terms of the audio–visual communications and the turn-taking process between therapist and patient.

The telehealth system applied in the Swedish trials is nevertheless an expensive investment (Fig. 16.3). Other groups have been researching the use of commercially available games controllers; for example, Chortis et al. [12] conducted a feasibility study with eight participants using the standard demonstration applications from a Novint Falcon, and the same group in 2010 [51] reported on the use of a virtual glove as a low-cost interface device, although again only a small feasibility trial was reported. Hand motion has also been investigated by Shefer Eini et al. [49] through the use of a camera-tracked hand grip—essentially two ping-pong balls illuminated by different colored LEDs—using a very simple vision algorithm. This paper conducted an extensive trial with 15 patients and 15 control subjects, concluding that this interface device was very reliable and a valid tool for assessing wrist range of motion during dynamic activities.

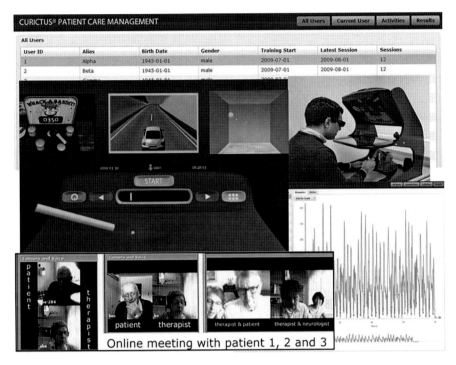

Fig. 16.3 Telehealth system: a desktop-sized immersive workbench, PCMS with activity data (velocity graph), and screen shots from the user interface, and video conferences. "Pictures showing subjects are approved for scientific publication by the person in the image" (Adapted from Ref. [4])

Brown et al. [8] also reported on a trial with 12 participants that used a bespoke target-reaching apparatus, the ULTrA, which was deployed in the home to guide upper-arm-reaching tasks for patients with cerebral palsy. After each session, data were sent to the research laboratory for further analysis. The initial results demonstrated an improvement in upper limb function with many participants being eager to continue similar training once the intervention was complete.

Cikajlo et al. [13] have conducted a pilot project to assess the use of a VR-based system for balance training. Six stroke patients performed therapy five times per week over a 3-week period, and the results showed improvement in all measures. The authors conclude that a telerehabilitation system could provide patients with the facility to continue therapy in the home over a longer rehabilitation period. Lange et al. [37] examined the feasibility of using off-the-shelf step-based exercise and dance video games to improve balance in older adults. Early results indicate that there is potential for use of these types of games in rehabilitation although the software requires modification to ensure that it is "fit for purpose" both for the target user population and to deliver controlled exercise tasks that are relevant to, and appropriate for, the rehabilitation exercises required. This research is opening up possibilities for new directions in telerehabilitation research that will focus on adaptation of existing computer programs rather than development of new software.

The resulting reduced cost of system development could lead to a great expansion in the availability and affordability of telerehabilitation programs.

16.7   Conclusion

This chapter brings up to date the authors' review of contributions to the ICDVRAT and ArtAbilitation conference series. Confinement of the articles cited to the conference series is deliberate and allows us to comment on the field as we are most familiar with it. We recognize that this might result in a confined view of the broader field of research engaged in development and application of VR, associated technologies, and other interactive technologies to medical research, assessment and diagnoses, rehabilitation, and accessibility. These are large research disciplines in their own right and represented sufficiently in specialist conferences and journals. Our objective, therefore, is not to provide a comprehensive state-of-the-art review of the field in general, but to offer comment on how we have seen one part of the research community develop over the last 15 years. Perhaps, most striking is the variety of participants on this community. Since its inception in 1996, ICDVRAT conferences have brought diverse groups together, pitching scientific research papers alongside technology feasibility demos, practitioner opinion, and questioning of the "added value" of such expensive, slow-to-realize technology alongside end-user presentations describing their involvement in research and the importance of developers listening directly to them. ArtAbilitation conferences took this a step further, hosting vast multimedia experience events and demonstrating fundamental principles of the "added value" that we believe is on offer. These technologies are not just gimmicks or entertainment. They can provide access to activities and communication for individuals for whom such affordances are otherwise restricted; they can make the process of rehabilitation more engaging and motivating. They *can* make a difference.

Summary

- The early 1990s witnessed the birth of a number of international conferences that focused on the use of emerging interactive technologies in the areas of disability, therapy, health, and rehabilitation.
- Since 1996, the focus of related conferences has been on how "virtual art" can be used as a creatively expressive tool to explain impairment and as a therapeutic tool for individuals in the most challenging circumstances.
- A key theme in the ArtAbilitation conferences is the relationship between sound, movement, and art, and how these can be used for rehabilitation and/or expression by individuals who may have limited access to conventional communication.
- There is a strong interest in developing wearable technologies to improve mobility and navigation for people with severe visual impairment or who are blind. Research has focused on the development of a wearable that monitors health status, detects potential problems, can provide activity reminders, and can also offer communication and alarm services.

- Although a VR rehabilitation workstation has been difficult to realize, recently some systems have successfully been placed in the home through which clinicians can remotely monitor patient performance. However, these still are affected by problems relating to cost and reliability of network services.
- These technologies can provide access to activities and communication for individuals for whom such affordances are otherwise restricted; they can make the process of rehabilitation more engaging and motivating.

Abbreviations/Acronyms

AAC	Augmentative and alternative communication
CNS	Central nervous system
HCI	Human-Computer Interaction
ICDVRAT	International Conference (series) on Disability, Virtual Reality and Associated Technologies
ICMC	International Computer Music Conference
ICT	Institute for Creative Technologies
ICVR	International Conference on Virtual Rehabilitation
ISVR	International Society for Virtual Rehabilitation
LEDA	Ludic Engagement Designs for All
MMVR	Medicine Meets Virtual Reality
MOOG	Massively multiplayer online game
PMLD	Profound and multiple learning disability
TVK	Therapeutic virtual kitchen
VAP-S	Virtual action planning supermarket
VIS	Virtual interactive spaces
VR	Virtual reality
VRAT	Virtual reality and associated technologies
VRCPAT	Virtual Reality Cognitive Performance Assessment Test

References

1. Almeida AP, Girão LM, Gehlhaar R, et al. SOUND=SPACE opera. In: Proceedings of the 7th international conference on disability, virtual reality and associated technologies with ArtAbilitation, Maia, Portugal, 8–11 Sept 2008, p. 347–54.
2. ArtAbilitation 2006 papers are available in full from the ICDVRAT. Available at: www.icd-vrat.rdg.ac.uk. Brooks AL. In: Proceedings of the 1st international conference on ArtAbilitation, Esbjerg, 19–20 Sept 2006.
3. Azeredo M. Real-time composition of image and sound in the rehabilitation of children with special needs: a case study of a child with cerebral palsy. In: Proceedings of the 1st international conference on ArtAbilitation, Esbjerg, 18–19 Sept 2006, p. 79–84.
4. Broeren J, Pareto L, Johansson B, et al. Stroke rehabilitation using m-Health Care and 3D virtual environments – work in progress. In: Proceedings of the 8th international conference on disability, virtual reality and associated technologies, Viña del Mar/Valparaíso, 31 Aug–2 Sept 2010.
5. Brooks AL. Towards a platform of alternative and adaptive interactive systems for idiosyncratic special needs. In: Proceedings of the 7th international conference on disability, virtual

reality and associated technologies with ArtAbilitation, Maia, Portugal, 8–11 Sept 2008, p. 319–28.

6. Brooks AL, Camurri A, Canagarajah N, et al. Interaction with shapes and sounds as a therapy for special needs and rehabilitation. In: Proceedings of the 4th international conference on disability, virtual reality and associated technologies, Veszprém, 18–20 Sept 2002, p. 205–12.

7. Brown DJ, Kerr S, Bayon V. The development of the virtual city: a user centred approach. In: Proceedings of the 2nd European conference on disability, virtual reality and associated technologies, Mount Billingen, Skövde, 10–11 Sept 1998, p. 11–5.

8. Brown SH, Langan J, Kern KL, et al. Remote monitoring and quantification of upper limb and hand function in chronic disability conditions. In: Proceedings of the 8th international conference on disability, virtual reality and associated technologies, Viña del Mar/Valparaíso, 31 Aug–2 Sept 2010, p. 147–54.

9. Burke JW, McNeill MDJ, Charles DK, et al. Designing engaging, playable games for rehabilitation. In: Proceedings of the 8th international conference on disability, virtual reality and associated technologies, Viña del Mar/Valparaíso, 31 Aug–2 Sept 2010, p. 195–202.

10. Cao X, Douguet AS, Fuchs P, et al. Designing an ecological virtual task in the context of executive functions: preliminary study. In: Proceedings of the 8th international conference on disability, virtual reality and associated technologies, Viña del Mar/Valparaíso, 31 Aug–2 Sept 2010, p. 71–8.

11. Challis B P, Challis K. Infrared sound and music controller for users with specific needs. In: Proceedings of the 7th international conference on disability, virtual reality and associated technologies with ArtAbilitation, Maia, Portugal, 8–11 Sept 2008, p. 339–46.

12. Chortis A, Standen PJ, Walker M. Virtual reality system for upper extremity rehabilitation of chronic stroke patients living in the community. In: Proceedings of the 7th international conference on disability, virtual reality and associated technologies with ArtAbilitation, Maia, Portugal, 8–11 Sept 2008, p. 221–8.

13. Cikajlo I, Rudolf M, Goljar N. Continuation of balance training for stroke subjects in home environment using virtual reality. In: Proceedings of the 8th international conference on disability, virtual reality and associated technologies, Viña del Mar/Valparaíso, 31 Aug–2 Sept 2010, p. 235–40.

14. Cobb SVG, Mallet A, Pridmore T, et al. Interactive flashlights in special needs education. In: Proceedings of the 1st international conference on ArtAbilitation, Esbjerg, 18–19 Sept 2006, p. 1–9.

15. Cobb SVG, Sharkey PM. A decade of research and development in disability, virtual reality and associated technologies: review of ICDVRAT 1996–2006. Int J Virtual Real. 2007;6(2): 51–68.

16. Côté I, Getty L, Gaulin R. Aphasic theatre or theatre boosting self-esteem. In: Proceedings of the 7th international conference on disability, virtual reality and associated technologies with ArtAbilitation, Maia, Portugal, 8–11 Sept 2008, p. 177–84.

17. Davies R C, Johansson G, Boschian K, et al. A practical example using virtual reality in the assessment of brain injury. In: Proceedings of the 2nd European conference on disability, virtual reality and associated technologies, Mount Billingen, Skövde, 10–11 Sept 1998, p. 61–8.

18. Flynn SM, Lange BS. Games for rehabilitation: the voice of the players. In: Proceedings of the 8th international conference on disability, virtual reality and associated technologies, Viña del Mar/Valparaíso, 31 Aug–2 Sept 2010, p. 185–94.

19. Frisoli A, Bergamasco M, Borelli L, et al. Robotic assisted rehabilitation in virtual reality with the L-EXOS. In: Proceedings of the 7th international conference on disability, virtual reality and associated technologies with ArtAbilitation, Maia, Portugal, 8–11 Sept 2008, p. 253–60.

20. Gehlhaar R, Rodrigues PM, Girão LM. CaDaReMi – an educational interactive music game. In: Proceedings of the 7th international conference on disability, virtual reality and associated technologies with ArtAbilitation, Maia, Portugal, 8–11 Sept 2008, p. 355–60.

21. Greenleaf WJ. Applying VR to physical medicine and rehabilitation. Commun ACM. 1997;40(8):43–6.

22. Grierson M. Making music with images: interactive audiovisual performance systems for the deaf. In: Proceedings of the 7th international conference on disability, virtual reality and associated technologies with ArtAbilitation, Maia, Portugal, 8–11 Sept 2008, p. 361–8.
23. Hasselblad S, Petersson E, Brooks AL. Interactivity in work with disabled. In: Proceedings of the 1st international conference on ArtAbilitation, Esbjerg, 18–19 Sept 2006, p. 25–34.
24. Herbelin B, Ciger J, Brooks AL. Customization of gaming technology and prototyping of rehabilitation applications. In: Proceedings of the 7th international conference on disability, virtual reality and associated technologies with ArtAbilitation, Maia, Portugal, 8–11 Sept 2008, p. 211–8.
25. Hummels C, van der Helm A, Hengeveld B, et al. Explorascope: an interactive, adaptive educational toy to stimulate the language and communicative skills of multiple-handicapped children. In: Proceedings of the 1st international conference on ArtAbilitation, Esbjerg, 18–19 Sept 2006, p. 16–24.
26. ICDVRAT papers are referenced by conferences below and are freely available in full from the online archive. Available at: www.icdvrat.rdg.ac.uk: Sharkey PM, editor. In: Proceedings of the 1st European conference on disability, virtual reality and associated technologies, Maidenhead, 8–10 July 1996. ISBN 070491140X; Sharkey PM, Rose FD, Lindström JI, editors. In: Proceedings of the 2nd European conference on disability, virtual reality and associated technologies, Mount Billingen, Skövde, 10–11 Sept 1998. ISBN 0704911418; Sharkey PM, Cesarani A, Pugnetti L, et al., editors. In: Proceedings of the 3rd international conference on disability, virtual reality and associated technologies, Algerho, Sardinia, 23–25 Sept 2000. ISBN 0704911426; Sharkey PM, Sik Lányi C, Standen PJ, editors. In: Proceedings of the 4th international conference on disability, virtual reality and associated technologies, Veszprém, 18–20 Sept 2002. ISBN 07049 11434; Sharkey PM, McCrindle RJ, Brown D, editors. In: Proceedings of the 5th international conference on disability, virtual reality and associated technologies, Oxford, 20–22 Sept 2004. ISBN 0704911442; Sharkey PM, Brooks AL, Cobb SVG, editors. In: Proceedings of the 6th international conference on disability, virtual reality and associated technologies, Esbjerg, 18–20 Sept 2006. ISBN 0704998653; Sharkey PM, Lopes-dos-Santos P, Weiss PL, et al., editors. In: Proceedings of the 7th international conference on disability, virtual reality and associated technologies with ArtAbilitation, Maia & Porto, Portugal, 8–11 Sept 2008. ISBN 0704915006; Sharkey PM, Sánchez J, editors. In: Proceedings of the 8th international conference on disability, virtual reality and associated technologies, Viña del Mar/Valparaíso, 31 Aug–2 Sepi 2010. ISBN 9780704915022.
27. ICF. The International Classification of Functioning, Disability & Health. 2000. Available at: http://www.who.int/classifications/icf/en/index.html.
28. ICIDH. The International Classification of Functioning, Disability & Health. 1980. Available at: http://www.who.int/classifications/icf/en/index.html.
29. ICIDH. The International Classification of Functioning, Disability & Health. 1995. Available at: http://www.who.int/classifications/icf/en/index.html.
30. Josman N, Klinger E, Kizony R. Performance within the virtual action planning supermarket (VAP-S): an executive function profile of three different populations suffering from deficits in the central nervous system. In: Proceedings of the 7th international conference on disability, virtual reality and associated technologies with ArtAbilitation, Maia, Portugal, 8–11 Sept 2008, p. 33–8.
31. Kirner C, Kirner TG, Wataya RS, et al. Using augmented reality to support the understanding of three-dimensional concepts by blind people. In: Proceedings of the 8th international conference on disability, virtual reality and associated technologies, Viña del Mar/Valparaíso, 31 Aug–2 Sept 2010, p. 41–50.
32. Kitani M, Hayashi Y, Sawada H. Interactive training of speech articulation for hearing impaired using a talking robot. In: Proceedings of the 7th international conference on disability, virtual reality and associated technologies with ArtAbilitation, Maia, Portugal, 8–11 Sept 2008, p. 293–302.
33. Klinger E, Chemin I, Lebreton S, et al. A virtual supermarket to assess cognitive planning. Cyberpsychol Behav. 2004;7(3):292–3.

34. Kuroda T, Yamamoto G, Yoshitake D, et al. PiTaSu: a wearable interface for assisting senior citizens with memory problems. In: Proceedings of the 8th international conference on disability, virtual reality and associated technologies, Viña del Mar/Valparaíso, 31 Aug–2 Sept 2010, p. 61–70.
35. Lahav O, Levy ST. Listening to complexity: blind people's learning about gas particles through a sonified model. In: Proceedings of the 8th international conference on disability, virtual reality and associated technologies, Viña del Mar/Valparaíso, 31 Aug–2 Sept 2010, p. 33–40.
36. Langdon P, Gonzalez MF, Biswas P. Designing studies for requirements and modelling of users for an accessible set-top box. In: Proceedings of the 8th international conference on disability, virtual reality and associated technologies, Viña del Mar/Valparaíso, 31 Aug–2 Sept 2010, p. 203–12.
37. Lange BS, Flynn SM, Chang CY, et al. Development of an interactive rehabilitation game using the Nintendo® WiiFit™ Balance Board for people with neurological injury. In: Proceedings of the 8th international conference on disability, virtual reality and associated technologies, Viña del Mar/Valparaíso, 31 Aug–2 Sept 2010, p. 249–52.
38. Lopes-dos-Santos P, Nanim A, Fernandes H, et al. Using immersion in a musical virtual space environment to enhance quality of body movement in young adults with hemiparesis. In: Proceedings of the 7th international conference on disability, virtual reality and associated technologies with ArtAbilitation, Maia, Portugal, 8–11 Sept 2008, p. 327–36.
39. Lo Priore C, Castelnuovo D, Liccione D. Virtual environments in cognitive rehabilitation of executive functions. In: Proceedings of the 4th international conference on disability, virtual reality and associated technologies, Veszprém, 18–20 Sept 2002, p. 165–72.
40. McCrindle RJ, Williams VM, Victor CR, et al. Wearable device to assist independent living. In: Proceedings of the 8th international conference on disability, virtual reality and associated technologies, Viña del Mar/Valparaíso, 31 Aug–2 Sept 2010, p. 17–26.
41. Merians AS, Fluet GG, Qiu Q, et al. Integrated arm and hand training using adaptive robotics and virtual reality simulations. In: Proceedings of the 8th international conference on disability, virtual reality and associated technologies, Viña del Mar/Valparaíso, 31 Aug–2 Sept 2010, p. 131–8.
42. Morie JF, Haynes K, Chance E. Warrior's Journey – a path to healing through narrative exploration. In: Proceedings of the 8th international conference on disability, virtual reality and associated technologies, Viña del Mar/Valparaíso, 31 Aug–2 Sept 2010, p. 165–74.
43. Pareto L, Broeren J, Goude D, et al. Virtual reality, haptics and post-stroke rehabilitation in practical therapy. In: Proceedings of the 7th international conference on disability, virtual reality and associated technologies with ArtAbilitation, Maia, Portugal, 8–11 Sept 2008, p. 245–52.
44. Parsons TD, Rizzo AA. Neuropsychological assessment using the virtual reality cognitive performance assessment test. In: Proceedings of the 7th international conference on disability, virtual reality and associated technologies with ArtAbilitation, Maia, Portugal, 8–11 Sept 2008, p. 47–52.
45. Rizzo AA. Virtual reality in psychology and rehabilitation: the last ten years and the next! Keynote. In: Proceedings of the 7th international conference on disability, virtual reality and associated technologies with ArtAbilitation, Maia, Portugal, 8–11 Sept 2008, p. 3–6.
46. Rizzo AA, Lange BS, Buckwalter JG, et al. SimCoach: an intelligent virtual human system for providing healthcare information and support. In: Proceedings of the 7th international conference on disability, virtual reality and associated technologies with ArtAbilitation, Maia, Portugal, 8–11 Sept 2010, p. 213–20.
47. Sánchez JH, Oyarzún CA. Mobile audio assistance in bus transportation for the blind. In: Proceedings of the 7th international conference on disability, virtual reality and associated technologies with ArtAbilitation, Maia, Portugal, 8–11 Sept 2008, p. 279–86.
48. Sánchez JH, Rodríguez A. Visual tracking and audio-based interfaces for the navigation of people who are blind. In: Proceedings of the 8th international conference on disability, virtual reality and associated technologies, Viña del Mar/Valparaíso, 31 Aug–2 Sept 2010, p. 51–8.

49. Shefer Eini D, Ratzon N, Rizzo AA, et al. Simple camera tracking virtual reality system for evaluation of wrist range of motion. In: Proceedings of the 8th international conference on disability, virtual reality and associated technologies, Viña del Mar/Valparaíso, 31 Aug–2 Sept 2010, p. 123–30.

50. Smith A C, Krause C. Providing disabled persons in developing countries access to computer games through a novel gaming input device. Proceedings of the 7th international conference on disability, virtual reality and associated technologies with ArtAbilitation, Maia, Portugal, 8–11 Sept 2008, p. 199–204.

51. Standen PJ, Brown DJ, Battersby S, et al. Study to evaluate a low cost virtual reality system for home based rehabilitation of the upper limb following stroke. In: Proceedings of the 8th international conference on disability, virtual reality and associated technologies, Viña del Mar/Valparaíso, 31 Aug–2 Sept 2010, p. 139–46.

52. Torres A. Cognitive effects of videogames on old people. In: Proceedings of the 7th international conference on disability, virtual reality and associated technologies with ArtAbilitation, Maia, Portugal, 8–11 Sept 2008, p. 191–8.

53. van Leeuwen L, Ellis P. Facilitating the experience of agency through an intersensory interactive environment. In: Proceedings of the 1st international conference on ArtAbilitation, Esbjerg, 18–19 Sept 2006, p. 62–8.

54. Vickers S, Bates R, Istance HO. Gazing into a second life: gaze-driven adventures, control barriers, and the need for disability privacy in an online virtual world. In: Proceedings of the 7th international conference on disability, virtual reality and associated technologies with ArtAbilitation, Maia, Portugal, 8–11 Sept 2008, p. 151–8.

55. Wilde D, Helmer RJN, Miles M. Extending body & imagination: moving to move. In: Proceedings of the 8th international conference on disability, virtual reality and associated technologies, Viña del Mar/Valparaíso, 31 Aug–2 Sept 2010, p. 175–82.

56. Williams C. Unintentional intrusive participation in multimedia interactive environments. In: Proceedings of the 7th international conference on disability, virtual reality and associated technologies with ArtAbilitation, Maia, Portugal, 8–11 Sept 2008, p. 205–10.

57. Williams C, Petersson E, Brooks AL. Picturing sound – an overview of its efficacy. In: Proceedings of the 1st international conference on ArtAbilitation, Esbjerg, 18–19 Sept 2006, p.70–8.

58. World Health Organization (WHO). The International Classification of Impairments, Disabilities and Handicaps (ICF 2000), Geneva. 2000. Available at: http://www.who.int/classifications/icf/en/index.html.

59. Yau D, McCrindle RJ. MusiCam – an instrument to demonstrate chromaphonic synesthesia. In: Proceedings of the 1st international conference on ArtAbilitation, Esbjerg, 18–19 Sept 2006, p. 85–90.

Chapter 17
Design, Construction, and Integration in Instrumented Walkways of a Portable Kit for the Assessment of Gait Parameters in Telerehabilitation

Daniele Giansanti, Sandra Morelli, Paco Dionisio, and Giovanni Maccioni

Abstract This chapter focuses on the use of telerehabilitation to assess gait in and outside the hospital. The work herein describes the design, construction, and integration of an innovative solution to create a new model of care concept in telerehabilitation. The complete system presents itself as a portable kit able to furnish feedback on parameters that are useful to both the patient and the trainer/therapist. This represents a novel approach for gait monitoring based simply on a step-counter (pedometer); photo-emitter/detectors (at the initial, intermediate, and final path stations); a central unit for collecting and processing the telemetrically transmitted data; and a software interface. The system is capable of integrating with the most common tools used in motion rehabilitation (e.g., handrails, scales, walkways), and can quantitatively assess and monitor patients' progress in rehabilitation. The portable kit can be used with different rehabilitation tools and on different ground rugosities. A case study provides data that the system is both feasible and well-accepted. Possible advantages include: (a) low costs, especially when compared to optoelectronic or other portable solutions; (b) high accuracy; (c) benefits to subjects with balance problems; and (d) integration (compatibility) with any rehabilitative tool.

17.1 Introduction

The present work is focused on the use of telerehabilitation to assess gait both within and outside the hospital environment. Measurements are obtained during daily rehabilitation exercise via sensorization of both the patient and rehabilitation tools.

D. Giansanti (✉) • S. Morelli • P. Dionisio • G. Maccioni
Technology and Health Department, The Italian National Institute of Health,
Via Regina Elena 299, Rome 00161, Italy
e-mail: daniele.giansanti@iss.it; sandra.morelli@iss.it; paco.dionisio@iss.it;
giovanni.maccioni@iss.it

S. Kumar, E.R. Cohn (eds.), *Telerehabilitation*, Health Informatics,
DOI 10.1007/978-1-4471-4198-3_17, © Springer-Verlag London 2013

This novel and simple approach to gait monitoring is based upon a step-counter; photo-emitter/detectors (at the initial, intermediate, and final path stations); a central unit for collecting and processing the telemetrically transmitted data; and a software interface.

The rationale for this system is that the sensorization of commonly used rehabilitation tools can furnish easy-to-process information about performance parameters that will be useful to patients, therapists and physicians. The system supplies quantitative information for gait assessment; these data can also be added to a qualitative interpretation of clinical exercise.

The solution must enable the daily assessment of a patient's physical and physiological conditions during a therapy session, wherever (e.g., hospital, gym, physiotherapy room, or home) the patient performs their exercise regimen. The general idea is thus (as the focus is the gait) to design a simple kit as an alternative to the complex and expensive instruments already in use, with an easy way to be interfaced or integrated within the clinical framework for both patient monitoring and clinical reporting needs. The kit herein presented can be implemented in a variety of settings and is designed for extensive use.

The requirements for the kit were as follows:

- *Simplicity* (for both set-up and use)
- *Low cost* (in terms of prototype design and construction, and maintenance)
- *Adaptability* to different environmental characteristics (hospital, home, outside, etc.)
- *Integrability* of different rehabilitation and measurement tools (from the hospital LAN to the WAN)
- *Portability*

The complete kit presents itself as a portable system that can collect data on relevant parameters and provide feedback to the patient via telerehabilitation. The system was designed to quantitatively assess and constantly monitor progress in rehabilitation care (i.e., generally for patient with wearable devices, using aids and supports, in a prescribed pathway). The implementation must be sufficiently simple to be integrated within a clinical setting for a typical set of exercises. The system can also be used in external areas, with specific path (i.e., curved, roughed, shaped surface, and multipath) or internal areas (e.g., home room with or without obstacles) to allow monitoring of daily motion exercise. The kit should be integrated with the mechanical tools used in gait rehabilitation:

- Assistive devices: canes, crutches, walkers
- Walkways: handrail systems, scales, equipped walkways
- Ankle–foot orthosis devices
- Reciprocating gait orthosis (RGO) and advanced reciprocating gait orthosis (ARGO)

In a previous report, we investigated possible solutions for designing and constructing the system [9]. The technical report presented an overview of the solutions available to obtain parameters relevant to gait and useful to be integrated in the design of rehabilitation walkways. The relevant emerging limits were described. In particular, the technical report assessed the current methodologies as:

- Too expensive and thus not adequate for the daily monitoring (e.g., optoelectronic or ultrasound-based methodologies [5])
- More suitable for the monitoring of the duration in a percentage of time of a motion task (e.g., activity-monitoring techniques [1, 2, 12])
- More suitable for the assessment of transitory tasks (e.g., wearable systems based on accelerometers and rate gyroscopes [4, 8, 14])
- Not adequate to be integrated with a walkway (e.g., scales, slides, etc.) or to assess the performance on a ground with different rugosities (e.g., baropodometric platforms [3])
- Not adequate for the monitoring of subjects with balance problems (e.g., as would be the case for step-counters in Parkinson's disease) [6, 7, 13]

In the same report, we proposed a preliminary solution based on a kit using a wearable step-counter called gastrocnemius expansion measurement unit (GEMU) [13] and photocells, and tested the solution with a healthy subject on a single walkway. To expand the methodology to environments for daily living and to subjects with a different degrees of motion ability, we proposed the integration of a cascade of walkways constructed on different grounds and differently equipped (handrail, scales, and slides), and use of a sensorized codivilla spring (SECOSP) [10] as an ankle–foot orthosis, integrated with a step-counter.

17.2 Methods

17.2.1 Definition of the Architecture (Hardware and Software Interface) of the System and Walkways

The functionalities of the system were as follows:

- Monitoring the steps performed during a rehabilitation task on the basis of a predefined protocol and an assigned cascade of walkways of a defined length, thus determining all relevant parameters of velocity and time. (We focused on a cascade of two walkways.)
- Formatting this information in a textual file that was easy to transmit to a communication center for post-processing and archiving, according to a specified database format.

The complete architecture (hardware and software) of the system was as follows:

- The hardware unit allows the telemetric acquisition of the row data from the subjects;
- The row data are sent by means of an acquisition card (NI-DAQ USB-6008 by National Instruments, USA) connected by USB connection to a PC;

- A software interface, designed by means of LabVIEW 8.2 (National Instruments, USA), preprocesses the information in the PC, rearranges it in an easy to manage ASCII textual file, and uploads it via a LAN or WAN connection for the final post-processing and archiving.

17.2.2   Design and Construction of the Hardware Solution and Software Interface

The minimum hardware solution was based on the following components:

- Step-counter
- Detectors positioned to detect the timing of the gait exercise
- One central unit for the collection of the row data
- The software interface for the data processing and handshaking with WAN

17.2.2.1   Step-Counter

In previous papers, we investigated novel solutions in step-counter design and construction [6, 7, 10, 13]. As a step-counter we used a SECOSP [10]. Thus, a codivilla spring (COSP) with sensors was proposed to obtain a SECOSP for telemonitoring daily rehabilitation to track step-count. The system is based on force-sensing resistors (FSRs) affixed in the plantar area of the COSP, and a wearable unit with the conditioning electronics and a micro-processor µP PIC 16 F877 (Microchip, USA). While ambulating, the FSRs CP0152 (interlink, USA) detect the pressure of the foot tip and the heel. This information is used by the PIC to increment the step-count based on an algorithm. The system is calibrated before use. The calibration is obtained by three consecutive bodyweight loadings on the heel and the foot tip. The algorithm calculates the step-count by recognizing the sequence heel to foot tip, which is used to increment the step-count. When the subject is still and standing, both FSRs are active, and this information is not used by the algorithm to increment the step-count. Small oscillations are eliminated using thresholds obtained during calibration. When the subject is sitting, the pressure is not sufficient to activate the calibrated FSR that runs as foot switches. The power supply is assured by 4 NI-MH rechargeable batteries with 3.6 V and capacity $I = 160$ mA×h (Extracell, USA). Figure 17.1 depicts the electronic components of the SECOSP. Figures 17.2 and 17.3 show the SECOSP after sensors are added.

17.2.2.2   Detectors of the Path

This study used a pathway that includes a cascade of two walkways. The assessment of the start, intermediate, and final position of the path is basic to detect the duration (in time) of the exercise associated at each walkway. This timing also acts as a temporal mask for the step-counting. Only the steps actually monitored during this timing interval

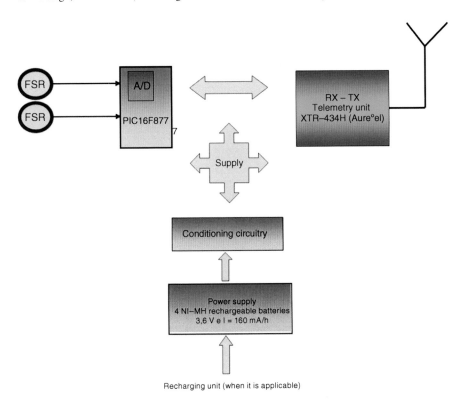

Fig. 17.1 The electronic components of the wearable unit. The *FSR*s are affixed on the COSP

are used to determine the total number of steps. Three pairs of photo-emitter/detectors PEM10D (Wellean, U.K.) and mirrors were used in a cascade of two consecutive walkways, positioned at the start; at the end of the first walkway; and at the end of the second walkway. The first pair allows the assessment of the Tstart of the task; the second pair allows the detection of the Tint at the end of the first (or intermediate) walkway (the starting of the second walkway); and the Tstop is the final timing of the task.

Figure 17.4 is a picture of the two towers with the pairs of photo-emitters/detectors. The importance of the design and construction of these towers cannot be underestimated, due to critical concerns for both patient safety and the required flexibility of the application.

17.2.2.3   Central Unit

The central unit is telemetrically connected with the other components of the equipment. It also provides the following functions:

- Assessment of the number of steps in real time
- Recharging of the step-counter
- Elaboration of the row data relevant to the timing

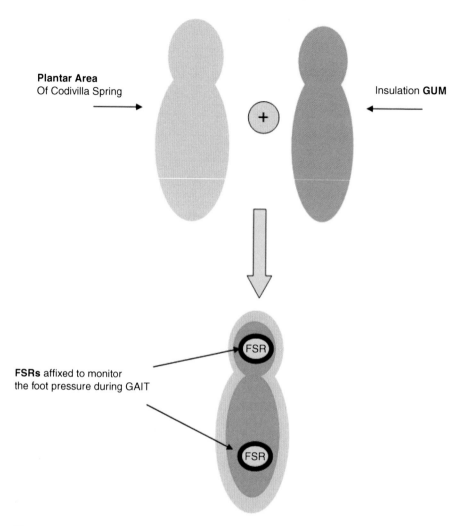

Plantar Area
Of Codivilla Spring

Insulation **GUM**

FSRs affixed to monitor
the foot pressure during GAIT

Fig. 17.2 Details of the affixation of the couple of the *FSR* at the level of the plantar area of the COSP

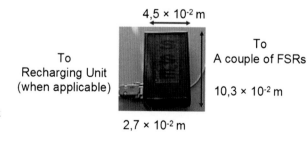

$4,5 \times 10^{-2}$ m

To
A couple of FSRs

To
Recharging Unit
(when applicable)

$10,3 \times 10^{-2}$ m

Fig. 17.3 The wearable unit
that can be affixed in a belt

$2,7 \times 10^{-2}$ m

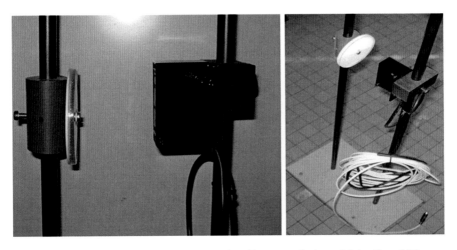

Fig. 17.4 A couple of towers with the photo-emitter/detector and mirror: (**a**) details and (**b**) complete view

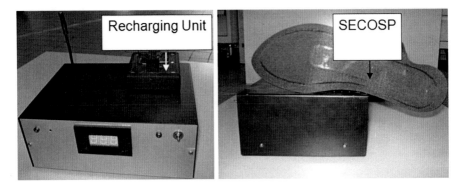

Fig. 17.5 The central unit (**a**) without and (**b**) with the *SECOSP*

- Biofeedback of seven-segment LED representation of the data
- Connection to send the timing parameters to a PC

Figure 17.5 depicts the central unit with and without the SECOSP.

17.2.2.4 Software Program

A software program was developed for monitoring the gait of patients wearing different step-counter sensors in a cascade of two different walkways (i.e., linear flat floor, without or with obstacles, slide, or stairs). The gait parameters were stored in a text ASCII file containing the patient's name and the features of the walkway (length, type of pathway, and gait aid type). The program was developed by LabVIEW programming language

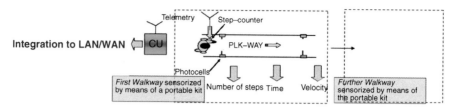

Fig. 17.6 The cascade of walkways

(*Laboratory Virtual Instrument Engineering Workbench*) version 8.2, accepting signals from different sensors. Customized user interfaces were designed to control the patient's gait and to configure the features of the walkway. The interface allows:

- Monitoring of a "gait session," consisting of one or more trials;
- Selection of a "step-counter type" from different wearable step-counter sensors such as GEMU and SECOSP, or based on accelerometers;
- Selection of a "gait aid type," a "pathway type," and the introduction of a "note." The "gait aid type" could be none, handrail, canes, and COSP. The "pathway type" could be a single walkway or a cascade with a linear flat floor, without or with obstacles, slide, or stairs. In the "note" it is also possible to add information about the rugosity of each component of the "pathway."

17.2.2.5   Cascade of Walkways and Clinical Trials

Figure 17.6 shows the approach of the methodology in the general case (i.e., a cascade of different walkways).

This study is limited to a cascade of two walkways: the first with the ground based on linoleum and with a length of 10 m, and the second on moquette, with a length of 10 m and an inclination of 15°.

A subject at the second level of the Tinetti test [11] wearing the SECOSP performed 10 repetitions of tasks of gait at three different speeds (low, medium, and fast).

17.3   Results

17.3.1   Case Study

As an example of application of a telerehabilitation-based methodology to one healthy subject at the second level of the Tinetti test [11] of motion imbalance disability (male; height 1.80 cm; weight 84 kg; age 69 years), we report an output of a single clinical application and the values relevant to 10 repetitions at the three different speeds for the two walkways in cascade (Table 17.1). The statistical significance was better than 1 %.

Table 17.1 Outcome of the study

Speed	Time (s) First walkway	Number of steps First walkway	Time (s) Second walkway	Number of steps Second walkway
Low	17	15	24	18
Mean	14	16	21	21
Fast	12	20	18	24

Table 17.2 Cost of the production (materials, test, and construction)

Description	No.	Price (€)
Mechanics (cases/boards/general mechanical hardware)		25
Microprocessor PIC	2	30
No. 1 SECOSP	1	130
Couple of photo-emitter/detectors	3	120
Transmitter/receiver	1	44
Cost associated to the time of construction and test 30 €/h	–	180
Other passive electronic components	–	57
Other active/integrated components	–	62
Total		648

Table 17.3 Acceptance of the methodology (3 = Maximum acceptance) subject

Item	Aspect	Score (mean)
1	User friendly	3
2	Help	2
4	Speed of operations	3
5	Failure rate (FR) of operations	3 (3 = no FR)

Table 17.4 Acceptance of the methodology (3 = Maximum acceptance) physician

Item	Aspect	Score (mean)
1	User friendly	3
2	Help	3
4	Speed of operations	3
5	Failure rate (FR) of operations	3 (3 = no FR)

17.3.2 Costs and Acceptance

Table 17.2 shows the detailed costs. The cost of production (montage, materials, and test) in the minimum setup was separated from the cost of the study to allow an estimation of a serial production. The complete cost of the prototype equipment is €648 for the materials, montage, and test. The cost of the software has not been included; in fact, the software LabVIEW 8.2 generates an executable file (no cost) for the interface. Because this software is currently available in biomedical laboratories for the design of a general bioengineering instrumentation, it does not make sense to include it in the forecasted costs of the study and the prototype. The final two tables portray the subject's (Table 17.3) and the physician's (Table 17.4) acceptance of the methodology.

17.4   Discussion and Future Perspectives

Today there is a continuous demand for easy, low-cost, and interoperative rehabilitation technology to promote and monitor health. One of the most commonly used motion monitoring technologies is the step-counter or pedometer. Step-counting is an important index of motion activity that can be useful for monitoring a patient's response to rehabilitation therapy, as well as for the management of both obesity and diabetes. Furthermore, when accompanied by other kinematic information (e.g., velocity, distance, and time), step-counting can provide physicians and therapists with useful quantitative information to assess a patient's progress. Step-counting biofeedback can also motivate a patient to continue therapy. In this paper, we have proposed a system that addresses both of these needs.

The kit includes a hardware unit that allows the telemetric acquisition of the row data from the subjects wearing a step-counter and the triggering of the task by means of photocells. The row data from the hardware unit are sent by means of a national instrument acquisition board NI-DAQ USB-6008 to a PC via an USB connection. A software interface, designed by means of LabVIEW 8.2, preprocesses the information in the PC and arranges it in an easy to manage text file that can be sent by LAN or WAN connection for final post-processing and archiving.

The kit has been successfully tested with a subject at the Level 2 of the Tinetti test in an application that included a cascade of two walkways with different inclinations and rugosities [11]. The acceptance of both the subject and the physician was high.

From a global point of view, the kit allows for easy monitoring of gait parameters via telerehabilitation and offers the following advantages:

- It allows the use of different properly designed step-counters. Even if we have used a SECOSP for illustrative purposes, different step-counters can be used in the hardware solutions [9].
- It can be used with different ground rugosities. This is an important parameter that can affect balance and most importantly, the fall risk.
- The equipment can be used with different rehabilitation mechanical equipments (i.e., from scales to slides).
- The customization of complex walkways is also possible for the daily monitoring. Properly designed walkways in a form of complex paths (also with obstacles) may be traced, for example, at a patient's home to assess daily progress and encourage motion activity.

In comparison to other solutions [9], the kit shows the following advantages:

- Very low costs, not only when compared to optoelectronic solutions but also when compared to other portable solutions such as the activity-monitoring commercial solutions (e.g., LifeGait) or portable gait analysis systems (e.g., GAITRite).
- Very high accuracy when using properly designed step-counters for subjects with balance problems, as compared to commercial step-counters or wearable systems with accelerometers, rate gyroscopes, and activity monitoring.

To date, three directions seem promising for the kit:

1. Integration with HIS: The equipment can be integrated with the hospital LAN and hospital information service (HIS).
2. Integration with homecare: The system's integration with homecare units assessing the most relevant medical parameters can provide a more complete profile of the rehabilitation care.
3. Integration with domotics (home automation): Walkways at home can be integrated in a manner that allows gait assessment of the daily preferred trajectories.

Summary

- There is increasing demand for easy, low-cost, and interoperative technology to promote and monitor health. One of the most commonly used technologies for motion monitoring is the step-counter or pedometer.
- Step-counting is an important index of motion activity that can be useful for monitoring a patient's response to rehabilitation therapy, as well as for the management of both obesity and diabetes. When accompanied by other kinematic information (e.g., velocity, distance, and time), step-counting provides useful quantitative information to assess patient progress.
- The authors describe a novel and simple telerehabilitation-based approach to gait monitoring that uses a step-counter; photo-emitter/detectors; a central unit for collecting and processing the telemetrically transmitted data; and a software interface.
- The sensorization of commonly used rehabilitation tools can furnish easy-to-process information about performance parameters that will be useful to patients, therapists, and physicians.

Abbreviations/Acronyms

ARGO	Advanced reciprocating gait orthosis
COSP	Codivilla spring
FSR	Force-sensing resistor
GEMU	Gastrocnemius expansion measurement unit
HIS	Hospital information service
LAN	Local area network
RGO	Reciprocating gait orthosis
SECOSP	Sensorized codivilla spring
WAN	Wide area network

References

1. Bussmann HB, Reuvekamp PJ, Veltink PH, et al. Validity and reliability of measurements obtained with an activity monitor in people with and without a transtibial amputation. Phys Ther. 1998;78(9):989–98.
2. Bussmann JB, Van de Laar YM, Neeleman MP, et al. Ambulatory accelerometry to quantify motor behaviour in patients after failed back surgery: a validation study. Pain. 1998;74(2–3):153–61.
3. Giacomozzi C, Macellari V, Leardini A, et al. Integrated pressure-force-kinematics measuring system for the characterisation of plantar foot loading during locomotion. Med Biol Eng Comput. 2000;38(2):156–63.
4. Giansanti D, Maccioni G. Comparison of three different kinematic sensors assemblies for the locomotion study. Physiol Meas. 2005;26(5):689–705.
5. Giansanti D, Maccioni G, Macellari V. The development and test of a device for the reconstruction of 3-D position and orientation by means of a kinematic sensor assembly with rate gyroscopes and accelerometers. IEEE Trans Biomed Eng. 2005;52(7):1271–7.
6. Giansanti D, Maccioni G, Macellari V, et al. A novel, user-friendly step counter for home telemonitoring of physical activity. J Telemed Telecare. 2008;14(7):345–8.
7. Giansanti D, Macellari V, Maccioni G. Telemonitoring and telerehabilitation of patients with Parkinson's disease: health technology assessment of a novel wearable step counter. Telemed J E Health. 2008;14(1):76–83.
8. Giansanti D, Macellari V, Maccioni G, et al. Is it feasible to reconstruct body segment 3-D position and orientation using accelerometric data? IEEE Trans Biomed Eng. 2003;50(4):476–83.
9. Giansanti D, Morelli S, Maccioni G, et al. Design and construction of a portable kit for the assessment of gait parameters in daily-rehabilitation. Rapporti ISTISAN 10/16, Istituto Superiore di Sanità, Roma; 2010.
10. Giansanti D, Tiberi Y, Silvestri G, et al. New wearable system for step-counting telemonitoring and telerehabilitation based on the codivilla spring. Telemed J E Health. 2008;14(10): 1096–100.
11. Kandel ER, Schwart RJ, Jessell TM. Principi di neuroscienze. Milano: CEA-Casa Editrice Ambrosiana Neuroscienze; 2000.
12. Lyons GM, Culhane KM, Hilton D, et al. A description of an accelerometer-based mobility monitoring technique. Med Eng Phys. 2005;27(6):497–504.
13. Maccioni G, Macellari V, Giansanti D. Design and construction of step counters for disable people: preliminary experience at the Italian Institute of Health. Conf Proc IEEE Eng Med Biol Soc. 2007;2007:4927–9.
14. Padgaonkar AJ, Krieger KW, King AI. Measurement of angular acceleration of a rigid body using linear accelerometers. ASME J Appl Mech. 1975;42:552–6.

Chapter 18
Design and Construction of a Wearable Tool for Fall-Risk Detection in Telerehabilitation

Daniele Giansanti, Paco Dionisio, and Giovanni Maccioni

Abstract Telerehabilitation services represent a promising option for patients undergoing home-based rehabilitation as a result of stroke or other pathologies. To facilitate recovery following stroke, prompt and constant neural and motion rehabilitation is essential. When a patient returns home after treatment, he or she may experience a high degree of imbalance. It can be challenging to remotely assess fall-risk in the home. This chapter describes a promising new telerehabilitation-based approach to fall-risk detection via a wearable tool, integrated to a global system for mobile communication (GSM) net. The technology is based upon an inertial measurement unit and two medical protocols (i.e., a sit-to-stand clinical application and a posturography clinical application). The approach incorporates a 4-point fall-risk score: 1, no fall- risk to 4, major fall-risk.

18.1 Introduction

Telerehabilitation services represent a promising option for patients undergoing home-based rehabilitation as a result of stroke or other pathologies [2]. After the first critical period at the hospital, it is important to plan programs for both neural and motion rehabilitation. And since motion and neural rehabilitation are highly related, prompt motion rehabilitation is essential to a rapid recovery. Therefore, remote therapists involved in a telerehabilitation program should monitor daily motion activity.

A comprehensive rehabilitation process that incorporates the patient's home is essential to a successful outcome. Additionally, a patient should have all possible

D. Giansanti (✉) • P. Dionisio • G. Maccioni
Technology and Health Department, The Italian National Institute of Health,
Via Regina Elena 299, Rome 00161, Italy
e-mail: daniele.giansanti@iss.it; paco.dionisio@iss.it; giovanni.maccioni@iss.it

S. Kumar, E.R. Cohn (eds.), *Telerehabilitation*, Health Informatics,
DOI 10.1007/978-1-4471-4198-3_18, © Springer-Verlag London 2013

means at their disposal to improve their rehabilitation care, such as a suitable prosthesis and/or instrumented walkways. During the telerehabilitation program, a patient may employ several different types of aids/prostheses.

When a patient returns home after treatment, he or she may experience a high degree of imbalance. A successful program should continuously move the patient to a lower level of imbalance and help them to progressively abandon assistive technologies. When the patient abandons the cane, he or she can use an aid such as the *codivilla spring* (COSP). This prosthesis helps in recovery of the fluidity of gait, helping the patient to avoid an equine step. The COSP can be tailored in an orthopedic laboratory according to the patient's need. With improvement, the patient abandons the use of the prosthesis and continues rehabilitation for further progress.

Because the conditions stemming from other disease consequences can inhibit rehabilitation, the rehabilitation path should be considered in two directions: the direction of the physical improvement and the direction of the detriment of the physical condition. When designing a complete motion telerehabilitation program, it should be noted that properly designed methodologies for step-counting should be furnished to the patient. In fact, step-counting is a useful parameter because it is related to daily motion activity [1, 24]. It should be noted that commercial pedometers fail to furnish suitable performances in subjects with a motion disability (this is caused by their more complex pattern of gait) [20]. Also, the integration of the pedometer with customized walkways could represent a valuable telerehabilitation strategy [21, 23]. However, a remote therapist, involved in a telerehabilitation program, could assign motion rehabilitation tools on the basis of fall-risk, and the tools may change with the patient's progress [25].

One of the major problems for the therapist is the assessment of fall-risk or the status of the imbalance. Telepresence by video camera connected to homecare does not allow correct and objective assessment of fall-risk using qualitative observation (or partially qualitative) tests such as the Tinetti test [25]. Thus, without sufficient information, it is not possible for the remote therapist to assign, for example, a particular cane or a COSP [1], or to allow the patient to abandon a specific aid/support. In a previous study [14], a methodology was used in motion laboratories that allows the quantitative assessment of fall-risk on the basis of posturography acquisitions with different constraints (eyes open; eyes open on foam; and eyes closed on foam) performed by means of an inertial measurement unit (IMU) with accelerometers, rate gyroscopes [15, 17], and a statistical clusterization process. Other studies using the same methodology followed other clustering algorithms, based on a neural network classification [16, 19]. Another study [18] focused on a dedicated protocol based on the sit-to-stand (STS) application [18] with different instructions of speed. In a previous paper, we described the integration in a telemedicine flow of the protocols based on the fall-risk and posturography protocols [15–17, 19, 22].

The purpose of this paper is to integrate the wearable telemedicine tool in a telerehabilitation application that remotely furnishes information to the therapist on fall-risk and imbalance accordingly to two different protocols (i.e., STS [18] and posturography [14]), to guide the therapist in assigning a therapy.

18.2 Materials and Methods

18.2.1 Tools for the Assessment of Fall-Risk and the Degree of Imbalance

18.2.1.1 Problems in Testing the Fall-Risk and Imbalance in Telemedicine

The test of Tinetti [25] is the gold standard for assessment of imbalance and fall-risk for subjects with a motion disability [15–17, 19]. It is well known that it allows the categorization of the subjects in four classes; the fourth class identifies the subjects with the highest level of imbalance and fall-risk. The major drawbacks of this test are that it is partially qualitative and is based partially on visual observation. Telepresence in telemedicine enabled by web video cameras (2D representation) is not sufficient to aid the therapist to a correct observation (and thus the correct execution of the test); 3D visualization is required.

18.2.1.2 A New Tool for the Assessment of Fall-Risk in Telemedicine

The proposed telemedicine tool is based on:

- An IMU
- A protocol based on the STS [18] called for the sake of clarity Prot-STS
- A protocol based on posturography [15, 17] called for the sake of clarity Prot-POST
- Off-line algorithms for the clusterization and the assignment of fall-risk on the basis of the IMU data posturography and STS acquisitions
- Kit for the integration with a global system for mobile communication (GSM) unit

The core element is thus the IMU used in the clinical application. It features three mono-axial accelerometers (3,031-Euro Sensors, USA) and three rate gyroscopes (Gyrostar ENC-03 J-Murata, Japan), which were assembled together and oriented according to an orthogonal reference system. A full description of the design and construction of the IMU (Fig. 18.1) has been published [15, 17]. The assessment of fall-risk and the degree of imbalance was made off-line in a personal computer and was based on the algorithms assigned to two protocols: Prot-STS and Prot-POST. The choice of the GSM communication components took into consideration the feasibility of integration to other possible wearable components for the position monitoring and the potential for monitoring other physiological parameters. This study focused on communication systems open to easy integration of third-party components and allowing the exact detection of the global positioning system (GPS) position. Many GPS/GSM systems fulfilled this requirement. The memory card Kingston (Kingston Technology Company, Inc., Fountain Valley, CA)

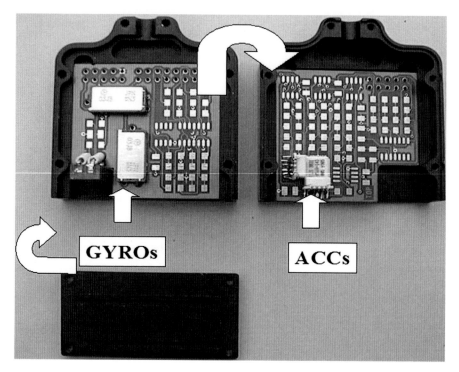

Fig. 18.1 Details of the IMU: 3D affixation of the rate-gyroscopes (*GYROs*) and accelerometers (*ACCs*)

with a capacity of 2 GB has also been integrated with the GPS/GSM unit for meta-data storing. A PIC micro-processor µP PIC 16 F877 (Microchip, USA) with the assembly language has been used for integration purposes. Figure 18.2 shows the system with the communication unit.

18.3   Results

Validation of the IMU as a standalone system [17] and a full description of the power of the test have been published [14, 16, 19, 22].

18.3.1   Weight and Sizes of the Telemedicine Tool

The use of a large number of electronic components (passive and active) with the packages for surface montage technology (SMT) allowed minimization of volume and weight. The complete telemedicine system developed using SMT was 1.49 N in

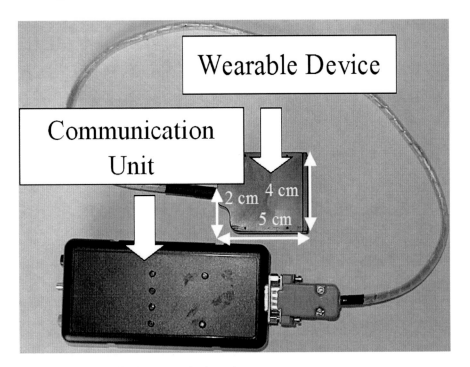

Fig. 18.2   The IMU with the communication unit

weight and 40 cm³ in volume for the sensor head, and 4.84 N in weight and 492 cm³ in volume for the other wearable components. Each component of the telemedicine system has been designed and integrated.

18.3.2   Agreement with Gold Standards

The system as a whole has been validated in standalone applications in previous studies [14, 16, 18, 19]. The output was similar to the Tinetti test for the three algorithms applied. A remote therapist may also use an approach that accounts for all three different clusterizations in the case of discordance.

18.3.3   Structure of SMS

Figure 18.3 shows the structure of the SMS. Three characters are used to map anonymously 0–999 subjects (or a higher number if a hexadecimal representation is used) in the section code of patient (COD-PAZ). For privacy reasons, we preferred to navigate a code without name and surname. Two characters are used in case

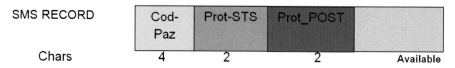

Fig. 18.3 Structure of the SMS: fall-risk assessed by means of Prot-STS; fall-risk assessed by means of *PROT-POST*; code of patient (*COD-PAZ*)

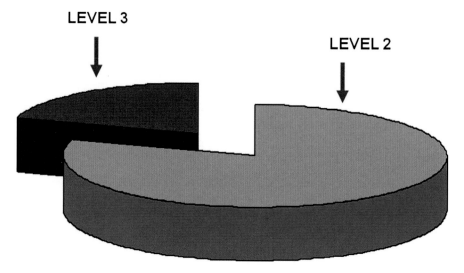

Fig. 18.4 Evolution in a subject undergoing stroke rehabilitation of the fall-risk index using the PROT-STS

of the fall-risk assessment using Prot-POST. Similarly, two characters are used in case of the fall-risk/imbalance assessment using Prot-STS.

18.3.4 Failure Rate Investigation

At the end of the application, the system sends one SMS. The application was repeated 20 times to investigate the success of the connection. The system did not show any failures.

18.3.5 Acceptance of the Telemedicine Tool

One volunteer was monitored for 20 days. Figure 18.4 specifically shows the evolution of the fall-risk index using the PROT-STS. Table 18.1 shows the high acceptance of both the subject and the therapist.

Table 18.1 Acceptance of the telemedicine application in the case study

Item	Aspect	Subject score	Therapist score
1	User-friendly application	3	3
2	Telephonic help	3	3
3	Encumbrance (4: high encumbrance)	1	1
4	Clearness of instructions	3	4

1 minimum, *4* maximum

18.4   Discussion and Conclusions

Telerehabilitation represents a valuable approach to service delivery for patients receiving home-based motion rehabilitation therapy. To facilitate recovery following stroke, for example, it is essential to have a prompt and constant program of both neural and motion rehabilitation. However, it can be challenging to remotely assess fall-risk in the home. Unfortunately, the 2-D telepresence function available in most telemedicine applications does not facilitate a complete and accurate qualitative evaluation. A novel tool has been proposed that allows assessment of the fall-risk according to two different protocols (PROT-POST and PROT-STS) and an SMS-based communication to the remote therapist on the basis of an IMU and a GSP/GPS unit. Each component of the wearable system has been designed and integrated. Each component in the system has been tested individually and in a closed loop. The test in a telemedicine link showed a high degree of acceptance.

From a global point of view, this study contributes three added values to the field of telerehabilitation. The first added value is the development of an accurate tool for the distant assessment of fall-risk and the degree of imbalance. The second added value is the availability of two different indices of fall-risk, suitable to construct an objective methodology, guiding the therapist to make a correct and objective decision. The third added value is the starting point of the design of a decision grid, based on a quantitative test useful to construct a legal and regulatory approach in telerehabilitation to protect the therapist.

18.5   Future Investigation

The system will be furnished to subjects along with a homecare device for daily monitoring of motion activity (and eventually for other physiological parameters useful for investigation in stroke telerehabilitation) along with different aids such as canes, COSPs, etc. With that deployment, it will be possible to monitor several parameters related to the success and failure of the telemedicine application along with clinical acceptance of the telerehabilitation application as a whole, embedding the tool for the fall-risk and imbalance assessment. At this moment, we are working toward the integration of this telemedicine tool with a portable kit for the sensorization/integration of walkways [21, 23].

These sensorized walkways have been discussed in Chap. 17 [21]. Along with the kit described in [21], the tool could find the applications as aid for the assessment of fall-risk and the degree of imbalance in the following three directions:

1. Integration with HIS: The first direction involves integration of the equipment with the hospital LAN and hospital information service (HIS).
2. Integration with homecare: The integration with homecare units assessing the most relevant medical parameters could allow a more complete record of the rehabilitation care.
3. Domotics: The third direction consists of the integration of walkways at home in domotics (home automation). It could be, for example, integrated in a manner that allows the assessment of gait of the daily preferred trajectories.

Other potentialities could be explored in the field of the integration with the wearable systems for monitoring the physical activity [1, 4, 6, 8–13, 26, 27, 29, 31, 32]. As the patient activates muscles for the control of motion and postures, they may change and configure a high number of positions as elucidated by posture and motion sciences. The assessment of fall-risk and the degree of imbalance may guide to the suggested motion activity, which could be monitored through properly designed wearable systems based, for example, on accelerometers [5, 7, 28, 30].

Summary

- Remote therapists who engage in telerehabilitation should monitor daily motion activity and employ motion rehabilitation tools, taking into account fall-risk.
- It is difficult to remotely assess fall-risk and the status of imbalance. Telepresence by video camera connected to a homecare system does not allow for objective and accurate assessment of fall-risk.
- A novel tool has been proposed that allows assessment of the fall-risk according to two different protocols (PROT-POST and PROT-STS) and an SMS-based communication to the remote therapist on the basis of an IMU and a GSP/GPS unit. The tool will be furnished to subjects along with a homecare device for daily monitoring of motion activity, along with different aids and monitoring tools.
- Other potentialities could be explored through integration of wearable systems for monitoring physical activity in a telerehabilitation application.

Abbreviations/Acronyms

COSP Codivilla spring
GPS Global positioning system
GSM Global system for mobile communication
HIS Hospital information service

IMU   Inertial measurement unit
LAN   Local area network
SMT   Surface montage technology
STS   Sit-to-stand

Acknowledgement   This work was funded by the Istituto Superiore di Sanità (The Italian NIH) in the 3-year long (2006–2008) program entitled "Design and Construction of Innovative Wearable Systems for the Monitoring of Kinematic Parameters." No competing financial conflicts exist.

References

1. Aminian K, Robert P, Buscher EE, et al. Physical activity monitoring based on accelerometry: validation and comparison with video observation. Med Biol Eng Comput. 1999;37(3): 304–8.
2. Available at: http://www.oposrl.it/pdf/molle_codivilla.pdf. Accessed Mar 2009.
3. Available at: http://www.stroke.org/site/PageNavigator/HOME. Accessed Mar 2009.
4. Busser HJ, Ott J, Uiterwaal M, et al. Ambulatory monitoring of children's activities. Med Eng Phys. 1997;19:440–5.
5. Bussmann HB, Reuvekamp PJ, Veltink PH, et al. Validity and reliability of measurements obtained with an activity monitor in people with and without a transtibial amputation. Phys Ther. 1998;78(9):989–98.
6. Bussmann JBJ, Tulen JHM, Van Herel ECG, et al. Quantification of physical activities by means of ambulatory accelerometry: a validation study. Psychophysiology. 1998;35: 488–96.
7. Bussmann JB, Van de Laar YM, Neeleman MP, et al. Ambulatory accelerometry to quantify motor behaviour in patients after failed back surgery: a validation study. Pain. 1998; 74(2–3):153–61.
8. Bussmann JBJ, Veltink PH, Koelma F, et al. Ambulatory monitoring of mobility-related activities: the initial phase of the development of an activity monitor. Eur J Phys Rehabil Med. 1995;5:2–7.
9. Dunne DM, Lyons GM, Grace PA. The feasibility of posture and physical movement detection using accelerometers. Ir J Med Sci. 2000;169:22.
10. Fahrenberg J, Foerster F, Mueller W, et al. Assessment of posture and motion by multi-channel piezoresistive accelerometer recordings. Psychophysiology. 1997;34:607–12.
11. Fahrenberg J, Muller W, Foerster F, et al. A multi-channel investigation of physical activity. J Psychophysiol. 1996;10:209–17.
12. Foerster F, Fahrenberg J. Motion pattern and posture: correctly assessed by calibrated accelerometers. Behav Res Methods Instrum Comput. 2000;32:450–7.
13. Foerster F, Smeja M, Fahrenberg J. Detection of posture and motion by accelerometry: a validation study in ambulatory monitoring. Comput Hum Behav. 1999;15(5):571–83.
14. Giansanti D. Investigation of fall-risk using a wearable device with accelerometers and rate gyroscopes. Physiol Meas. 2006;27:1081–90.
15. Giansanti D, Maccioni G. Comparison of three different kinematic sensor assemblies for locomotion study. Physiol Meas. 2005;26:689–705.
16. Giansanti D, Maccioni G, Cesinaro S, et al. Assessment of fall-risk by means of a neural network based on parameters assessed by a wearable device during posturography. Med Eng Phys. 2008;30:367–72.
17. Giansanti D, Maccioni G, Macellari V. The development and test of a device for the reconstruction of 3-D position and orientation by means of a kinematic sensor assembly with rate gyroscopes and accelerometers. IEEE Trans Biomed Eng. 2005;52:1271–7.

18. Giansanti D, Maccioni G, Macellari V, et al. Towards the investigation of kinematic parameters from an integrated measurement unit for the classification of the rising from the chair. Conf Proc IEEE Eng Med Biol Soc. 2006;1:1742–5.
19. Giansanti D, Macellari V, Maccioni G. New neural network classifier of fall-risk based on the Mahalanobis distance and kinematic parameters assessed by a wearable device. Physiol Meas. 2008;29:N11–9.
20. Giansanti D, Macellari V, Maccioni G. Telemonitoring and telerehabilitation of patients with Parkinson's disease: health technology assessment of a novel wearable step counter. Telemed J E Health. 2008;14:76–83.
21. Giansanti D, Morelli S, Dionisio P, et al. Design, construction and integration in instrumented walkways of a portable kit for the assessment of gait parameters in tele-rehabilitation. In: Cohn E, Kumar S, editors. Telerehabilitation. London: Springer; 2012.
22. Giansanti D, Morelli S, Maccioni G, et al. Toward the design of a wearable system for fall-risk detection in telerehabilitation. Telemed J E Health. 2009;15(3):296–9.
23. Giansanti D, Morelli S, Maccioni G, et al. Design and construction of a portable kit for the assessment of gait parameters in daily-rehabilitation. Rapporti ISTISAN 10/16, Istituto Superiore di Sanità, Roma; 2010.
24. Giansanti D, Tiberi Y, Maccioni G. Integration of motion sensor monitoring units in stroke gait telerehabilitation programs of continuity of care. Telemed J E Health. 2009;15:105–11.
25. Kandel ER, Schwart RJ, Jessell TM. Principi di neuroscienze. Milan, Italy: CEA; 2000.
26. Kiani K, Snijders CJ, Gelsema ES. Computerised analysis of daily life motor activity for ambulatory monitoring. Technol Health Care. 1997;5:307–18.
27. Kiani K, Snijders CJ, Gelsema ES. Recognition of daily motor activity classes using an artificial neural network. Arch Phys Med Rehabil. 1998;79:147–54.
28. Lyons GM, Culhane KM, Hilton D, et al. A description of an accelerometer-based mobility monitoring technique. Med Eng Phys. 2005;27(6):497–504.
29. Uiterwaal M, Glerum EB, Busser HJ, et al. Ambulatory monitoring of physical activity in working situations, a validation study. J Med Eng Technol. 1998;22:168–72.
30. Van den Berg-Emons HJ, Bussmann JB, Balk AH, et al. Validity of ambulatory accelerometry to quantify physical activity in heart failure. Scand J Rehabil Med. 2000;32(4):187–92.
31. Veltink PH, Bussmann HBJ, de Vries W, et al. Detection of static and dynamic activities using uniaxial accelerometers. IEEE Trans Rehabil Eng. 1996;4:375–85.
32. Veltink PH, Bussmann HBJ, Koelma F, et al. The feasibility of posture and movement detection by accelerometry. In: Proceedings of the 15th annual international conference of the IEEE, engineering in medicine and biology society, San Diego, 1993. p. 1230–1.

Chapter 19
Professional Associations, State Licensure, and the Reimbursement of Telerehabilitation

Janet E. Brown

Abstract Professional associations and state licensing boards play important roles in the credentialing and practice standards for occupational therapists, physical therapists, and speech-language pathologists in the United States. The policies and regulations developed by these groups play a role in educating and influencing others about telerehabilitation. This chapter will describe how the emerging area of telerehabilitation is being handled by national and international professional associations and will address the role and variability of state licensing boards. The current status of telerehabilitation reimbursement will be discussed.

19.1 Introduction

The credibility of health professionals is founded on the standards that underlie their training and competencies to practice their respective professions. The three rehabilitation professions recognized by the Centers for Medicare and Medicaid Services (CMS)—occupational therapy, physical therapy, and speech-language pathology—have somewhat different processes and relationships between their professional associations, credentialing organizations, and state licensing boards. Their respective associations, the American Occupational Therapy Association (AOTA), American Physical Therapy Association (APTA), and American Speech-Language-Hearing Association (ASHA) have a number of commonalities. They are all member-driven organizations that provide resources for their members, build public awareness, and advocate for political action and reimbursement on behalf of their respective professions. Most relevant for the purposes of this chapter is that the

J.E. Brown
American Speech-Language-Hearing Association,
2200 Research Boulevard, Rockville, MD, 20850-3289, USA
e-mail: jbrown@asha.org

S. Kumar, E.R. Cohn (eds.), *Telerehabilitation*, Health Informatics,
DOI 10.1007/978-1-4471-4198-3_19, © Springer-Verlag London 2013

associations establish policies for professional practice and guide the evolution of the profession, including emerging areas of practice such as telerehabilitation.

State licensure is independent of professional associations and credentialing organizations. Statutes passed by state legislators stipulate the makeup of the state licensing board and the essential elements of that state's licensure law. Regulations may be passed by the board to expand or interpret the law in a specific area. The objective of state boards is to protect the citizens of their state through the licensing process; however, in fulfilling this obligation they may approach their task in ways that demonstrate considerable variation and that reflect the unique nature of their state laws and procedures.

A brief summary of the three professions is included in the following sections.

19.2 Professional Associations, Credentialing, and Licensure in the United States

19.2.1 Speech-Language Pathology

The ASHA is unique in that it serves as both a professional membership organization and an accrediting body for speech-language pathologists (SLPs). Earning the Certificate of Clinical Competence (CCC) in speech-language pathology requires graduating from a master's or doctoral-level graduate program accredited by the Council on Academic Accreditation in Audiology and Speech-Language Pathology, passing a national examination, and completing a 36-week clinical fellowship under the mentorship of a certified SLP [10].

ASHA provides opportunities for professional specialization through special interest groups (SIGs). In addition, specialty recognition is awarded to applicants who demonstrate a higher level of achievement and focus in the following areas of practice: fluency, child language, and swallowing [16].

Almost all states (and the District of Columbia) license the practice of speech-language pathology. Some states exempt SLPs working in school settings from licensure because they are subject to educational requirements instead. Other states require licensure for all SLPs regardless of setting (e.g., universal licensure).

The definition and scope of the licensure law may or may not be consistent with ASHA's current standards, since licensure and certification requirements are developed independent of each other. Through the Council for Clinical Certification, ASHA periodically reviews and may update standards for certification. Licensure boards may change standards by introducing new legislation. States may require that the licensure law be "sunset" at specified intervals, creating opportunities to make changes when the law is reintroduced. Changes can also be made through regulations promulgated by the licensure board. Each state differs in terms of requirements that are statutory (e.g., in the law) and those that are regulatory; these differences are important when it comes to how professionals can advocate for changes. To change the statute may mean that other provisions in the law are open to challenge or revision, whereas regulatory changes may be made without opening the entire law for review.

19.2.2 Occupational Therapy

The National Board for Certification in Occupational Therapy (NBCOT) administers the national certification examination for occupational therapists. Occupational therapists in the United States must graduate with a master's or doctoral degree from an accredited program, including 24 weeks of full-time supervised fieldwork, and pass the certification examination. The Accreditation Council for Occupational Therapy Education (ACOTE) accredits the academic programs.

State licensure or registration is required to practice in all states, including the District of Columbia, Puerto Rico, and Guam; these requirements include graduation from an accredited occupational therapy education program, completion of supervised fieldwork, and passing the certification examination administered by NBCOT. Some states may require applicants to complete a jurisprudence examination.

The AOTA offers 11 special interest sections, four areas of board certification (i.e., gerontology, mental health, pediatrics, and physical rehabilitation), and four areas of specialty certification (driving and community mobility; environmental modification; feeding, eating, and swallowing; and low vision) [40].

19.2.3 Physical Therapy

The APTA is the national professional organization for physical therapists. Membership in APTA also includes membership in a state chapter. APTA has 18 special interest sections for members; it also recognizes eight areas of advanced clinical practice in a specialty area, which require passing an examination.

Effective in 2015, the Commission on Accreditation in Physical Therapy Education (CAPTE) requires that all accredited programs award the Doctor of Physical Therapy (DPT) as the professional entry level. Until that time, physical therapists may obtain a master's or doctoral degree.

State licensure is required for physical therapists to practice in all states and territories. The Federation of State Boards of Physical Therapy comprises member licensing boards from all states and the District of Columbia, Puerto Rico, and Virgin Islands. It develops the National Physical Therapy Exam (NPTE) that serves as a national entry-level examination for physical therapists [41].

19.3   Professional Associations and Telerehabilitation

The application of technology for medical practice at a distance was initially explored in aeronautics and in the private sector from the 1950s through the 1980s [19]. With the improvement of technology, a renewed wave of interest in telemedicine began in the 1990s [19]. As early as 1997, ASHA, APTA, and the NBCOT participated in an Interdisciplinary Telehealth Standards Working Group with other professional organizations, various nursing and physicians' organizations, and federal agencies [5]. The focus of their meetings was to discuss issues that would arise in the further development of telehealth, including licensure and standards of practice. ASHA developed an internal telehealth issues brief in 1998 outlining the various issues that would need to be addressed, including practice, credentialing and licensing, ethics and legal considerations, and reimbursement [6]. Over a decade later, these issues are still being addressed by professional associations, licensure boards, and payers.

APTA was the first to draft an official position on telehealth, which was approved in 2001 and later revised in 2006 [3]. A guidelines document was originally drafted in 2003 and amended in 2006 [4]. APTA's amended document makes some specific recommendations on the subject of licensure and telehealth, including the development of mechanisms to regulate and monitor inter- and intrastate telehealth practice, including endorsement or reciprocity for consultations. The document stipulates that a provider physical therapist must be "… licensed in the state and jurisdiction where the patient/client receives the care" [4].

In 2002, the AOTA Commission on Practice developed a white paper on telehealth and occupational therapy; its focus was to ensure that practice remained consistent with face-to-face intervention and in keeping with evidence-based practice and the domain and framework of occupational therapy practice [1].

AOTA's Commission on Practice approved a telerehabilitation position paper in 2005, defining telerehabilitation as "…the clinical application of consultative, preventative, diagnostic, and therapeutic services via two-way interactive telecommunication technology" [2]. It discussed the current status of telerehabilitation with respect to current research and topics such as diagnosis, intervention, monitoring and related technology, and addresses practitioner qualifications and ethics. It urged further research on the effectiveness of telerehabilitation in all aspects of its use.

In 2002, ASHA fielded a survey of telepractice use among audiologists and SLPs [7]. ASHA adopted the term *telepractice* to encompass services that are not exclusively health-related because many SLPs are employed in education settings. Of the 1,667 responses, 11 % reported using telepractice to deliver services based on a very broad definition that was provided. Respondents most frequently reported that they conducted telepractice via telephone (93 %), e-mail (74 %), web-based information/resources (40 %), web-based conferencing (13 %), and video teleconferencing (8 %). Only 15 % of telepractice users reported being reimbursed for their services. In retrospect, it is likely that the majority of these reported telepractice encounters were adjunct services (particularly counseling, follow-up, and equipment checks) in support of in-person services.

In 2003, ASHA appointed a telepractice working group that developed a position statement, technical report, and knowledge and skills document on telepractice for audiologists and SLPs [8, 9, 11, 12, 35, 36]. In the position statements, ASHA defined telepractice as "…the application of telecommunications technology to delivery of professional services at a distance by linking clinician to client, or clinician to clinician, for assessment, intervention, and/or consultation" [8, 36]. A very important component of ASHA's position statement is the following proviso: "The use of telepractice does not remove any existing responsibilities in delivering services, including adherence to the Code of Ethics, Scope of Practice, state and federal laws (e.g., licensure, HIPAA, etc.), and ASHA policy documents on professional practice. Therefore, the quality of services delivered via telepractice must be consistent with the quality of services delivered face-to-face" [8, 36].

ASHA also became engaged in ongoing advocacy to include SLPs and audiologists as eligible providers by Medicare. As interest among members has developed, ASHA's website added a page on telepractice (www.asha.org/telepractice) with policy documents and articles featuring member activities and research in telepractice. In 2010, ASHA members petitioned to create an 18th SIG on telepractice, which began in 2011. Formation of a SIG established a means for members interested in telepractice to communicate with each other through a quarterly publication and electronic forums.

The professional organizations collaborate with telehealth organizations such as the American Telemedicine Association (ATA), the Center for Telehealth and e-Health Law, and the Association of Telehealth Service Providers. The ATA has a SIG on telerehabilitation whose members largely come from the three rehabilitation professions. A subcommittee of the telerehabilitation SIG developed a blueprint for telerehabilitation guidelines (2010) with core administrative, clinical, technical, and ethical principles built on ATA's *Core Standards for Telemedicine Operations* [17].

19.4   State Licensure and Telerehabilitation

Telehealth affords the potential to deliver services anywhere. However, obtaining a state license in every state in which one might practice imposes a daunting barrier of time and expense to maintain 50 or more licenses. Regardless of the profession, licensure has been proved to be a potential barrier that has not been satisfactorily addressed even by professions that have dealt with telemedicine since its earliest days.

The Federation of State Medical Boards (FSMB) published a report of its Ad Hoc Committee on Telemedicine in 1996, including a model act to establish a special license for practicing across state lines [27]. Subsequently, the FSMB has passed several resolutions to make recommendations about license portability and to develop common and consistent policies with regard to telemedicine. However, to date, even physician organizations have not developed a national solution for providing telemedicine across state lines.

Along with physicians, nurses have struggled with the issue of licensure portability for decades. The National Council of State Boards of Nursing (NCSBN) sought to address the problem through a nurse licensure compact (NLC) [33]. Nurses who live in a state that has passed legislation to authorize the NLC may practice without restriction in other states that participate in the NLC. Thus, it is less restrictive than the model special license proposed by the FSMB, which was intended solely for telemedicine. To date, 24 states have enacted the NLC.

Awareness of telerehabilitation has prompted much discussion and a range of actions at the level of state licensing boards and their national boards. In 2003, the National Council of State Boards of Examiners for Speech-Language Pathology and Audiology (NCSB) adopted a position statement recommending that states develop statutory language about telepractice [32]. The position statement provides sample language stating that licensure is required to practice in the state via electronic or telephonic means. With respect to providing services across state lines, the statement suggests that states consider issuing a temporary or restricted license.

In speech-language pathology, states that developed statutes or regulations on telepractice demonstrated considerable variability, from Delaware's prohibition against practice via telecommunications to Maryland's definition of service delivery models and equipment and guidelines for telepractice. By the end of 2010, less than 25 % of the state licensure boards had passed any language, but it was under discussion in other states [13]. The majority of states that have adopted language have followed NCSB's recommendations to consider telepractice as an activity requiring licensure in the state; however, none to date has adopted a limited license for interstate practice. In 2010, ASHA developed model regulations for telepractice and model language for a limited license for interstate telepractice [14, 15].

19.5   Role of Associations and Licensure in Reimbursement

As of this writing, the reimbursement of telerehabilitation in the United States is still limited by the relatively recent introduction of this form of service delivery in occupational therapy, physical therapy, and speech-language pathology. However, the statements or actions of professional associations and licensure boards can be influential in advocating with payers. When new areas of practice or service delivery are introduced, payers look for policies or regulations that define, endorse, or specify conditions or competencies that meet professional standards. The professional associations may work collaboratively in their advocacy toward a common reimbursement goal; in addition, they may collaborate with professional/trade organizations such as the ATA that employ a lobbyist dedicated to telehealth issues and sponsor interdisciplinary telerehabilitation SIGs for professionals working in telerehabilitation.

19.5.1   Private Health Plans

One of the earliest documented reimbursement successes was by a SLP in North Dakota who worked in a hospital supported by a telemedicine network. With the telemedicine infrastructure already in place, she advocated with Blue Cross/Blue Shield of North Dakota to reimburse speech-language pathology services that she delivered from the main hospital hub to a stroke patient at a satellite clinic in a remote area of the state. Upon being denied, she asked ASHA to write a letter to Blue Cross/Blue Shield of North Dakota stating its support of telepractice. Ultimately, the insurance company agreed to reimburse such services that were then provided to patients at other satellite locations [29]. However, at present, the same process must be repeated to win acceptance by Blue Cross/Blue Shield in other states, or by other private health plan insurers. The exception is in states that have passed legislation mandating that all private health plans' covered services must be reimbursed if delivered via telehealth [39]. States such as Maine were able to advocate for passing of comprehensive legislation to this effect by demonstrating the cost effectiveness of timely intervention compared to subsequent remedial treatment (Towey, personal communication).

19.5.2   Medicaid

Medicaid is a joint state and national entitlement program established in 1965 to cover medical care to eligible low-income Americans. Unlike Medicare, Medicaid is administered by each state, resulting in great variability from state to state in terms of eligibility criteria, covered services, and reimbursement rates [23]. Like state licensure, the variability creates challenges in tracking regulations across states. However, some state Medicaid programs are ahead of the national Medicare program by reimbursing telerehabilitation services. A 2002 survey of telerehabilitation reimbursement by Medicaid programs yielded 35 responses; of those respondents, only four states—Hawaii, Louisiana, Minnesota, and Nebraska—reimbursed any occupational therapy, physical therapy, or speech-language pathology services delivered remotely [34].

More state Medicaid programs may now reimburse for telerehabilitation services, but the exact status is difficult to track. As with Medicare, the decision needs to include authorization of specific Current Procedural Terminology (CPT) codes that will be reimbursed.

Another distinction between Medicare and Medicaid is that Medicaid programs may reimburse providers for their travel time or mileage. Thus, Medicaid has additional incentives to cover telerehabilitation for its savings on travel costs. Providers seeking verification of telerehabilitation within their state are advised to contact the Medicaid office directly and confirm approved CPT codes and any other requirements for providing services remotely.

19.5.3   Medicare

Perhaps due to concerns that utilization of Medicare services via telehealth would explode beyond its already-stretched funding, legislation authorizing telehealth reimbursement has rather narrowly constrained the scope of covered services. Bills passed in 1997 and 2000 authorized reimbursement of telehealth services to specific providers: physicians, nurse practitioners, physician assistants, nurse midwives, clinical nurse specialists, clinical psychologists and social workers, and registered dietitians or nutrition professionals. In addition, the Medicare beneficiary was required to receive services only from an originating site in a rural health professional shortage area or outside a metropolitan statistical area. Further, only specific CPT codes were identified as reimbursable and required the modifier GT to indicate that they were delivered via an interactive telecommunications system [24]. Ongoing advocacy is needed to expand the providers, originating sites, and CPT codes that will be reimbursed by Medicare.

19.6   International Telerehabilitation

Countries that lack a sufficient pool or distribution of qualified providers to provide services to extensive rural areas may embrace telerehabilitation as one possible solution to these challenges. In 1998, Kully reported her use of telepractice in Canada to deliver speech-language pathology services to children who stutter [30, 31]. Several Canadian professional associations have adopted policy documents on telerehabilitation. One of the earliest was the Canadian Association of Occupational Therapists (CAOT), which developed a position statement in 2000 stating the potential value of teleoccupational therapy in expanding access to occupational therapy services [20]. The College of Audiologists and Speech-Language Pathologists of Ontario (CASLPO) approved a 2004 position statement, which asserts that practitioners may use telepractice as long as the treatment is consistent with existing standards and the code of ethics. It further states that the primary amount of treatment should be delivered in a "face-to-face" condition, which can include electronic form if the following conditions are met: audio, visual, in real time, and interactive [25]. It also comments on other key features such as patient consent, provider competencies, and confidentiality.

The Canadian Association of Speech-Language Pathologists and Audiologists (CASLPA) approved a position statement in 2006. It endorses the use of telepractice when applied in the best interest of the client. This statement includes both live and store-and-forward services in its definition, unlike CASLPO, but reiterates the need for informed consent, confidentiality, and competencies on the part of the provider [21].

Australia has been the source of a significant amount of interdisciplinary research on telerehabilitation. A position statement on telerehabilitation was written by the

Australian Physiotherapy Association in 2009 [18], but nothing to date has been developed by Speech Pathology Australia [37].

Telehealth initiatives have been embraced in countries such as Brazil and South Africa for collaborations involving teleaudiology [28, 38]. In Brazil, the national association for SLPs and audiologists adopted a 2009 statement on the use of tele-health (telessaude) [26].

19.7 Conclusion

Professional associations' widespread support of telerehabilitation in the United States and internationally attests to their vision of making services accessible to individuals who otherwise may be limited by distance, disability, or unavailability of providers. Their policy statements and guidelines share similar themes of maintaining the quality of service, ensuring competence in telerehabilitation as a form of service delivery, and advocating for further research. Acceptance of telerehabilitation by state licensure boards and payers has been a slow ongoing process, perhaps attributable to the legal and financial implications of such changes. For licensure boards, acceptance involves regulatory and/or statutory change and the unresolved challenge of achieving national consensus on licensure portability across state lines. For payers, the challenges include defining reimbursable services within this model of service delivery and clarifying documentation and/or coding protocols for those services. In light of the positive momentum toward using technology to provide timely and efficient services, it is expected that associations, licensure boards, and payers will continue to develop more unified solutions to these remaining issues.

Summary

- Professional associations and state licensing boards play important roles in the credentialing and practice standards for occupational therapists, physical therapists, and speech-language pathologists in the United States.
- State licensure or registration is required for physical/occupational therapists or SLPs to practice in different U.S. states and territories.
- Telehealth has the potential to deliver services anywhere. However, licensure has been a potential barrier that has not been satisfactorily addressed even by professions that have dealt with telemedicine since its earliest days. Physicians and nurses have struggled with the issue of licensure portability for decades.
- Acceptance of telerehabilitation by state licensure boards, which involves regulatory and/or statutory change and the unresolved challenge of achieving national consensus on licensure portability across state lines, has been a slow ongoing process.

- The reimbursement of telerehabilitation in the United States is still limited by the relatively recent introduction of this form of service delivery in occupational therapy, physical therapy, and speech-language pathology. However, the statements or actions of professional associations and licensure boards can be influential in advocating with payers.
- In light of the positive momentum toward using technology to provide timely and efficient services, it is expected that associations, licensure boards, and payers will continue to develop more unified solutions to overcome any issues.

Abbreviations/Acronyms

ACOTE	Accreditation Council for Occupational Therapy Education
AOTA	American Occupational Therapy Association
APTA	American Physical Therapy Association
ASHA	Speech-Language-Hearing Association
ATA	American Telemedicine Association
CAOT	Canadian Association of Occupational Therapists
CAPTE	Commission on Accreditation in Physical Therapy Education
CASLPA	Canadian Association of Speech-Language Pathologists and Audiologists
CASLPO	College of Audiologists and Speech-Language Pathologists of Ontario
CCC	Certificate of Clinical Competence
CMS	Centers for Medicare and Medicaid Services
CPT	Current Procedural Terminology
DPT	Doctor of Physical Therapy
FSMB	Federation of State Medical Boards
NBCOT	National Board for Certification in Occupational Therapy
NCSB	National Council of State Boards of Examiners for Speech-Language Pathology and Audiology
NCSBN	National Council of State Boards of Nursing
NLC	Nurse licensure compact
NPTE	National Physical Therapy Exam
SIG	Special interest group
SLP	Speech-language pathologist

References

1. American Occupational Therapy Association Commission on Practice. Board approves white paper on telehealth. Occup Ther Pract. 2002;7(6):3–4.
2. American Occupational Therapy Association Commission on Practice. Telerehabilitation position paper. Am J Occup Ther. 2005;59(6):656–60.

3. American Physical Therapy Association. Telehealth BOD P03-06-10-20 [position statement]. 2009. Available at: www.apta.org. Accessed 14 Mar 2011.
4. American Physical Therapy Association. Telehealth – definitions and guidelines BOD G03-06-09-19 [guideline]. 2009. Available at: www.apta.org. Accessed 15 Mar 2011.
5. American Speech-Language-Hearing Association. Inter-professional perspectives on telehealth standards of practice, May 29 [internal memorandum]; 1997.
6. American Speech-Language-Hearing Association. Telehealth issues brief. A report to the ASHA Executive Board from the Issues in Credentialing Team [unpublished]; 1998.
7. American Speech-Language-Hearing Association. Survey of telepractice use among audiologists and speech-language pathologists. 2002. Available at: http://www.asha.org/uploaded-Files/practice/telepractice/SurveyofTelepractice.pdf. Accessed 15 Mar 2011.
8. American Speech-Language-Hearing Association. Audiologists providing clinical services via telepractice: position statement [position statement]. 2005. Available at: www.asha.org/policy. Accessed 15 Mar 2011.
9. American Speech-Language-Hearing Association. Audiologists providing clinical services via telepractice: technical report [technical report]. 2005. Available at: www.asha.org/policy. Accessed 15 Mar 2011.
10. American Speech-Language-Hearing Association. Background information and standards and implementation for the certificate of clinical competence in speech-language pathology. 2005. Available at: http://www.asha.org/certification/slp_standards_new.htm. Accessed 27 Dec 2010.
11. American Speech-Language-Hearing Association. Speech-language pathologists providing clinical services via telepractice: position statement [position statement]. 2005. Available at: www.asha.org/policy. Accessed 15 Mar 2011.
12. American Speech-Language-Hearing Association. Speech-language pathologists providing clinical services via telepractice: technical report [technical report]. 2005. Available at: www.asha.org/policy. Accessed 15 Mar 2011.
13. American Speech-Language-Hearing Association. State licensure trends. 2009. Available at: http://www.asha.org/advocacy/state/StateLicensureTrends.htm. Accessed 17 Mar 2011.
14. American Speech-Language-Hearing Association. Model language for interstate telepractice. 2010. Available at: http://www.asha.org/uploadedFiles/ModLangInterstatPract.pdf .Accessed 29 Dec 2010.
15. American Speech-Language-Hearing Association. Model language for telepractice. 2010. Available at: http://www.asha.org/uploadedFiles/ModRegTelepractice.pdf. Accessed 29 Dec 2010.
16. American Speech-Language-Hearing Association. Clinical specialty recognition: introduction. Available at: http://www.asha.org/certification/specialty/. Accessed 28 Dec 2010.
17. American Telemedicine Association. A blueprint for telerehabilitation guidelines. 2010. Available at: www.americantelemed.org. Accessed 14 Mar 2011.
18. Australian Physiotherapy Association. Telerehabilitation and physiotherapy [position statement]. 2009. Available at: http://www.physiotherapy.asn.au/images/Document_Library/Position_Statements/2012%20telerehabilitation.pdf. Accessed 7 Feb 2011.
19. Bashshur RL, Reardon TG, Shannon GW. Telemedicine: a new health care delivery system. Annu Rev Public Health. 2000;21:613–37.
20. Canadian Association of Occupational Therapists (CAOT). CAOT position statement telehealth and tele-occupational therapy. 2000. Available at: http://www.caot.ca/pdfs/telehealthPS.pdf. Accessed 7 Feb 2011.
21. Canadian Association of Speech-Language Pathologists and Audiologists (CASLPA). Position paper on the use of telepractice for CASLPA speech-language pathologists and audiologists. 2006. Available at: http://www.caslpa.ca/PDF/position%20papers/telepractice.pdf. Accessed 7 Feb 2011.
22. Centers for Medicare and Medicaid Services. Medicare benefit policy manual, Chapter 15, section 230.3. 2010. Available at: http://www.cms.gov/manuals/downloads/bp102c15.pdf. Accessed 27 Dec 2010.

23. Centers for Medicare and Medicaid Services. Medicaid program – general information. 2010. Available at: http://www.cms.gov/MedicaidGenInfo/. Accessed 28 Dec 2010.

24. Centers for Medicare and Medicaid Services. Medicare learning network. Telehealth Services [factsheet].n.d.Availableat:http://www.cms.gov/MLNProducts/downloads/TelehealthSrvcsfctsht. pdf. Accessed 28 Dec 2010.

25. College of Audiologists and Speech-Language Pathologists of Ontario (CASLPO). Use of telepractice approaches in providing services to patients/clients. 2004. Available at: http:// www.caslpo.com/Portals/0/positionstatements/mptelepractice.pdf. Accessed 7 Feb 2011.

26. Conselho Federal de Fonoaudiologia. Dispoe sobre a reulamentacao do uso do sistema telessaude em fonoaudiologia. Resolucao CFFa numero 366. 2009. Available at: http://www.fonoaudiolo-gia.org.br/legislacaoPDF/Res%20366-09%20Telessaude.pdf. Accessed 7 Feb 2011.

27. Federation of State Medical Boards of the United States. Report of the Ad Hoc Committee on Telemedicine. 1996. Available at: http://www.fsmb.org/pdf/1996_grpol_Telemedicine.pdf. Accessed 15 Mar 2011.

28. Ferrari DV, Bernardez-Braga GRA. Remote problem microphone measurement to verify hearing aid performance. J Telemed Telecare. 2009;15:122–4.

29. Houn B, Trottier K. Meeting the challenge of rural service delivery. The ASHA Leader. 2003. Available at: http://www.asha.org/Publications/leader/2003/031118/031118d.htm. Accessed 15 Mar 2011.

30. Kully D. Telehealth in speech pathology: applications to the treatment of stuttering. J Telemed Telecare. 2000;6 Suppl 2:S2:39–41.

31. Kully D. Venturing into telehealth: applying interactive technologies to stuttering treatment. The ASHA Leader. 2002. Available at: http://www.asha.org/Publications/leader/2002/020611/ f020611_2/. Accessed 7 Feb 2011.

32. National Council of State Boards of Examiners for Speech-Language Pathology and Audiology (NCSB). Position statement on the regulation of telepractice. 2003. Available at: http://www. ncsb.info/position-statements. Accessed 29 Dec 2010.

33. National Council of State Boards of Nursing. Nurse licensure compact. Available at: https:// www.ncsbn.org/nlc.htm. Accessed 15 Mar 2011.

34. Palsbo S. Medicaid payment for telerehabilitation. Arch Phys Med Rehabil. 2004;85:1188–91.

35. Speech-Language-Hearing Association. Knowledge and skills needed by audiologists providing clinical services via telepractice [knowledge and skills]. 2005. Available at: www.asha.org/ policy. Accessed 15 Mar 2011.

36. Speech-Language-Hearing Association. Knowledge and skills needed by speech-language pathologists providing clinical services via telepractice [knowledge and skills]. 2005. Available at: www.asha.org/policy. Accessed 15 Mar 2011.

37. Speech Pathology Australia. Available at: http://www.speechpathologyaustralia.org.au/. Accessed 5 Feb 2011.

38. Swanepoel DW, Koekemoer D, Clark J. Intercontinental hearing assessment: a study in teleaudiology. J Telemed Telecare. 2010;16(4):248–52.

39. Towey M. Maine advocacy wins telepractice coverage. The ASHA Leader. 2009. Available at: http://www.asha.org/Publications/leader/2009/090901/090101a1/. Accessed 15 Mar 2011.

40. U.S. Bureau of Labor Statistics. Occupational therapists. Occupational outlook handbook. 2010–11 ed. Available at: http://www.bls.gov/oco/ocos078.htm. Accessed 5 Feb 2011.

41. U.S. Bureau of Labor Statistics. Physical therapists. Occupational outlook handbook. 2010–11 ed. Available at: http://www.bls.gov/oco/ocos080.htm. Accessed 5 Feb 2011.

Chapter 20
Making a Business Case for eHealth and Teleservices

Suzanne Paone and Grant Shevchik

Abstract Telemedicine is emerging as a critical solution to some challenging problems of our current health-care system: access to care, cost-effective delivery, and distribution of limited providers. With Internet connectivity and decreasing computer costs, online health-care services are increasingly available. Now, more than ever, patients expect personalized connectivity and communication with health-care providers along with self-service access to their personal health information. Teleservices and e-Health are therefore being deployed to provide medical management to consumers of various ages and health statuses through secure e-mail, websites, and online home medical devices. This chapter describes the application of Return on Investment (ROI) models to shape Teleservices and e-Health.

20.1 Introduction: Concept of eHealth and Teleservices in Medicine

The use of the Internet for both health information and alternative methods of care is being embraced by consumers in all sectors of the health economy. Approximately 113 million people or 80 % of adults in the United States report using the Internet to seek out health information [13]. Internet-based solutions, called *eHealth or teleservices*, have offered consumers of various ages and health statuses an assortment of help, including secure e-mail, websites, and online home medical devices

S. Paone (✉)
eHealth Services Information Services Division,
University of Pittsburgh Medical Center, Pittsburgh, PA, USA
e-mail: PaoneSJ@upmc.edu

G. Shevchik
Health-UPMC, University Center at Level Green,
101 Orchard Drive, Level Green, PA 15085, USA

S. Kumar, E.R. Cohn (eds.), *Telerehabilitation*, Health Informatics,
DOI 10.1007/978-1-4471-4198-3_20, © Springer-Verlag London 2013

since early 2000. Research studies have shown benefits for patients, health providers, and payer organizations who participate in eHealth for the self-management of chronic disease, whether conditions are newly identified or previously diagnosed [15, 21]. Furthermore, improved Internet connectivity and decreasing computer costs make online health-care services increasingly available [18].

Teleservices represents the entirety of applications and processes that utilize information and communication technologies (ICT) to provide health-care services using non-traditional methods. This encompasses a broad spectrum of applications that offer both clinical and administrative functions such as diagnosis and treatment, administration of therapies, prescription refill management, and scheduling of services. In the context of broad teleservices, telerehabilitation is defined as the delivery of rehabilitation services using ICT [6]. Telemedicine is emerging as a critical component of the health-care crisis solution. Telemedicine holds the promise to impact significantly some of the most challenging problems of our current health-care system: access to care, cost-effective delivery, and distribution of limited providers. Telemedicine can change the current paradigm of care and allow for improved access and improved health outcomes in cost-effective ways.

20.1.1   Societal Drivers and Factors Affecting the Development of eHealth and Teleservices

Health-care entities that offer innovative programs using eHealth and teleservices position themselves as leadership organizations. Historically, technology leadership arose from sectors of the economy that drove measurable economic growth, such as manufacturing, entertainment, finance, and retail services [12]. As discussed by Meyer et al. [26], *eServices*, or transactions over the Internet, evolved with vendors such as IBM during growth in the business sectors of Fortune 400 and 500 firms in the early 1990s. eServices is a new market concept in the health-care industry. To date, specialized health information technology vendors who have minimal experience in the design of eServices are struggling to deliver eServices to providers and patients in the framework of current health-care business models. Likewise, teleservices such as telerehabilitation are provided using ICT; yet for the most part they lack not only succinct cost-based economic models but often strategic fit in the providing organization. While research on value chain analysis and cost modeling for telerehabilitation identifies structural and execution costs, there is little emphasis on providing a holistic business strategy for the implementation and sustaining needs of the program [14]. Demographic trends and economic challenges in the delivery of traditional health care compel organizations that embrace technology to acquire, deliver, and maintain these programs in a fashion that sustains and complements the overall strategy of the organization.

Patient self-management is part of most chronic care models in the United States and involves an evolving role for ICT, such as the Internet, in patient–provider communication [29, 33]. Telemedicine increases access to health care. Likewise, chronic disease growth at the national and international level supports the need for cost-effective ICT designs to manage chronic illness along with the global impetus toward evolving consumerism in health-care markets. Estimates place the cost of managing the disease burden of elder care at more than $1.3 trillion by 2014 or 13 % of the gross domestic product [5]. This increase in disease burden with implied increases in costs enumerates the need for low-cost technology solutions that are readily available to all segments of the population. Without technologies such as e-mail, instant messaging platforms, cellular devices, and telephonic automation in eHealth development, neither of health services providers, payers, or pharmaceutical companies can reach broad populations, given the magnitude of chronic illness in the United States.

Advances in the globalization of consumer health markets are happening outside of the United States as well. For example, in Sweden a mix of national and private entities comprise health services and consumer preferences are being studied in the areas of education and health services as a part of reforms. Informatics researchers have reported the development of online communities and public portals as indicative of an advancing agenda toward active preferences in both education and health services [20]. Similar trends are seen in the United Kingdom relative to diabetes groups advancing to online medical venues as well as the advancement of consumers' online health communities [23]. Thus, advancements in global connectivity and trends toward consumerism are expanding eHealth markets outside of the United States.

Payers in the United States are reticent to recognize reimbursement models for eHealth services outside of small pockets of activity [35]. However, there is increasing movement in the market toward a broad business model for eHealth and teleservices, as evidenced by the entry of large technology suppliers into advanced ICT development focused on health care. Industry strategies indicate that information technology suppliers such as Microsoft are readily approaching the large chronic disease consumer market in the United States. The U.S. government continues to invest considerably in eHealth developmental initiatives to improve the probability of managing chronic disease cost effectively in populations for which they are liable such as Medicare, Medicaid, and military programs.

20.2 Strategic Considerations for eHealth and Teleservices

Over 10 years ago, Christensen and colleagues at the Harvard Business School discussed the concept of disruptive innovations as a solution for the change-averse industry known as health care. Disruptive technologies, as seen in other industries, are those that come from ground-up markets and focus on simple solutions needed to ignite slow, non-responsive, overly complex industries. The personal computer, for example, is described as a disruptive innovation in the technology industry [10]. Today's evidence-based medical models use increasingly complex technologies such as electronic health records and varied specialist interventions to manage medically complex persons with the primary goal of minimizing catastrophic medical incidents. For example, targeted rehabilitation delivered in the United Kingdom through the SMART program allows users to self-manage by picking exercises and also attain immediate feedback using a teleservice-based technology application. Sensors allow movements to be recorded and clinicians to view the progress of stroke survivors' progress remotely and in a more timely fashion [6]. This relatively straightforward telerehabilitation program completely changes the paradigm for access to therapy in this environment. Generally speaking, most eHealth and teleservices models that change access to health care and promote self-management are disruptive to current models of traditional brick-and-mortar health care.

Repeated implementations of eHealth and teleservices across the United States led by innovative organizations will have an impact on the management of both chronic disease and rehabilitation science by creating markets of consumers and family members as leaders in defining the delivery of health care. Many telemedicine applications that can use live interactive telemedicine are available now. In California, live interactive telemedicine has been used for over 50 specialty services. In 2008, the California Telemedicine & eHealth Center (CTEC) began to consider the impact that reimbursement and other factors have on the full deployment of telemedicine and telehealth in California. This effort included a collaborative policy development with major telemedicine stake holder groups from health care, government, and industry [7]. There is an opportunity to establish consumer-led models in health care in the United States, as employer groups and insurers look toward member input for decision making regarding insurance coverage and the configuration of plans that focus on health maintenance. The ability to engage populations of persons with conditions that lend themselves to using ubiquitous tools like eHealth will allow societies to define effective self-management in health care and to adapt both economic and social aspects of health-care delivery to create ways of accessing health services.

Although access improvements and eHealth proliferation in the United States are important, the interconnected nature of international markets today implies a more global view of eHealth services relevant to the discussion of overall global economic health. Likewise, virtualized disease management practices allowed for the ability to manage globally certain aspects of population health related to the advancement of therapies for chronic illness that are the topic of world health dialogue. For example, international management standards that existed for conditions such as diabetes, as described by Cederholm et al. [8], demonstrated that data could be aggregated across many countries to formulate population health management plans as well as approaches for targeting specific demographics of persons with the aim of early intervention.

Numerous opportunities exist in both private and public sectors to develop leader organizations to execute these virtual national and international disease management constructs. Vendors who produce health information system applications as well as consumer technology vendors who design health-specific web applications (e.g., Microsoft, Google, and Web MD) can facilitate connected communities across geographic and political boundaries. Vast social networks of individuals who are self-managing diseases can interact and can drive entire markets for both goods and services in a connected health economy. Although some researchers in management and leadership are critical of the diminishing role of innovative leadership in U.S. firms in the last 10 years, the progression of consumer-driven health models grounded in self-management can catalyze innovation in health services across the United States and international markets [27].

Like any newly developed medical intervention, ICT-based eHealth and teleservices applications should be incorporated into the overall strategy of the organization sponsoring these technologies. While grant-funded pilot and feasibility projects are important methods to test the efficacy of the technology, provider processes, and user experience, the development of the business strategy for eHealth and teleservices programs must occur early in the conceptual and initiation phases to ensure adoption and the ability of the program to be sustained with ongoing health-care economies. Often, there is early emphasis in eHealth and teleservices programs on the details of clinical practice and technology. Standards in both practice and technology are evolving and assist in establishing a basis for the broad implementation of these programs across health-care sectors. The establishment of best practice guidelines by organizations such as the American Telemedicine

Association for teleservices such as telerehabilitation is important; however, before performing design, organizations should initiate a business planning process [1].

The following questions assist in the planning process when examining new ideas for eHealth and teleservices. They are best discussed and executed within the context of multidisciplinary stakeholder groups with input from functional areas such as executive management, physicians, non-physician providers, operational administration, technology leaders, finance, and legal councils.

- What is the organizational imperative driving the eHealth/teleservices program?
- What are the implications to the current leadership structures with the organization/organizations?
- Who are the operational leaders responsible for program outcomes and what are their expectations?
- What are the risks associated with developing and maintaining the technology, and what factors mitigate that risk?
- What is the value proposition to the users of the eHealth/teleservices program?
- How are other stakeholders are involved—payers, suppliers, or governing agencies?
- How will the qualitative and quantitative outcomes of the program be measured?
- How will the measurement of outcomes tie to the annual program planning process?
- What are the initiation/start-up costs of the program?
- What are the annual operating costs inclusive of program maintenance?
- What is the business model for quantitative cost recovery?
- How will any competitive advantages or strategic outcomes of the program be measured?

20.2.1   Applications of eHealth and Teleservices

Consumer demand for convenient service has brought electronic transactions into almost every aspect of daily living. Banking can be handled online and bills can be paid with the click of a mouse. Shopping via computer, whether for groceries, clothes, books, or just about any other product available in stores is routine for millions of Americans. Consumers are looking for the same convenience when it comes to communicating with their health-care providers. Now, more than ever, patients expect personalized connectivity and communication with health-care providers along with self-service access to their personal health information. Patients who use personal health records to improve interactions with health-care providers make more informed health-related decisions and experience higher quality of care and outcomes. Technology is being used to bring together information and services in new and patient-friendly ways.

In health care, a myriad of applications in the form of pilot programs, academic studies, and corporate access-based solutions have been deployed. The focus on the electronic medical record (EMR) provided the basis for providers and payers to offer some eHealth solutions that are integrated into suites of EMR products. Generally, patients use eHealth to manage processes such as appointment scheduling, prescription management, and chronic disease care compliance [28, 30]. The types of services doctors can offer vary from appointment scheduling and prescription refills to communicating test results or discussing other sensitive subject matter. Integrated patient portals, for example, offer computer applications that run from the same databases as the EMR and are generally available to sites with EMRs. These eHealth programs improve communication between the provider and the consumer. Patient demand for these services exists today. A September 2006 Wall Street Journal Online/Harris Interactive poll found that 74 % of respondents would like to use e-mail to communicate with their physicians directly. About 67 % would like to get diagnostic test results via e-mail, according to the online survey of 2,600 American adults [34].

Selected reimbursement for online services and pressures on physicians to manage chronic conditions in larger patient populations are increasing the amount of eHealth activity in the United States as providers install comprehensive EMRs with secured patient portals [2]. According to Bob Carroll, Vice President and Chief Operating Officer for Cigna Healthcare, e-visits will improve access for members who may have limited mobility and transportation options. E-visits allow patients who have a relationship with a health-care provider to consult with their physicians about non-urgent medical needs, such as follow-ups on chronic conditions, allergies, or cough or cold symptoms [31].

A host of eHealth and teleservices applications exist that are not integrated into provider and/or payer electronic health records. These may include teleservices applications such as remote patient home health monitoring, telerehabilitation video-supported occupational therapy consultations, and provider-to-provider telestroke video consultations. Some of these teleservices models provide consumer-to-provider offerings and other applications focus on provider-to-provider consultative offerings. Where therapists and medical specialists are not available, such as critical access hospitals and rural settings, teleservices modalities that use ICT such as video conferencing and Internet data exchange can bring specialized expertise to outreach settings or smaller providers within large networks.

20.3   Concept of the Business Case for Teleservices

20.3.1   Considerations for the Business Case

20.3.1.1   Competitive Considerations

There are opportunities for organizations in all aspects of the health services sector to differentiate themselves using eHealth and teleservices. It is important that these programs be fully incorporated into competitive organizational strategies to ensure that they sustain. For example, the onslaught of retail-based primary care and urgent care offerings in the market allows for organizations that have an electronic health record and an integrated ICT-based portal offering to provide value-added services to consumers with the support of online treatment such as electronic visits. In this example, known patients use structured questionnaires to access non-urgent care for episodic illness at their convenience over the Internet. As reported by Albert et al., patients report high satisfaction and pay out of pocket when insurance does not cover the service. This eHealth program allows primary care physicians who are part of a large health system to compete, in a highly differentiated manner, with emerging urgent care models in their market [3]. With some commercial payers covering the service and data gathering for federal policy support, services such as ICT-based care allow for increased competition and choice in the market place.

Another type of competitive advantage to eHealth and teleservices offerings is the ability for complex, specialty programs to extend their offerings to the community. In this model, specialists of all disciplines can offer technology-based outreach programs using video or by the passing of data. This approach, store and forward, is used when a face-to-face visit is not necessary. Store-and-forward systems allow a provider or technician at the patient site to capture diagnostic information using clinical instruments and send the digital image of the information to a clinician at a remote site. The remote-site clinician retrieves the digital images, reviews them, and sends a report back to the patient site. It is commonly used for dermatology, diabetic retinopathy screenings, radiology, and pathology [32]. Store and forward allows specialists to review patient findings at convenient times without depending on the presence of the patient. Since there is no requirement to meet face to face with the patient, store and forward maximizes the time a clinician spends reviewing and reporting on findings. It also saves the patient travel time and expense. While provider systems need to be attuned to potential Stark law issues and consult legal experts, in general, the presence of extended expertise in the community can be offered in a fair and consistent manner such that specialists of all types can gain increased patient referrals and activity in specialty services.

20.3.1.2 Outcomes

The direct impact of eHealth and teleservices program to improved medical management outcomes is more difficult to measure than referrals, customer satisfaction, or service volumes. Some groups have demonstrated efficacy in the improvement of medical measures in populations such as persons with diabetes by augmenting existing medical management processes with eHealth technologies [21]. A recent study finds that remote online visits with dermatologists achieved equivalent clinical outcomes for patients with acne. Also, doctors and patients ranked the e-visits as convenient and time saving, and said that they could be used as a model for chronic conditions such as diabetes and hypertension. Alice Watson, MD, Corporate Manager, Center for Connected Health, and the study's lead author commented, "This study is among the first to examine the clinical effectiveness of online visits between specialists and patients without them needing to communicate simultaneously" [9]. Likewise decreased hospital costs have been reported in Veteran's Administration users of a telerehabilitation program [5]. The potential of telerehabilitation and other teleservices programs has not yet been thoroughly evaluated.

20.3.2 Leadership Implications for the Evolution of eHealth and Teleservices

Evolving eCommerce strategies for health care requires executive and strategic leadership prowess, defined by Bass [4], as essential in organizations' ability both to be differentiated and to improve on delivery to a complex set of stakeholders. Telemedicine is emerging as a critical component of the health-care crisis solution. Telemedicine holds the promise to impact significantly some of the most challenging problems of our current health-care system: access to care, cost-effective delivery, and distribution of limited providers. Telemedicine can change the current paradigm of care and allow for improved access and improved health outcomes in cost-effective ways.

There is a host of leader provider and payer organizations in the United States that have made the investments in electronic health records that are necessary to facilitate access to the data and communications platforms to execute eHealth at a strategy level. These organizations realize that innovation is the ability to see change as an opportunity—not a threat.

Inherent in this health services leadership progression is a sense of social responsibility driven through sound business management and the ability to improve struggling health-care models [24]. Internal to the industry, health-care organizations continued to struggle with formalized leadership development and increasingly ambiguous leadership roles between stakeholders within health organizations [25]. Physicians' roles as leaders were the most challenging in many cases. Despite the fact that the medical literature was full of articles on patient self-management for chronic care, the concept of directly engaging patients through technology was still relatively new and novel to the industry [22]. Organizations that enable consumer engagement in chronic care will lead in local and possibly national markets as costs shift toward members who are information seekers. eHealth programs offer a strategic opportunity to health care, and, as in many innovations in popular consumer electronics such as Apple, sometimes people do not know what they want until it is offered to them [19].

Researchers have suggested that organizations with consumers who benefit from eHealth are likely to have innovative leaders who facilitate technology adoption and drive organizational change by challenging existing norms [17]. Innovative leader models are indicated in transformational leadership thinking and often are facilitators of advancement in both product and process development [16]. Acceptance of the risks associated with innovation-based leadership is essential in the advancement of programs such as eHealth that do not have existing business process or technology models [11].

20.4 Measures and Metrics for Teleservices

It is important to identify adequately all costs associated with the development, implementation, and ongoing operation of any eHealth or teleservices program. Table 20.1 details the projected costs over 5 years for a sample program. Programs such as telerehabilitation, telestroke, eVisits, and others all have associated start-up or capital expenses in addition to ongoing operational expenses. Interdisciplinary teams of leaders in the operations, medicine, technology, and finance areas can work together to develop cost estimates through request-for-proposal (RFP) processes in the market place and other activities such as research pilots and collaboration with other sites. Program estimates should be re-evaluated annually and also be adjusted for progressive cost increases according, at minimum, to an index such as the Consumer Price Index.

20.4.1 Cost and Benefit Assessment

Formal return on investment (ROI) models can be used to evaluate eHealth and teleservices programs. In general, after the costs are established, stakeholders must provide estimates as to measurable metrics for organizational benefits. These may be quantitative and revenue based, such as appointments scheduled, or they may represent cost avoidance, such as decreased emergency room visits. Provider, payer,

Table 20.1 Sample program costs

	Year 1	Year 2	Year 3	Year 4	Year 5	Total
Capital or structural costs						
Consulting services or third parties ($)	100,000	100,000	0	0	0	200,000
Implementation salaries ($)	200,000	200,000	150,000	150,000	0	700,000
Database software ($)	300,000	0	0	0	0	300,000
Hardware (server/end-user devices) ($)	50,000	5,000	5,000	5,000	5,000	70,000
Network costs ($)	40,000	0,000	5,000	5,000	5,000	75,000
Licensed software ($)	30,000	0	0	0	0	30,000
Capital total ($)	720,000	325,000	160,000	160,000	10,000	1,375,000
Operating or execution costs						
Software support or subscription fees ($)	6,000	6,000	6,000	6,000	6,000	30,000
Hardware maintenance/support ($)	0	2,000	2,000	2,000	2,000	8,000
Physician salary support ($)	50,000	50,000	50,000	50,000	50,000	250,000
Support/post-production salaries ($)	0	60,000	60,000	120,000	120,000	360,000
Travel/training ($)	5,000	5,000	5,000	5,000	5,000	25,000
Materials/supplies costs for operations ($)	2,000	2,000	2,000	2,000	2,000	10,000
Operating total ($)	63,000	125,000	185,000	185,000	185,000	683,000
Grand total (capital and operating) ($)	783,000	450,000	345,000	345,000	195,000	2,058,000

and/or other for-profit constituents in various health-care sectors may look at benefits differently depending on core business models for the organization and the proposed value proposition of the eHealth and teleservices program to the customer. Table 20.2 shows an example of a simple ROI for an eHealth application called eVisits—Internet visits for episodic, non-urgent illness—in a primary care physician practice. The main assumption in this example is that due to demand analyzed from existing office information technology systems, there was additional capacity to take on more office visits while freeing up physician time with eVisits. A pilot eVisit study, office time studies, and data analysis from existing information systems allow for the business case assumptions to be formulated.

It is clear that consumerism, increasing aging, chronic illness demographics, and advances in information technology are making the development of ICT technologies in health care more prevalent. Organizations must establish leadership in this realm to advance both clinical and business objectives. Multidisciplinary teams of stakeholders can work toward aligning eHealth and teleservices programs with existing and evolving organizational strategies to pilot work that does not sustain in the form of operationally lead programs. Identifying start-up as well as ongoing costs, both capital and operational, is crucial at the onset of a program. Information analysis of existing information systems can be important in establishing returns on

Table 20.2 Sample ambulatory practice return on investment analysis

	Office visits versus eVisit/eHealth				
	Office visit		eVisit		eVisit
	ROI based on 581 visits		ROI based on 581 visits		ROI based on 1,824 visits[a]
	$ per visit	Total $	$ per visit	Total $	Total $
Revenue	62	36,022	43	24,983	78,447
Expense	43	24,983	30	17,430	54,730
Net Income	19	11,039	13	7,553	23,716
		A		B	C
Business assumptions					
581 office visits are replaced with electronic visits	(3,486)	B – A			
581 office visits converted and 581 office visits backfilled	18,592	A + B			
1,824 eVisits replace 581 office visits (3:1 ratio)	12,677	C – A			
1,824 eVisits and backfill 581 office visits	34,755	A + C			

[a]1824 eVisits are based on 3:1 eVisit to office visit ratio as calculated per the time study analysis

investment. Return or value to the organization can be measured in quantities and qualitative metrics and consider both revenue opportunities as well as cost avoidance in the case of improved safety and compliance.

Summary

- eHealth and teleservices offer medical management to consumers of various ages and health statuses through secure e-mail, websites, and online home medical devices. Improved Internet connectivity and decreasing computer costs make online health-care services increasingly available.
- Teleservices offered through ICT provide health-care services such as diagnosis and treatment, administration of therapies, prescription refill management, and scheduling of services using non-traditional methods.
- Increase in disease burden and cost of treatment enumerates the need for low-cost technology solutions that are readily available to all segments of the population. There is increasing movement in the market toward a broad business model for eHealth and teleservices, as evidenced by the entry of large technology suppliers into advanced ICT development focused on health care.
- Telemedicine is emerging as a critical solution to some challenging problems of our current health-care system: access to care, cost-effective delivery, and distribution of limited providers.

- Consumerism, increasing aging, chronic illness demographics, and advances in information technology are making the development of ICT technologies in health care more prevalent. Organizations and stakeholders can work together toward aligning eHealth and teleservices programs with existing and evolving organizational strategies.

Abbreviations/Acronyms

CTEC	California Telemedicine & eHealth Center
ICT	Information and communication technologies
EMR	Electronic medical record
RFP	Request for proposal
ROI	Return on investment

References

1. ATA's new practice guidelines seek to make telemedicine a standard of care. 2011. A blueprint for telerehabilitation guidelines. Business Wire, Retrieved 8 Jan 2011, from ABI/INFORM Complete (Document ID: 2187041831).
2. Adler K. Making a case for online physician–patient communication: it can improve communications, practice efficiency and maybe even the bottom line. Just don't expect all your patients to join you online…yet. Fam Pract Manag. 2008;15(5):A3.
3. Albert S, Shevchik G, Paone S, et al. Internet-based medical visit for and diagnosis for common medical problems: experience of first user cohort. Telemed J E Health. 2011;17(4):304–8. doi:10.1089/tmj.2010.0156.
4. Bass B. Executive and strategic leadership. Int J Bus. 2007;12(1):33–52.
5. Bendixen R, Levy C, Olive E, et al. Cost effectiveness of a telerehabilitation program to support chronically ill and disabled elders in their homes. Telemed J E Health. 2009;15(1):31–8.
6. Brennan D, Mawson S, Brownsell S. Telerehabilitation: enabling remote delivery of healthcare, rehabilitation, and self management. In: Gaggioli A et al., editors. Advanced technologies in rehabilitation. Washington, D.C.: IOS Press; 2009.
7. California Telemedicine and eHealth Center. 2010. Available at: www.cteconline.org. Accessed 10 Jan 2011.
8. Cederholm J, Erg-Olofsson K, Eliasson B, et al. Risk prediction of cardiovascular disease in type 2 diabetes. Diabetes Care. 2008;31(10):2038–43.
9. Center for Connected Health. 2010. Available at: www.connected-health.org. Accessed 10 Jan 2011.
10. Christensen C, Bohmer R, Kenagy J. Will disruptive innovations cure health care? Harv Bus Rev. 2000;78(5):102–12. September–October:1–10.
11. Collins J. Level 5 leadership. Harv Bus Rev. 2001;79:66–77.
12. Cusmano MA, Glawer A. The elements of platform leadership. MIT Sloan Manag Rev. 2002; 43:51–9.
13. Fox S. The engaged e-patient population. 2008. Available at: http://www.pewinternet.org/~/media//Files/Reports/2008/PIP_Health_Aug08.pdf.pdf. Accessed 26 Mar 2009.
14. Gamble J, Savage G, Icenogle M. Value-chain analysis of a rural health program: toward understanding the cost benefit of telemedicine applications. Hosp Top. 2004;82(1):10–7.

15. Gustafson DH, McTavish FM, Stengle W, et al. Reducing the digital divide for low-income women with breast cancer: a feasibility study of a population-based intervention. Gender-specific epidemiology of diabetes: a representative cross-sectional study. J Health Commun. 2005;10: 173–93.
16. Ham C. Improving the performance of health services: the role of clinical leadership. Lancet. 2003;361:1978–81.
17. Herzlinger RE. Consumer driven health care: implications for providers, payers and policy-makers. San Francisco: Jossey-Bass; 2004.
18. Homer J, Hirsch G, Milstein B. Chronic illness in a complex health economy: the perils and promises of downstream and upstream reforms. Syst Dyn Rev. 2007;23:313–43.
19. Jobs S. Business Week, May 25 1998. Available at: www.wired.com/gadgets/mac.
20. Josefsson U, Ranerup A. Consumerism revisited: the emergent roles of new electronic intermediaries between citizens and the public sector. Inform Policy. 2003;8:167–80.
21. Kwon HS, Cho JH, Kim HS, et al. Establishment of blood glucose monitoring system using the Internet. Diabetes Care. 2004;27:478–83.
22. Lanseng E, Andreassen T. Electronic healthcare: a study of people's readiness and attitude toward performing self-diagnosis. Int J Serv Ind Manag. 2007;18(4):394–409.
23. Loader BD, Muncer S, Burrows R, et al. Medicine on the line? Computer-mediated social support and advice for people with diabetes. Int J Soc Welf. 2002;11:53–65.
24. Maak T, Pless N. Responsible leadership in a stakeholder society: a relational perspective. J Bus Ethics. 2006;66:99–115.
25. McAlearney A. Leadership development in health care: a qualitative study. J Org Behav. 2006;27:967–82.
26. Meyer MH, Azani M, Walsh G. Innovation and enterprise growth. Res Technol Manag. 2005;48:34–44.
27. Miles R. Innovation and leadership values. Calif Manag Rev. 2007;50(1):192–201.
28. Moody LE. E-health web portals. Holist Nurs Pract. 2005;19:156–60.
29. Morewitz SJ. Chronic diseases and healthcare. New York: Springer; 2006.
30. Nguyen HQ, Kohlman V, Rankin SH, et al. Supporting cardiac recovery through eHealth technology. J Cardiovasc Nurs. 2004;19:200–8.
31. Phoenix Business Journal. Cigna expands e-Visit options. 2010. Available at: http://www.bizjournals.com/phoenix/stories/2007/04/09/daily14.html. Accessed 28 Mar 2012.
32. Sidorsky T, Huang Z, Dinulous G. A business case for shared medical appointments in dermatology. Arch Dermatol. 2010;146(4):374–81.
33. Siminerio L, Zgibor J, Solano FX. Implementing the chronic care model for improvements in diabetes practice and outcomes in primary care: the University of Pittsburgh Medical Center experience. Clin Diab. 2004;22:54–8.
34. The Wall Street Journal Online. Harris Interactive Poll, 5:16. 2006 Available at: http://www.schedulemd.com/WSJOnline_HI_Health-CarePoll2006vol5_iss16.pdf. Retrieved 28 Mar 2012. p. 1–7.
35. Whitten P, Buis L, Love B. Physician-patient e-visit programs, implementation and appropriateness. Dis Manag Health Outcomes. 2007;15(4):207–14.

Chapter 21
Speech-Language Pathology and Telerehabilitation

Deborah Theodoros

Abstract Speech-language pathology services are eminently suited to delivery via telerehabilitation owing to the audio–visual nature of the interaction between the clinician and the client. An increasing need for alternate modes of service delivery in this profession is evident because of the growing demand and cost of health care, a changing society, and rapid developments in technology. Equitable access to services, improvement in quality of care, ongoing intervention, and the promotion of self-management are several benefits to be derived from telerehabilitation. The evidence base supporting the use of telerehabilitation in speech-language pathology continues to grow, with research conducted in neurogenic communication disorders, stuttering, voice disorders, dysphagia, laryngectomy, and pediatric speech, language, and literacy disorders. A variety of technologies are now available to support a continuum of care for people with chronic communication and swallowing disorders. The future of telerehabilitation in speech-language pathology is promising, although several challenges such as clinician confidence, education and training, professional portability, reimbursement, and economic evaluation need to be addressed.

21.1 Introduction

Speech-language pathology has been a leading profession in the use of telerehabilitation for the delivery of services to children and adults with communication and swallowing disorders. Early reports of the use of technology to deliver services date back to the 1970s when Vaughn [45] used the telephone, and printed materials

D. Theodoros
Division of Speech Pathology, Telerehabilitation Research Unit,
School of Health and Rehabilitation Sciences, The University of Queensland,
St. Lucia, Brisbane, QLD, Australia
e-mail: d.theodoros@uq.edu.au

S. Kumar, E.R. Cohn (eds.), *Telerehabilitation*, Health Informatics,
DOI 10.1007/978-1-4471-4198-3_21, © Springer-Verlag London 2013

mailed to the patient, to provide speech and language therapy. The American Speech and Hearing Association (ASHA) endorses the use of telepractice, where telecommunications technology is used to deliver professional services [1]. This broader term encompasses all aspects of professional services in speech-language pathology across various clinical settings, and may be used interchangeably with the term "telerehabilitation."

By nature of the interaction between a speech-language pathologist (SLP) and a client, services can be readily translated into an online or technology-based environment. Essentially, the majority of consultations involve an audio–visual interaction between the SLP and the client where auditory and visual stimuli are used to facilitate communication in its various forms. For consultations in which physical contact is required (e.g., oromotor examination and dysphagia assessment), adjustments to the assessment procedure may need to be included to achieve a valid and reliable assessment. Since the early foray into the use of telerehabilitation in speech-language pathology, a growing number of studies reported in the literature have evaluated the feasibility, reliability, and validity of this method of service delivery. The benefits and challenges associated with telerehabilitation can readily be identified and provide a basis for informing the implementation of technology-based services into mainstream practice.

21.2   The Need for Telerehabilitation in SLP

The impetus for the use of telerehabilitation in SLP has accelerated in recent years owing to a number of worldwide imperatives. These factors include the ever-increasing demand and cost of health care, the changing structure and demography of society, the impact of rapidly developing technology on a clinician's capacity to deliver services, and clients' expectations of access to such service. By 2030, 72.1 million people who are 65 years and older will represent 20 % of the population of the United States [32]. The "baby boomer" generation will constitute a large proportion of this population, with people in this age group (born between 1946 and 1964) beginning to turn 65 years old in 2011 [29]. This older generation is likely to live longer and, with chronic disabilities, placing increasing demands on already over-committed health-care systems.

Equitable access to SLP services continues to challenge current service delivery models. The tyranny of distance and the ongoing difficulties with recruitment and retention of SLPs in rural and remote areas remains a vexing issue for service providers and clients alike [35]. Furthermore, many individuals with a communication disorder have co-occurring physical difficulties that preclude ready access to face-to-face (FTF) intervention. The increased effort involved in attending FTF therapy services may result in the person being in a less-than-optimal physical and cognitive state for the consultation.

Changes in the structure and demography of society over time will create an unprecedented need to alter traditional service delivery methods. The aging population alone will require new and innovative ways to meet their expectations of living independently in their own homes [29]. With reduced capacity to drive and mobilize easily within the community, the elder generation will need services that accommodate this change [29]. In concert with changing demographics, people are experiencing extended time in employment and longer working hours, which have impacted negatively on work–life balance [17]. The capacity to commit to FTF SLP services has become increasingly difficult for many families. The need for more time and cost-effective methods of service delivery are paramount.

Rapid developments in telecommunication technologies in recent years have resulted in greater access to information and services for people worldwide [3]. With increasing sophistication of technology users both young and old, and the ubiquity of Internet connectivity, the expectation to access SLP services at a distance will grow with successive generations.

21.3 Benefits of Telerehabilitation

While the advantages of telerehabilitation are obvious with respect to reducing costs and improving equitable access to SLP services, the benefit of this mode of service delivery in improving the *quality of care* to people with communication and swallowing disorders is understated. The capacity to deliver SLP services to a child or an adult in their own home, school, or local community where they communicate on a daily basis is considered best practice in many areas of rehabilitation [28]. Positive effects have been seen in the generalization of behavior, functional outcomes, patient satisfaction and self-management in conditions such as stroke [25], and severe brain injury [56] when treated in their own environment. This approach is also consistent with the World Health Organization intervention framework, which promotes a person's functioning within the context of their environment [55]. Telerehabilitation enables the SLP to optimize the timing, intensity, and sequencing of intervention [54] such that a continuum of care may be implemented and maintained over time. Intensive neurorehabilitation regimens may be more readily implemented through the use of telerehabilitation [2], while the capacity to monitor communication and swallowing function in a client remotely enables the clinician to optimize the timing of intervention and avoid, or at least reduce, morbidity and functional limitation.

Maximizing communication and swallowing in children and adults with chronic disorders requires long-term management, which is difficult to sustain FTF. The importance of ongoing management was emphasized by Bruins et al. [5] who noted that sustained treatments were needed to reduce isolation, dependency, and depression in patients post-stroke. Furthermore, self-management is considered a crucial component of the overall management of chronic conditions [23]. Telerehabilitation has the potential to provide sustained intervention, and facilitate self-management, across a continuum of care in SLP through the use of various technologies combined with innovative clinical management programs.

21.4 Current Evidence for Telerehabilitation in SLP

Research involving the use of telerehabilitation in SLP has focused primarily on the validity and reliability of assessment and treatment protocols, and client satisfaction [39]. The quantity and quality of research have improved significantly in recent years, with more rigorous research designs and more advanced technologies underpinning the various studies. There has been a predominance of research in the health services domain, with a paucity of evidence supporting the use of telerehabilitation in the educational sector [39]. Despite this, numerous SLPs are known to use technology successfully to deliver services to children in schools in the public and private sectors. Client and clinician satisfaction has been remarkably positive across the majority of studies [39], a finding consistent with other areas of telehealth research [6]. However, cost–benefits of telerehabilitation services in SLP in various settings remain undetermined [39].

Research into the use of telerehabilitation in SLP has been conducted across the areas of adult neurogenic communication disorders, voice disorders, stuttering, dysphagia, laryngectomy, and speech, language, and literacy disorders in children. Overall, these studies have demonstrated comparability in outcomes between FTF and telerehabilitation modes of service delivery.

21.4.1 Adult Neurogenic Communication Disorders

Research in adult neurogenic communication disorders has focused predominantly on the assessment and treatment of aphasia, dysarthria, and apraxia of speech. Researchers in Australia have assessed over 40 participants with mild to moderate-severe dysarthria [18, 19], 32 participants with mild to severe aphasia [20, 41], and 11 participants with mild to severe apraxia of speech [21] in a laboratory setting using a custom-made PC-based multimedia videoconferencing system. Assessments were conducted simultaneously online and FTF. Overall, the findings from these studies revealed high levels of agreement between the online and FTF assessors for ratings of speech, language, and oromotor performance, and standardized test scores. Similarly, intra- and inter-rater reliability between the online and FTF assessors was found to be good to very good for the majority of parameters [18–21, 41]. Across these studies, participant satisfaction with online assessment was notably high (>80 %). Using a similar methodology and an integrated acoustic analyzer to measure vocal sound pressure level (SPL) and frequency in real time across the Internet, Constantinescu et al. [12] assessed the speech and voice of 61 people with Parkinson's disease (PD) online and FTF. They found comparable agreement between the two assessment environments for the majority of perceptual and acoustic measures of voice, oromotor function, articulatory precision, and speech intelligibility.

Other researchers have assessed the language comprehension and expression of 40 participants following either traumatic brain injury or stroke on a story-retelling task, using a custom-built PC-based telerehabilitation system [4, 15]. The participants were assessed in the online and FTF environments on two separate occasions. No significant differences in story-retelling performance between the FTF and online environments were identified [4, 15]. High participant satisfaction was also recorded during these studies [4, 15]. A subsequent study examined the validity of assessing functional communication online in people post-stroke [33]. High levels of agreement were achieved between online and FTF assessments.

Treatment studies reported in the literature have focused on dysarthria in PD and on aphasia. Tindall et al. [43] used the videophone to deliver LSVT® to 24 patients with PD and demonstrated significant improvements in SPL for voice and speech tasks pre- to post-treatment. Using a web camera and videoconferencing via Skype®, Howell et al. [22] delivered LSVT® to three people with PD in combination with FTF treatment. Participants received one treatment session per week FTF and the remaining three sessions via Skype®. Results revealed gains in SPL across voice and speech tasks that were consistent with data from previous FTF treatment studies. Technologies such as videophones and Skype® have some limitations, however, including the inability to record SPL accurately and frequency, and the need for participant training and specific computer requirements where Skype® is used.

By using a specifically designed integrated multimedia videoconferencing system, other researchers have overcome some of the limitations of off-the-shelf technology [11, 13, 40]. A randomized controlled trial involving 34 people with PD revealed significant improvements in acoustic and perceptual measures following treatment in both the online and the FTF treatment groups [13]. No significant differences in treatment outcomes were identified for participants across the treatment environments. A further study examined the effectiveness of LSVT® online in the home with substantial improvements in SPL and overall speech intelligibility in a single case following the treatment [11].

Other researchers have developed software to enable people with PD to practice LSVT® techniques, independently [16]. This software may be used in conjunction with FTF treatment, or autonomously, following 16 sessions of treatment. The software includes calibrated measurement of SPL and frequency of the voice, interactive verbal feedback on patient performance, a facility for the clinician to adjust treatment goals, and data analysis. In a treatment study by Halpern et al. [16], 16 people with PD received 50 % of their sessions at home using the software and the remaining sessions FTF. Positive outcomes similar to previously published data for LSVT® were obtained.

In the treatment of aphasia, a number of computer-based interventions have been developed which allow the patient to practice at home independently. Studies have found little or no difference in outcomes between computer-based and FTF treatment of word retrieval [30, 36], difficulties in the production of grammatical structures [26, 44], oral reading [8], and conversational speech [9]. A new web-based technology (web-Oral Reading for Language in Aphasia—web-ORLA™) allows for client practice independently as well as direct contact with the therapist via the Internet [10].

21.4.2   Voice Disorders and Stuttering

There has been limited research in the use of telerehabilitation for the management of voice disorders. In a study by Mashima et al. [27], 23 participants with a voice disorder were treated online using a secure Internet-based videoconferencing system integrated with speech analysis software. Pre- and post-treatment assessments were conducted in the traditional FTF manner. Positive treatment effects were achieved in the online group, with outcomes being similar to those obtained for 28 people treated FTF. Further research involving the treatment of different types of voice disorders and the use of technology for self-management is required to promote telerehabilitation in this area of practice.

The strongest evidence to date for the use of technology in the management of stuttering has been provided by Onslow and colleagues [7, 53] who have developed telephone-based applications for the delivery of the Lidcombe program for children [53] and the Camperdown program for adults [7]. Four of the five children who received the Lidcombe program scored a mean of less than 2.0%SS at 12 months post-intervention [53]. No statistically or clinically significant difference in %SS was recorded between the 20 participants who engaged in the Camperdown program via the telephone and the 20 participants who received this treatment FTF, when assessed immediately post-intervention, or at 6 and 12 months later [7].

21.4.3   Dysphagia and Laryngectomy

A limited number of studies have so far been conducted to determine the feasibility and validity of managing patients with dysphagia, and others following head and neck surgery, via telerehabilitation. The feasibility of doing so seems less plausible than for clients with common communication disorders. Recent studies, however, have challenged traditional expectations in these areas of practice. Myers [31] reported on the successful use of videoconferencing to provide speech rehabilitation, voice prosthesis management, psychosocial support, and family education to a patient's post-laryngectomy in rural areas.

More recent experimental studies by Ward and colleagues [50, 52] have validated the assessment of oromotor, swallowing, and communication outcomes of patients following laryngectomy using a customized videoconferencing system. In a laboratory setting, 20 laryngectomy patients were assessed online and FTF simultaneously [52]. Results revealed greater than 80 % agreement between the online and FTF assessors for all variables relating to oromotor function, swallowing status, and communication ability. Patients were 100 % satisfied with the usability of the system and the quality of service received. In a subsequent study, Ward et al. [50] investigated the assessment of 10 laryngectomy patients remotely over a distance of 1,700 km with connection via a mobile phone network. Excellent levels of agreement were achieved between the two assessors for swallowing, stoma, and communication status. Satisfaction of both patient and clinician was high.

The clinical evaluation of swallowing involves close observation of the patient, and a greater degree of "hands-on" interaction from the clinician, compared to other areas of SLP practice. As such, this process may at first seem difficult to accomplish via telerehabilitation. The first attempt to validate a clinical bedside swallowing assessment via telerehabilitation was conducted by Sharma et al. [38] who assessed 10 simulated patients presenting with a range of dysphagia severity levels. Each "patient" was simultaneously assessed online and FTF using a clinical swallowing examination (CSE) protocol. The CSE was administered with the support of an assistant at the patient end. High to excellent levels of agreement between the online and FTF assessors for all parameters of the CSE were obtained. In a subsequent study, Ward et al. [51] investigated the online assessment of 40 patients with dysphagia caused by various neurological and structural etiologies. Results revealed high levels of exact agreement (83–100 %) between the online and FTF assessors for oromotor ratings, food and fluid trials, and diagnosis and recommendations for future management. The results of these studies have provided the initial evidence for the feasibility and validity of online assessment of swallowing.

21.4.4 Pediatric Speech, Language, and Literacy Disorders

Few studies have addressed the feasibility and validity of telerehabilitation in the management of speech, language, and literacy disorders in children. This dearth of research is somewhat surprising in view of the fact that these communication disorders constitute a major proportion of SLP practice. Waite and colleagues [46–49], in a series of studies, investigated the validity of online assessment of speech, language, and literacy disorders in children. In a study involving the online evaluation of the speech of 20 children with suspected or identified speech impairment, a high level of agreement overall (84–100 %) was achieved between the FTF and online assessments for single-word articulation, speech intelligibility, oromotor function, phonological processes, phonetic transcription accuracy, and speech severity ratings [46]. Assessment of the language abilities of 25 children online and FTF simultaneously using the *Clinical Evaluation of Language Fundamentals*, 4th edition (CELF-4) [37] revealed no significant differences between the online and FTF total raw scores and scaled scores for each subtest [48]. Very good agreement for individual test item scores and severity level was obtained for the two raters, while intra- and inter-rater reliability for online ratings was very good across all measures. A further study by Waite [49] investigated the online assessment of literacy skills of 20 children who were assessed on standardized literacy, spelling, and reading tests. Percentage levels of agreement between the online and FTF assessors were above 80 % for most measures. Intra- and inter-rater reliability was very good for all online parameters. To date, there is no strong evidence to support the online treatment of pediatric speech, language, and literacy disorders. Research is urgently required to address this gap in the evidence base for the pediatric population.

21.5   Telerehabilitation Technology in SLP

A range of technologies may be used in the delivery of SLP services. Such technology may be categorized under two main types: synchronous and asynchronous. Synchronous technology enables real-time audio or visual interaction between a client and a clinician [1], and includes the telephone, networked videoconferencing, free Internet videoconferencing services, and integrated multimedia videoconferencing systems [13, 34]. Asynchronous technology includes store-and-forward mechanisms such as audio and video recordings, photos, and e-mail where the client's performance data are collected, stored, and retrieved, and responded to at a later time by the SLP [1].

Different types of technology may be used during various stages of a client's management program. For example, synchronous technology such as videoconferencing may be used for the assessment and initial phase of treatment while specialized software programs may be used asynchronously to complement real-time therapy sessions, e.g., LSVT®LOUD Companion, web-ORLA [10, 16]. Following a period of treatment, the client may continue to use asynchronous technologies such as e-mail, telephone, and specific software programs to self-manage their communication disorder while remaining in contact with the clinician. For example, a person with a dysarthric speech disorder may digitally record their speech onto a Smartphone, measure SPL and frequency of their voice via dedicated Smartphone applications, and e-mail this information to the clinician for review. The clinician may subsequently provide advice regarding an upgrade of speech exercises or forward a video recording of a specific technique to the client for viewing and practice. In another example, a clinician may use free Internet videoconferencing to observe a client with a swallowing difficulty during a meal and provide online advice.

In addition to the various technologies for delivering treatment programs, the proliferation in electronic therapy resources has resulted in speech-language therapy being transformed from paper- and pencil-based activities to digital applications that are smart, engaging, and ubiquitous. The vast array of applications that are currently available provides the clinician and the client with a wealth of resources that may be used innovatively and flexibly to achieve communication goals.

The choice of technologies for use in delivering SLP services is determined by the client population being served, the cost of equipment, available training and technology support, and the level of connectivity available within the area of service. Rapid advances in technology, however, complicate decision making even further, with many technologies being quickly superseded and replaced by cheaper and smarter technologies. The choice of technology for a specific SLP activity ultimately remains dependent upon the clinical reasoning skills of the clinician.

21.6   Challenges of Telerehabilitation in SLP

Although the evidence base for telerehabilitation in SLP continues to grow, and the benefits of this mode of service delivery can be readily identified, there are a number of challenges facing the profession in the implementation of telerehabilitation into mainstream practice. These challenges include professional issues (clinician confidence, education and training, professional portability), reimbursement, and economic evaluation.

On a professional level, clinician confidence and adaptability in delivering SLP services via technology are key factors underpinning the implementation of telerehabilitation. For some clinicians, the perception that FTF interaction with a client is the "gold standard" of service delivery is difficult to modify despite the potential of telerehabilitation to enhance a client's communication in their natural environment. In concert with this perception is the clinician's concern that some clients, in particular the elderly, will be unable to adapt to the online environment. Many of the research studies in telerehabilitation to date effectively dispel this assumption, with participant cohorts consisting of older people reporting high levels of satisfaction with the online environment [6]. Clinician perceptions are likely to change in due course with increasing evidence for the ecological validity and benefits of this mode of service delivery in its various forms. Education and training of SLPs in the use of technology-enabled practice by educational institutions and professional bodies will also facilitate clinician confidence in telerehabilitation and prepare future SLPs to engage in this method of service delivery. Another major challenge to the uptake of telerehabilitation is the issue of professional portability. Currently in the United States, for example, such portability is restricted with SLPs needing to be licensed in the state or territory where the client receives the service. For many clinicians, this barrier presents a logistical and financial disincentive in moving forward with telerehabilitation. Changes to policy and legislation at state and federal levels will be needed to address this challenge.

Reimbursement continues to be a major barrier to the provision of SLP telerehabilitation services. There is a need for strong evidence to support the effectiveness and cost–benefits of the service before reimbursement becomes a reality across all areas of practice. The importance of ongoing lobbying to policy makers on this issue cannot be underestimated and requires support from professional organizations. The American Telemedicine Association and ASHA are proactive in this arena.

The economic attributes of telerehabilitation are critical to sustainability in today's health-care and educational systems. The limited economic evidence currently available for SLP services remains a key obstacle to reimbursement, program funding, and widespread adoption of telerehabilitation. Economic analysis of any SLP service via telerehabilitation requires detailed information regarding the costs of technology, facilities, personnel, time expended by the client/family members and service provider, client and provider travel expenses, as well as the benefits to the client/family, and the effects on quality of life [14, 24]. The most comprehensive form of economic evaluation is a benefit–cost analysis that compares economic costs and monetized economic benefits (outcomes of service converted to monetary values) to determine if the service is economically justified and better than alternative uses of same resources [14].

To date, only two examples of economic evaluation of an SLP telerehabilitation service have been reported in the literature. Tindall et al. [43] compared the client-reported costs and time for 16 sessions of treatment via videophones to costs incurred for FTF treatment. The videophone treatments involved 16 h of time, no mileage, and no other costs compared to the FTF treatments, which required 51 h of time (travel and therapy time), $953 for mileage, and $269 for other costs. An additional analysis of the impact of videophone treatment on caregiver burden for 11 caregivers of people with PD revealed average savings of 48 h of time, more than 92 h of work time, and just over $1,000 per caregiver as a result of videophone treatment [42].

Despite the challenges of telerehabilitation, there are prevailing circumstances that will impel the use of this method of service delivery in SLP. Ongoing research in the field will ultimately provide the economic evidence to inform policy makers and service providers leading to the implementation of telerehabilitation into mainstream SLP practice. The ever-increasing range of technology available will transform everyday practice and provide alternate service delivery options that are applicable across a continuum of care.

Summary

- SLP services can be readily translated to technology-based practice.
- Telerehabilitation in SLP is driven by the increasing demand and cost of health care, a changing society, and rapid developments in technology.
- Benefits of telerehabilitation include equitable access to services, improvement in quality of care, sustained intervention, and promotion of self-management across a continuum of care.
- Evidence exists to support the validity of telerehabilitation in adult neurogenic communication disorders, voice disorders, stuttering, dysphagia, laryngectomy, and articulation, language, and literacy disorders in children.
- Synchronous and asynchronous technologies may be used in SLP.
- Challenges of telerehabilitation in SLP include clinician confidence, education and training, and professional portability, reimbursement, and economic evaluation.

Abbreviations/Acronyms

ASHA	American Speech-Language-Hearing Association
CELF-4	Clinical Evaluation of Language Fundamentals 4th edition
CSE	Clinical swallowing examination
FTF	Face to face
PD	Parkinson's disease
SLP	Speech-language pathologist
SPL	Sound pressure level

References

1. American Speech-Language-Hearing Association. Professional issues in telepractice for speech-language pathologists [Professional Issues Statement]. 2010. Available at: http://www.asha.org/policy/PI2010-00315.htm, doi:10.1044/policy.PI2010-00315HY.
2. Bach-y-Rita P. Conceptual issues relevant to present and future neurologic rehabilitation. In: Levin H, Grafman J, editors. Neuroplasticity and reorganization of function after brain injury. New York: Oxford Press; 2000. p. 357–79.
3. Bednarz A. The network world. 2011. Available at: http://www.networkworld.com/supp/2011/25thanniversary/050911-anniversary.html. Accessed 19 Jun 2011.
4. Brennan DM, Georgeadis AC, Baron CR, et al. The effect of videoconference-based telerehabilitation on story retelling performance by brain-injured subjects and its implications for remote speech-language therapy. Telemed J E Health. 2004;10:147–54.
5. Bruins Slot K, Berge E, Dorman P, et al. Impact of functional status at six months on long term survival in patients with ischaemic stroke: prospective cohort studies. BMJ. 2008;336:376–9.
6. Cardoso L, Steinberg J. Telemedicine for recently discharged older patients. Telemed J E Health. 2010;16:49–55.
7. Carey B, O'Brian S, Onslow M, et al. Randomized controlled non-inferiority trial of telehealth treatment for chronic stuttering: the Camperdown program. Int J Lang Commun Disord. 2010;45:108–20.
8. Cherney LR. Oral reading for language in aphasia (ORLA): evaluating the efficacy of computer delivered therapy in chronic nonfluent aphasia. Top Stroke Rehabil. 2010;17:423–31.
9. Cherney LR, Holland AL, Cole R. Computerized script training for aphasia: preliminary results. Am J Speech Lang Pathol. 2008;17:19–34.
10. Cherney LR, Kaye RC, Hitch RS. The best of both worlds: combining synchronous and asynchronous telepractice in the treatment of aphasia. Perspect Neurophysiol Neurogenet Speech Lang Disord. 2011;21:78–129.
11. Constantinescu G, Theodoros DG, Russell T, et al. Home-based speech treatment for Parkinson's disease delivered remotely: a case report. J Telemed Telecare. 2010;16:100–4.
12. Constantinescu G, Theodoros D, Russell T, et al. Assessing disordered speech and voice in Parkinson's disease: a telerehabilitation application. Int J Lang Commun Disord. 2010; 45:630–44.
13. Constantinescu G, Theodoros DG, Russell T, et al. Treating disordered speech and voice in Parkinson's disease online: a randomised controlled noninferiority trial. Int J Lang Commun Disord. 2011;46:1–16.
14. Davalos M, French MT, Burdick AE, et al. Economic evaluation of telemedicine: review of the literature and research guidelines for benefit-cost analysis. Telemed J E Health. 2009; 15:933–48.
15. Georgeadis A, Brennan D, Barker LM, et al. Telerehabilitation and its effect on story retelling by adults with neurogenic communication disorders. Aphasiology. 2004;18:639–52.
16. Halpern A, Matos C, Ramig L, et al. LSVTC – a PDA supported speech treatment for Parkinson's disease. Paper presented at the 9th international congress of Parkinson's disease and movement disorders, New Orleans, 2005.
17. Hayes A, Qu L, Weston R, et al. Families in Australia 2011: sticking together in good and tough times. Melbourne: Australian Institute Family Studies; 2011. p. 1–23.
18. Hill AJ, Theodoros DG, Russell TG, et al. An internet-based telerehabilitation system for the assessment of motor speech disorders: a pilot study. Am J Speech Lang Pathol. 2006; 15:1–12.
19. Hill AJ, Theodoros DG, Russell T, et al. The re-design and re-evaluation of an internet-based telerehabilitation system for the assessment of dysarthria in adults. Telemed J E Health. 2009;15:840–50.
20. Hill AJ, Theodoros DG, Russell T, et al. The effects of aphasia severity upon the ability to assess language disorders via telerehabilitation. Aphasiology. 2009;23:627–42.

21. Hill A, Theodoros DG, Russell T, et al. Using telerehabilitation to assess apraxia of speech in adults. Int J Lang Commun Disord. 2009;44:731–47.
22. Howell S, Tripoliti E, Pring T. Delivering the Lee Silverman voice treatment (LSVT®) by web camera: a feasibility study. Int J Lang Commun Disord. 2009;44:287–300.
23. Jones F, Riazi A. Self-efficacy and self-management after stroke: a systematic review. Disabil Rehabil. 2011;33:797–810.
24. Krupinski E, Dimmick S, Grigsby J, et al. Research recommendations for the American Telemedicine Association. Telemed J E Health. 2006;12:579589.
25. Legg L, Langhorne P. Rehabilitation therapy services for stroke patients living at home: a systematic review of clinical trials. Lancet. 2004;363:352–6.
26. Linebarger MC, Schwartz MF, Kohn SE. Computer-based training of language production: an exploratory study. Neuropsychol Rehabil. 2001;11:57–96.
27. Mashima PA, Birkmire Peters DP, Syms MJ, et al. Telehealth: voice therapy using telecommunications technology. Am J Speech Lang Pathol. 2003;12:432–9.
28. McCue M, Fairman A, Pramuka M. Enhancing quality of life through telerehabilitation. Phys Med Rehabil Clin N Am. 2010;21:195–205.
29. Morris J, Mueller J, Jones M. Tomorrow's Elders with disabilities: what the wireless industry needs to know. J Eng Des. 2010;2:131–46.
30. Mortley J, Wade J, Davies A, et al. An investigation into the feasibility of remotely monitored computer therapy for people with aphasia. Adv Speech Lang Pathol. 2003;5:27–36.
31. Myers C. Telehealth applications in head and neck oncology. J Speech Lang Pathol Audiol. 2005;2:125–9.
32. Older Americans. Key indicators of well-being. Federal Interagency Forum on Aging-Related Statistics. Washington, D.C.: U.S. Government Printing Office; 2010. Available at: http://www.agingstats.gov. Accessed 13 Sep 2011.
33. Palsbo SE. Equivalence of functional communication assessment in speech pathology using videoconferencing. J Telemed Telecare. 2007;13:40–3.
34. Parmanto B, Saptono A, Pramana G, et al. VISTYER: versatile and integrated system for telerehabilitation. Telemed J E Health. 2010;16:939–44.
35. Pickering M, McAllister L, Hagler P, et al. External factors influencing the profession in six societies. Am J Speech Lang Pathol. 1998;7:5–17.
36. Ramsberger G, Marie B. Self-administered cued naming therapy: a single-participant investigation of a computer-based therapy program replicated in four cases. Am J Speech Lang Pathol. 2007;16:343–58.
37. Semel E, Wiig EH, Secord WA. Clinical evaluation of language fundamentals, 4th edn (CELF-4). Toronto: The Psychological Corporation; 2003.
38. Sharma S, Ward EC, Russell T, et al. Assessing swallowing disorders online: a pilot telerehabilitation study. Telemed J E Health. 2011;17:688–95.
39. Theodoros DG. Telerehabilitation: current status and needs. San Antonio, TX: Paper presented at the American Telemedicine Conference; 2010.
40. Theodoros DG, Constantinescu G, Russell T, et al. Treating the speech disorder in Parkinson's disease online. J Telemed Telecare. 2006;12 Suppl 3:88–91.
41. Theodoros DG, Hill AJ, Russell T, et al. Assessing acquired language disorders in adults via the Internet. Telemed J E Health. 2008;14:552–9.
42. Tindall LR, Huebner RA. The impact of an application of telerehabilitation technology on caregiver burden. Int J Telerehab. 2009;1:3–7.
43. Tindall LR, Huebner RA, Stemple JC, et al. Videophone-delivered voice therapy: a comparative analysis of outcomes to traditional delivery for adults with Parkinson's disease. Telemed J E Health. 2008;14:1070–7.
44. Thompson CK, Choy JW, Holland A, et al. Sentactics: computer-automated treatment of underlying forms. Aphasiology. 2010;24:1242–66.
45. Vaughn GR. Tel-communicology: health-care delivery system for persons with communicative disorders. Am Speech-Lang Hear Assoc. 1976;18:13–7.

46. Waite M. Online assessment and treatment of childhood speech, language, and literacy disorders. Doctoral dissertation, University of Queensland, Queensland; unpublished 2010.
47. Waite M, Cahill L, Theodoros D, et al. A pilot study of online assessment of childhood speech disorders. J Telemed Telecare. 2006;12 Suppl 3:92–4.
48. Waite M, Theodoros DG, Russell T, et al. Internet-based telehealth assessment of language using the CELF-4. Lang Speech Hear Serv Sch. 2010;41:445–58.
49. Waite M, Theodoros DG, Russell T, et al. Assessing children's literacy via an internet-based telehealth system. Telemed J E Health. 2010;16:564–75.
50. Ward E, Crombie J, Trickey M, et al. Assessment of communication and swallowing post-laryngectomy: a remote telerehabilitation trial. J Telemed Telecare. 2009;15:232–7.
51. Ward EC, Sharma S, Burns C, et al. Using telerehabilitation to assess clinical dysphagia status. San Antonio, TX: Paper presented at the Dysphagia Research Society; 2011.
52. Ward L, White J, Russell T, et al. Assessment of communication and swallowing function post laryngectomy: a telerehabilitation trial. J Telemed Telecare. 2007;13 Suppl 3:88–91.
53. Wilson L, Onslow M, Lincoln M. Telehealth adaptation of the Lidcombe program of early stuttering intervention: five case studies. Am J Speech Lang Pathol. 2004;13:81–93.
54. Winters JM, Winters JM. A telehomecare model for optimizing rehabilitation outcomes. Telemed J E Health. 2004;10:200–12.
55. World Health Organization. ICF: international classification of functioning, disability and health. Geneva: WHO; 2001.
56. Ylvisaker M. Context-sensitive cognitive rehabilitation after brain injury: theory and practice. Brain Impair. 2003;4:1–16.

Index

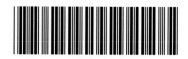